DR. VLASSARA'S
A.G.E. LESS DIET

HOW CHEMICALS IN THE FOODS WE EAT PROMOTE DISEASE, OBESITY, AND AGING AND THE STEPS WE CAN TAKE TO STOP IT

HELEN VLASSARA, MD
SANDRA WOODRUFF, MS, RD
GARY E. STRIKER, MD

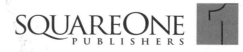

SQUAREONE
PUBLISHERS

The information and advice contained in this book are based upon the research and the professional experiences of the authors, and are not intended as a substitute for consulting with a healthcare professional. The publisher and authors are not responsible for any adverse effects or consequences resulting from the use of any of the suggestions discussed in this book. All matters pertaining to your physical health, including your diet, should be supervised by a healthcare professional who can provide medical care tailored to meet individual needs.

COVER DESIGNER: Jeannie Tudor
TYPESETTER: Gary A. Rosenberg
IN-HOUSE EDITOR: Joanne Abrams

Square One Publishers
115 Herricks Road
Garden City Park, NY 11040
(516) 535-2010 • (877) 900-BOOK • www.squareonepublishers.com

Library of Congress Cataloging-in-Publication Data
Names: Vlassara, Helen, author. | Woodruff, Sandra L., author. | Striker, Gary E., 1934- author.
Title: Dr. Vlassara's A.G.E.-less diet : how chemicals in the foods we eat promote disease, obesity, and aging and the steps we can take to stop it / Helen Vlassara, MD, Sandra Woodruff, MS, RD, Gary E. Striker, MD.
Description: Garden City Park, NY : Square One Publishers, [2017] | Includes bibliographical references and index.
Identifiers: LCCN 2016031406 (print) | LCCN 2016036061 (ebook) | ISBN 9780757004209 (pbk) | ISBN 9780757054204 (Epub) | ISBN 9780757054204
Subjects: LCSH: Glycoproteins—Physiological effect. | Glycosylation.
Classification: LCC QP552.G59 V53 2017 (print) | LCC QP552.G59 (ebook) | DDC 572/.68—dc23
LC record available at https://lccn.loc.gov/2016031406

Printed in the United States of America

10   9   8   7   6   5   4   3   2   1

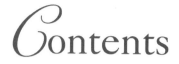

Contents

$\mathscr{P}$reface

In 1974, with a background in both medicine and biology, I began my work as a medical researcher at The Rockefeller University of New York. Although I originally studied genetic diseases of the blood, my focus shifted as my colleagues and I became aware of a fascinating group of complex substances that accumulated in the tissues of people with diabetes. Little did we know at that time that we were on the way to making several revolutionary discoveries. As our research progressed over the next couple of decades, we found that these compounds—called advanced glycation end products, or AGEs—were a cause not just of diabetes and its many complications, but also of a far wider range of devastating conditions, including cardiovascular disease; kidney disease; Alzheimer's disease; obesity; and bone, joint, and skin problems. Moreover, while these conditions were all common in older age, clearly, they had begun to affect much younger people as well. The question was: Why?

Our understanding took a mighty leap when we discovered that the most important source of these damaging substances is our diet, which has changed over the years to include more AGEs. At fault is not just the excessive consumption of favorite foods like beef and poultry, but also our favorite methods for preparing them, such as grilling, roasting, and frying (all high-dry-heat techniques). Because AGEs define much of the deliciousness of foods—taste, color, and aroma—people now prefer to use the high-dry-heat techniques that increase AGEs. In addition, to cater to the public's tastes, there has been a sea change in the food industry toward the development and marketing of industrially made heat-processed foods. The result has been an explosion of packaged foods that are high in AGEs. In other words, whether we cook our food at home or pick up commercially prepared foods, we are in effect eating our way to poor health.

Over our decades-long journey, prominent scientists and health care professionals across the world have been keen to embrace our new insights and accumulating data. But alas, the translation of science into clinical practice often moves at a snail's pace. The only discussion of the significant harm that cooking might have on our food has been the acknowledgment that extremely high temperatures can result in carcinogens or neurotoxins in foods (such as grilled meats or fried potatoes). It is important to state up front that these differ from the far more prevalent AGE compounds discussed in this book. An earnest discussion about the widespread effects of dry-heat cooking and food processing has been largely absent from public debate and health recommendations.

As I write these words, cooking schools, cookbooks, culinary magazines, and television shows continue to extol the joys of grilling, frying, roasting, barbecuing, and other high-dry-heat methods—practices that have now been scientifically shown to promote the production of large amounts of AGEs. As you have already read, this is true because most people prefer foods prepared using these methods. To most of us, high-AGE foods simply taste, look, and smell better. (Consider how everyone likes fried bacon, steaks with a "good sear," and chicken that's "golden brown"—sure signs of excessive AGE production.) For this reason, America has long been conditioned to welcome these health-damaging substances to the table.

Even though it's gratifying to have your work recognized by your peers and academic institutions, this isn't enough. If we are to ever stop the spread of the epidemics of chronic disease in our country, *everyone* has to become aware of the health risks posed by AGEs. *Everyone* must realize not only that we have invited AGEs to the table, but also that we can push back at these destructive invaders . . . and secure astonishing gains. For just as we unequivocally showed that a diet high in AGEs has devastating effects, our clinical studies also showed that when we limit dietary AGEs to a level that the body can handle, we can regain and enjoy greater health.

Despite the wealth of sound and in-depth scientific evidence supporting the association between a high-AGE diet and chronic illness, most people still don't know what AGEs are and how much damage they cause. After many years of research, thought, and inspiration, this book was written to alert everyone to the dangers of AGEs and, just as important, to show how easy it is to live the AGE-less way. In Part One, we explain what AGEs are, how they are formed, how they damage your body, and what you can do to minimize your exposure to these toxic substances. Then in Part Two, we present over one hundred AGE-less recipes. You will see how easy it is to prepare food that is not just low in AGEs, but also delicious and satisfying. By choosing the foods you eat with a little care and by mainly using simple AGE-less preparation techniques, you can enjoy a wide range of flavorful dishes and at the same time safeguard or even improve your well-being, without ever feeling hungry.

We hope that this book raises awareness of the threat AGEs pose to everyone and, just as important, that it inspires you to make simple but essential changes to how you select and prepare your diet. While you can't control every aspect of your environment, you do have the power to change your food environment—which is no small feat. And it's never too late to start. Regardless of your age, regardless of your past consumption of AGE-rich foods, the AGE-less diet will improve your ability to fight the debilitating conditions that plague our society and to enjoy greater health for many years to come.

Introduction

For centuries, and indeed as far back as Hippocrates, countless leaders in the field of health have warned us that what we eat can greatly affect our mental and physical well being. Since then, hundreds of fad diets have come and gone. From low-fat to low-carb, vegan to Paleo, and everything in between, seemingly every possible eating plan has been devised and touted. And yet, with all the promises of good health, weight control, and longer life, we are not getting any healthier. In fact, the number of degenerative diseases continues to explode. What have we been missing? Is there some strategy that could actually provide us with more vitality, greater health, and even a longer lifespan? Fortunately, the answer is a resounding *yes.*

Forty years ago as a young researcher, I worked with a team of other scientists to examine a class of destructive substances that accumulate in people with diabetes. These toxic substances were found to hasten many dangerous complications of diabetes, such as vascular disease and nerve damage. The aim of the research team was to understand the nature of these compounds. Were they a direct cause of the diabetes? Were they by-products of another process? Exactly how did they damage the body? There was much to learn. And what we discovered was something completely unexpected and surprising.

These destructive substances were not related to a deficiency or excess of vitamins or minerals, nor were they contaminants in the same sense that heavy metals, pesticides, and industrial waste are. Yet their path of damage was clear. The compounds were found to be directly linked to virtually every aspect of aging and degenerative disease, including cardiovascular and kidney diseases, bone loss, cognitive and neurological issues, and the weight gain and wrinkles that creep up on us as we age.

We called these toxic substances *advanced glycation end products,* or *AGEs.* The acronym AGE was actually coined to remind us that these compounds are linked to the accelerated aging that is part of diabetes and other chronic diseases. It was already clear that having high blood sugar levels caused more AGEs to form in the body. What we did not suspect until much later was that most AGEs actually enter the body with our food—and that they have the potential to affect many more people than was previously believed!

Over the past two decades, studies in both animals and humans have strengthened the case for AGEs as key players in many of the diseases that plague the modern world. A striking realization throughout these studies was that food AGE intake goes hand in hand with markers of inflammation, which has long been known to underlie most chronic degenerative diseases.

Unfortunately, the existence and nature of AGEs remain largely unknown to the general public—and, for that matter, to many health care professionals, as well. The translation of research into clinical practice is notoriously slow in the medical community, even in today's information-obsessed world. Meanwhile, our modern health predicament is all too clear: We may now live longer, but we struggle with poorer health.

The intention of this book is to open your mind to a whole new way of thinking about food and health. It exposes a root cause of the modern "lifestyle diseases," including obesity, cardiovascular disease, diabetes, arthritis, osteoporosis, Alzheimer's, and many more. But it also shares exciting and inspiring news: We have found that as people adopt the AGE-less diet, regardless of age or health status, indicators of inflammation and disease quickly plummet. This book will show you how you, too, can reap the benefits of AGE-less eating.

The book is divided into two parts. Part One helps you understand AGEs and how you can minimize your exposure to these harmful compounds. Chapter 1 provides a brief but illuminating look at the groundbreaking research that led to our current understanding of AGEs. In this chapter, you will get a sense of how long, difficult, and, yes, fascinating the history of AGE science has been.

Chapter 2 focuses on the science of AGEs. What exactly are these compounds? How do they form in the body? Why are they so prevalent in the modern diet? And how do they cause us so much harm? Chapter 2 answers these questions and more, all while making AGE science easy to understand.

Chapter 3 takes a closer look at the many health problems that are linked to excess exposure to AGEs. You will find that AGEs are intertwined with virtually every aspect of chronic disease and aging, from arthritis to diabetes; from Alzheimer's to cardiovascular disease. While this may seem disheartening, it also provides a simple key to better health—improving diet to provide fewer AGEs.

By the time you reach Chapter 4, you will know that the main source of AGEs in the body is the food you eat. In this chapter, you will learn exactly which foods provide large amounts of AGEs, and which foods offer good nutrition without burdening the body with an excess of these substances. Best of all, Chapter 4 presents the three basic principles of healthy AGE-less eating.

At this point, you may wonder if you have to abandon your current diet to eat the AGE-less way. Fortunately, AGE-less principles can be applied to *any* type of diet. Chapter 5 focuses on five of the most popular diet philosophies: low-carbohydrate diets, low-fat diets, the Mediterranean diet, the Paleolithic diet, and various forms of the vegetarian diet. You will see how simple it is to integrate AGE-less principles into these and other diets—including your own—to make them even more healthful.

Once you've learned the basics of eating the AGE-less way, it will be time to stock your pantry with healthy foods. Chapter 6 highlights foods that can fit into an AGE-less eating plan, offers smart substitutions for high-AGE foods and ingredients, and provides additional tips for selecting and preparing foods. You will find that AGE-less food can be tasty, easy to prepare, and economical.

Although it's important to center your diet on low-AGE foods, the way in which you prepare your foods is just as important as the foods you choose. This is because while some cooking methods promote the formation of large amounts of AGEs, other methods greatly minimize AGE formation. Chapter 7 guides you in the use of simple AGE-less cooking techniques, including braising, boiling, poaching, pressure cooking, slow cooking, simmering, stewing, and steaming. In addition, it offers practical tips for preparing some of your favorite foods with fewer AGEs.

Increasingly, people are eating away from home or picking up take-out fare rather cooking meals in their kitchen. Besides being generally higher in calories and lower in nutrition, food prepared outside the home often makes AGE-overload a near certainty. But it doesn't have to be that way. Chapter 8 guides you to the best choices whenever eating out, enabling you to make the most of the menu's offerings in a wide variety of settings while keeping your AGE load at a modest level.

Throughout this book, we assure you that AGE-less food can be delicious and satisfying. But tasting is believing. That's why Part Two of *Dr. Vlassara's AGE-Less Diet* offers over a hundred recipes that emphasize low-AGE foods and employ AGE-less cooking techniques. From breakfasts to desserts, from main courses to sides, these dishes are not just easy to make, but also easy to love. Just as important, each includes Nutrition Facts—calorie, carbohydrate, fiber, protein, fat, saturated fat, cholesterol, sodium, and calcium counts—so you can be sure that the recipes you choose are in tune with your dietary needs and restrictions.

Beyond a doubt, research has shown that AGEs are the "missing link" which explains why our modern diet is so strongly associated with inflammation and a wide range of chronic diseases. While this may strike you as just one more piece of bad news, the truth is that AGEs pose a problem which you can control with ease and at no extra cost. It is our hope that you will use the information provided in this book to introduce small but important changes that can make a real difference to your health and that of your loved ones. We wish you greater health and many satisfying meals to come.

PART ONE

Understanding AGEs

1.

The Missing Link

It was a fine summer afternoon in 1974, when I landed at The Rockefeller University of New York as a newly minted medical doctor, ready to try my luck as a researcher. I had grown up in Athens, Greece, right under the Acropolis, in an ancient—and now touristy—neighborhood called Plaka. It was there that I attended medical school, and with the help of strong letters from my professors, I secured a position at one of The Rockefeller's research laboratories.

The Rockefeller University is a small but prestigious research institute ranking among the very top few in the United States and around the world. Its famous independent laboratories attract scientists from every corner of the world to learn and to investigate cutting-edge scientific issues, most of them disease related. The university, although very small in overall size, also has its own hospital, which is devoted solely to clinical research. It works closely with the laboratories, where important discoveries in heart disease, obesity, immune disorders, tropical diseases, and other health conditions have been brought to light. It was at The Rockefeller University Hospital that clinical (human) studies took place, leading to the development of the hemoglobin A1C test, which allows us to monitor overall glucose control. This was a major step forward in the treatment of diabetes (more about this later). It was in this laboratory and hospital that I would live and work for the next twenty years.

When I arrived, the university was teeming with Nobel laureates and had the finest scientific faculties in the world. It had been credited with making countless inroads in areas such as protein biochemistry, cell biology, immunology, brain physiology, and physics. Needless to say, I was exceedingly lucky to find myself working with some of the best minds in American medicine and science. It was like a dream come true.

Armed with curiosity and enthusiasm, I was to start working on certain genetic diseases of the blood that are very common in Mediterranean countries. I envisioned all of the same things that other young, idealistic, ambitious doctors dream about—helping the sick, finding new cures, and eradicating diseases. Who would have guessed that forty years later, I would be writing a book about food?

THE DANCE OF SUGAR

The late 1970s was a time of many exciting scientific breakthroughs. In the first few years of my career, I witnessed first-hand several "aha!" moments. For example, there was the revolutionary discovery that aging-related problems might not be due simply to "wear and tear," and that heart disease was not caused just by bad genes. As for diabetes, it continued to be life-threatening despite the discovery of insulin therapy, but no one knew exactly why. So it was a real breakthrough when a connection was made between the high blood sugar of diabetes and the complications it brings, such as heart attacks, kidney failure, and blindness.[1-4] Now, of course, this is taken for granted.

These breakthroughs all transpired as medical scientists in both my lab and other labs began to tease out odd pieces of information from our research into blood disorders. Although we did not know it at the time, this information would ultimately give us new insights into diabetes, heart disease, and a wide array of other serious chronic disorders. Our first clue came as we were studying hemoglobin, the protein in red blood cells that transports oxygen. We recognized that sugar in the blood could bond with hemoglobin in a process that's known as glycation.[5] The more glucose in the blood, the more glucose molecules attached to hemoglobin, and as levels of these glucose-hemoglobin complexes increased, so did the risk for health problems in diabetes. We soon developed a blood test to assess this risk, which became widely known as the glycated hemoglobin, or hemoglobin A1C, test. This discovery radically changed our ability to control the complications of diabetes. It also was clearly important enough to force a shift in the direction of our research team. From that point on, my research was focused on diabetes and its effects on the body. As I reflect on those days, I am proud that I was part of the team that brought to light and established the A1C test, which remains an essential tool in the care of people with diabetes.

It was not long before we confirmed that sugar could latch onto many other proteins besides hemoglobin—and that important changes take place in both the sugar and the protein, causing them to transform into complex substances that we had not been aware of before.[3,4,6] Moreover, these substances accumulated in older people and were present in even higher amounts in those with diabetes.[7] We wondered if they might be at the root of the problems associated with diabetes and older age. As we soon learned, these couplings of sugar with proteins—and with fat, as we later discovered—spelled trouble.

THE COMING OF AGEs

This new phase of discovery was most intriguing and of far greater consequence than we expected. It became evident that once glucose attached itself to a protein, through a series of elaborate transformations, it changed the protein so that it no longer had its normal function and also evolved into an end product that could be toxic. Based on the process we had witnessed, we called these substances *advanced glycation end products,* or *AGEs.* This acronym seemed appropriate, since we found more of these substances in older people. The name also seemed to fit well with the notion that diabetes is a form of "accelerated aging."

Our task was to figure out how AGEs worked, and we were in for a rude awakening. AGEs cause trouble in seemingly inexhaustible ways.[6] For instance, the first thing we learned was that acting like glue, AGEs bind proteins together, causing joints to become stiff and blood vessels to become narrow or blocked. We also learned that

AGEs work as oxidants, damaging tissues much like acid rusts metal. They also overstimulate the immune system, turning it against body tissues instead of protecting them. These changes cause the cells and organs of the body to malfunction, as we'll learn in more detail in Chapter 2.

At first, it did not all come together in a neat package. But eventually, we discovered that the most insidious effect of AGEs was that they caused a low-grade, body-wide inflammation.[8] Acute inflammation is a perfectly normal, healthy response that's meant to help fight infections or repair damaged tissues. However, when inflammation persists and becomes chronic, it is almost always harmful. This finding provided a crucial insight. Low-grade almost "silent" inflammation appeared to be associated with many different diseases, including diabetes, cardiovascular disease, kidney disease, arthritis, and brain disease. But the cause of this "silent" inflammation was unknown. All laboratory evidence pointed to AGEs as a culprit. But how could we prove it?

It was time for us to get to the heart of the matter. We needed to develop clinical tests for AGEs, find their source, and search for an agent—a drug—that blocked AGEs from forming. If this agent successfully stopped the creation of AGEs and also avoided the harm caused by diabetes, we would have both proof of the missing link and a cure.

THE QUEST FOR ANTI-AGE DRUGS

The first anti-AGE drug, aminoguanidine, found by our team around 1981, blocked AGEs from forming, and when we tested it in mice, it prevented many of the problems related to diabetes and aging.[9] The substance was hailed as a potential "cure" and a "fountain of youth." That was a rare moment of victory, since it provided the first definitive evidence that AGEs—not just high sugar—were the culprits in the development of diabetes. Testing of more and better anti-AGE drugs followed. We could taste hope. We almost believed that soon, many health problems due to diabetes would be history.

Not quite. Despite their enormous promise, when it came to clinical trials, the benefits of our anti-AGE drugs were less effective than we had hoped. The same disappointing fate was befalling many unrelated but equally "smart" drugs being tested to reverse diabetes, heart disease, and other disorders.[10,11] In spite of the huge efforts and enormous costs, we were going nowhere. Rather than being pushed back, diabetes seemed to be gaining in momentum, joined by obesity. Similar trends were noted in other chronic diseases affecting the heart, brain, and kidneys.[12,13]

Some tried to make light of these new epidemics by claiming that because we now lived longer, we would naturally develop more diseases. But since these diseases also involved the younger generation, that reasoning did not hold up. New theories attempted to link these disorders to our genes. A single inborn genetic defect can certainly be the key to a rare disease like cystic fibrosis or sickle cell anemia. This type of genetic defect passes from parent to child, but it affects a relatively small number of people and could not explain the sudden explosive growth of chronic diseases such as diabetes within just one generation. On the other hand, some gene defects, or mutations, are not inborn but occur during a person's lifetime. Many of these *epigenetic* changes have been linked to environmental factors such as viruses, bacteria, hormones, pesticides, plastics, and the like. Some of these factors have recently ended up in our food. Food, in essence, seemed to pop up in connection with each chronic disease. Could changes in our food cause epigenetic defects? Clearly, there was much to learn.

Over the next several years, my team and I continued our efforts, well aware that the rate of diabetes—the subject of our research—was growing unabated, linked intimately with obesity, cardiovascular disease, and kidney disease, as well as aging and Alzheimer's. What was it that we were missing?

A BLIND SPOT

Although we did not recognize it at the time, a simple experiment conducted in the early 1900s would be crucial to our own research. In 1912, a professor of chemistry by the name of Louis Camille Maillard had discovered a complex chemical reaction that occurs between certain amino acids (the building blocks of proteins) and sugars during cooking. This reaction is accompanied by the appearance of brown-colored compounds on the food.[14,15] Everyone is well acquainted with these brown substances, because they impart enticing color, aroma, and flavor to foods such as roasted turkey and toasted bread. The chemical reaction was known as the *Maillard reaction,* and the compounds, which Maillard first described as "browning products" or "melanoidins," came to be called *Maillard products.*

We were well aware of what Maillard had described in foods, since Maillard products are formed by the same chemical reaction that leads to the formation of AGEs in the body. An inside joke was that "all of us are slowly cooking." But as medical scientists, we were focused on human disease and not on what cooking did to food. We simply did not link Maillard products—which, for all we knew, simply made food taste better—to the harmful AGEs found in the body. This was true for a few reasons. First, the early studies—which were based on methods of quantifying AGEs that would not be considered reliable today—failed to show that the Maillard products in food were absorbed into the body in significant quantities. Second, the then standard tests of toxicity focused on rapidly occurring dramatic effects such as liver failure, hemorrhage, certain tumors, or death. Scientists of the day found that they had to administer massive doses of food AGEs to animals before they saw any kind of recognizable acute changes or gross toxicity. Since they did not see any adverse effects within a short time when "normal" amounts of AGEs were used, it was concluded that Maillard products were not absorbed to levels worth worrying about.

A major clue, which was missed for a very long time, was that AGEs are indeed absorbed in significant quantities, but accumulate slowly over time and cast a very wide net, affecting most organs in the body. As often happens, science moved in a lopsided manner. Food, nutrition, and medical scientists worked in parallel but separate universes, neither talking with nor listening to one another.

AN UNEXPECTED FINDING

Often, when dealing with vexing questions, you must think outside the box to move science forward. Perhaps this is what transpired on a day in 1995, when a breakthrough moment occurred at, of all places, a banquet reception. By then, I was an American citizen and a professor of medicine and science at The Rockefeller University. Invited to speak at an international diabetes conference in Japan, I was pleased to attend a spectacular banquet reception—a testament to Japanese hospitality. Looking at the stunning display of Western-style food, I whispered to my German colleague and friend Dr. Theodor Koschinsky, "Look at all these AGEs! At a diabetes event? Really!" Theodor replied, "Why not? We don't absorb AGEs from food, isn't it so? So enjoy!" How wrong we were!

It was, in fact, widely believed that food AGEs were not absorbed. But even as we made these lighthearted comments, I was aware of my own hidden doubt and dawning insight. "Just a second," I said. "What if we *do* absorb them?" Theodor responded, "Let's test it, then. You have the tools, I can help!"

The tools to which he was referring was the modern-day sensitive test we had developed in my laboratory in New York City.[16,17] We and others were by then able to measure levels of AGEs both in blood and in tissues. But no one had thought of using the test to analyze foods or AGE absorption from foods.

Days later, over a transcontinental phone line, we "cooked" up a simple test—egg whites heated together with a lot of table sugar to make a meringue, a prototypical AGE-rich meal. After happily consuming this delicious dish, Dr. Koschinsky collected samples of his own blood and sent them to me. In a few days, we had the results. The levels of AGEs in his blood had unmistakably skyrocketed within minutes after he ate the meal, revealing the passage of AGEs from my friend's stomach into his blood. Soon, this simple experiment, together with the first proper clinical trial, demonstrated for the first time that AGEs are, in fact, absorbed from the foods we eat.[18]

A new chapter had begun in our research on AGEs. AGEs from food were absorbed into the body and, if absorbed in large enough quantities and over a longer period of time, this could make a compelling argument that AGEs played a role in the development of complications related to diabetes and aging. Perhaps we had finally found a clue to the missing link.

SCIENCE GETS TURNED UPSIDE DOWN

Although we had made the mental leap necessary to link AGEs in the body with AGEs in food, it would take another couple of decades of testing food AGEs and their chemistry, biology, and pathology to show that Maillard products in foods could be a source of the harmful AGEs found inside the body. Whether working with laboratory animals or conducting new "pilot" clinical studies, this was a long, fascinating, oftentimes tedious exploration. We had to pinch ourselves to believe that no aspect of this process had ever been explored before—that no one had tackled it, certainly not from this perspective and not in this depth and detail.

As time went on, we learned a great deal, much of which overturned some of the claims that we had made only a few years before, when there was still little available in terms of technical capability. We had originally believed that AGEs built up imperceptibly over a lifetime and were not greatly affected by our diet. Having an easy and sensitive method to track levels of AGEs in the bloodstream around the clock, we discovered that in general, AGE blood levels bounce up after meals, just as sugar and fat levels do. We also learned that, astoundingly, AGE levels in the blood can vary, based not only on ingredients and nutritional composition, but also on how the food is cooked. Next, we learned that AGE levels could be quite high even in people who believed themselves to be healthy but had been consuming a high-AGE diet for a long time.

Just as important, we found that if certain cooking methods are employed—methods that used less heat and more water—AGEs in the body could actually be *decreased*. (To learn more about this, turn to Chapter 4.) Only after acquiring large amounts of scientifically rigorous evidence were we convinced that our long-held ideas about AGEs had been wrong, or at best, incomplete.

We were struck by the implication that food AGEs, if ingested regularly and liberally, could easily surpass those produced inside the body in both quantity and impact. We also made another critical observation. The body has a finite capacity for handling AGEs. In large part, it uses the kidneys to flush out these harmful substances. This means that, assuming you have healthy kidneys, a "reasonable" amount of AGEs can be removed. But if either too many AGEs are consumed or the kidneys' function is decreased, the excess AGEs remain behind, and those deposits in the tissues are like "bad" deposits in a bank—a truly toxic asset.

While it was long in coming, a wealth of extremely useful new information was our reward. For a good many years, we studied countless laboratory mice, feeding them a diet that, although perfectly balanced in nutrients and vitamins, was designed to be either rich in AGEs or low in AGEs. We watched the animals closely over their lifespan, with an eye to even minute changes in their metabolism, heart, kidney, bone, and even brain function. The findings were very exciting, especially since they closely matched what we had observed in our patients. There was no question that AGEs brought about vascular, kidney, bone, and brain disease. Moreover, beyond our wildest expectations, AGEs caused profound metabolic disturbances, such as insulin resistance and diabetes, in these animals.[19] Up to that moment, remember, the dogma was that AGEs followed and were the result of uncontrolled diabetes, not the other way around.

But most astonishing of all was the effectiveness of reducing the intake of foodborne AGEs. There was no doubt that lowering the intake of AGEs by just 50 percent could slow down or prevent every single one of these conditions from developing. The mice on the low-AGE diet also lived longer and healthier lives.[19]

UNCHARTED TERRITORY— MEASURING AGES IN HUMAN FOOD

These revelations were in many ways thrilling. But since our ultimate area of interest was human AGE consumption and its effect on health, we once again were face-to-face with unknowns. How do you count the AGEs in food? Which foods are highest in AGEs? *Why* are AGEs high in these foods? There are hundreds of thousands of food products, and since we needed this data, we had no option but to take up the task of determining their AGE levels. It took over ten years to develop new tools to bridge the gaps in our knowledge. Hundreds of thousands of tests later, we published the first reliable database listing the AGE levels in hundreds of the most commonly consumed foods.[20,21]

A fascinating pattern emerged: The items most heavily laden with AGEs were among the most popular foods in the United States. Many—such as steaks, bacon, fried chicken, French fries, and pizza—were regularly prepared using high-dry heat, such as grilling, frying, or baking. In addition, foods high in animal fat—cheese and butter, for instance—were AGE-rich even in their uncooked state. These findings strengthened our suspicion that toxic amounts of AGEs could slip into the body with large meals. But the surprise was that the same could happen even when eating a moderate-sized "healthy" meal. This is because although some foods are high in AGEs before cooking, certain cooking methods can create even higher amounts of AGEs. The higher the heat and the longer the cooking time, the more AGEs end up in the food. (We'll cover this in further detail in Chapter 4.)

DO WE GAIN ANYTHING BY LOWERING THE AGES IN FOOD?

We had made great progress, but much work still remained to be done, not the least of which was research that would assess if any benefit was to be gained by reducing AGEs in daily diets. This, too, was a completely new notion. As usual, more studies were needed.

Our next step was to earn the funds required for the studies. Funding from the National Institutes of Health (NIH) is a real lifeline for academic career scientists like me and my colleagues. It is also the most prestigious, and thus, the most competitive and difficult to win. Fortunately, the NIH placed a high priority on our research and proved to be a keen and faithful supporter of this herculean investigation. With this support in place, a wealth of promising insights from animal studies prepared the way for human trials. These would take another eight to ten years to materialize.

The easy part was completed in two short trials, both conducted in "normal" adults. Reducing the ingestion of food AGEs clearly led to lower levels of AGEs in the human body.[22,23] Importantly, this also happened in people with diabetes—something that no one expected.

These findings provided unprecedented support for our developing theory that AGEs from food were an important source of AGEs in the body, regardless of the presence of diabetes. These small clinical studies also showed solid evidence of a marked reduction in inflammation. But could restricting foods high in AGEs also turn the disease clock back? As you will see, the answer was a resounding "yes." Without a doubt, this was the most exciting and gratifying aspect of this journey, and you will have the opportunity to follow it in more detail in Chapters 2 and 3.

WHAT CAN YOU BELIEVE?

Randomized controlled clinical trials, especially involving a new drug or diet as a therapeutic intervention, are the litmus test for all sound medical scientific discoveries. This type of rigorous research has unfortunately not been the rule across many nutritional studies. With this in mind, after decades of groundbreaking basic science work, we were determined to put our AGE-less program through such clinical trials in order to secure the proof needed to establish the human value of the principles presented in this book. Unlike most other "diets," the AGE-less diet offers protection from several major health threats without the need to cut calories, unless you choose to do so, since it is not based on the restriction of nutrients. Rather, it is based on changing the way foods are prepared. It does not require drugs or doctors. Moreover, because of the positive results and "feedback" collected after observing many participants, we can assure you that you, too, can achieve these goals without making major changes in your daily life.

In this chapter, we wanted to give you a sense of how long, difficult, and, yes, fascinating the history of AGE science has been. Excitement about the huge health implications of the AGE-less diet is exactly what led to this book. We grant you that the world of agribusiness and food conglomerates will not provide the help we need. It is up to us. It comes down to a few simple steps that we can each take to deal with those "toxic assets" that are embedded in our food.

The following chapters are set up to help you understand what AGEs are, how they form, and how they do their damage. We predict that as you learn more about the solid science behind this concept, you will embrace the message. Soon, you will find yourself eager to learn the simple ways that you and your family can keep excess amounts of AGEs at arm's length so that they never threaten your life or well-being.

CONCLUSION

As our studies ran the entire gamut from the laboratory workbench to the clinic, they provided abundant evidence and solid proof that food AGEs are a huge health hazard. Albeit, this is a hazard that can be swiftly and decidedly dealt with, since by simply consuming fewer food AGEs, you can delay, stop, or reverse dangerous disease processes. What can this mean for you? If you have stubborn diabetes, you can expect to live a longer life, better protected against common predicaments such as a heart attack or stroke. If you have prediabetes, you may be able to correct the key underlying problem—insulin resistance—and should be able to prevent it from turning into full-blown diabetes and heart disease. The same applies to dementia, kidney disease, arthritis, and numerous other age-related maladies. Remember that today, many of these diseases begin in childhood and appear in young adulthood, so you can certainly trust your new knowledge about AGEs to safeguard your children's health. The simple message is that while these diseases can easily develop and progress when you consume an excess of AGEs with food, simply lowering "the heat" and making smarter low-AGE food choices can keep your health blooming for the rest of your life.

2.

$\mathscr{T}$he Science of AGEs

Researchers have known about AGEs for decades. A search for AGEs at the National Library of Medicine's PubMed website yields over 8,000 links to scientific articles. Why, then, does the public, and even many healthcare professionals, know so little about their health hazards? One example that can help us answer this question is that of cigarette smoking. It took many years of research and countless human lives to raise public and professional awareness of the risks of smoking due to toxic substances hidden in cigarettes. For decades, smoking had been associated with enjoyment and enhancement of personal image and was aggressively marketed. Changes in public policy were slow to come. Because the health problems related to smoking develop very slowly, while marketing campaigns were quickly effective, too many people became addicted to tobacco at a young age,[1] only to suffer huge consequences.

The primary goal of this chapter is to reveal a similar phenomenon of toxic substances, namely AGEs, that are hidden in your daily diet. You will learn what AGEs are, how they form, and how they do their damage. It will become clear how these insidious toxins can underlie virtually every aspect of aging and chronic disease, including cardiovascular and kidney diseases, bone loss, dementia, and even the weight gain and wrinkles that creep up on us as we get older. Just as important, you will begin to understand simple ways to control AGEs so that you can avoid or delay these conditions.

WHAT ARE AGES?

In Chapter 1, we touched on the fact that AGEs are compounds that form when proteins or certain types of fats react with sugars. It all starts when, in a process called *glycation,* a sugar molecule latches onto certain amino acids of proteins or fats (also called lipids), or

---

AGEs as Oxidants

We all have heard of free radicals—those scary sounding compounds that run wild in the body, wreaking havoc as they go. Put more scientifically, *free radicals* are highly reactive, unstable molecules that have one or more unpaired electrons in the outer ring. They run around snatching electrons from other molecules in a process known as *oxidation.*

Free radicals usually take electrons from nearby molecules that have electrons to spare, so no harm is done. But in other cases, free radicals attack molecules that have no electrons to spare. In this case, these molecules become free radicals themselves. This exchange of electrons between molecules is known as *oxidant stress* (also known as *oxidative stress*), and it is an essential part of all normal cell functions—as long as it is brief and tightly controlled. But oxidant stress can become excessive in the constant abundance of too many free radicals. This can cause damage to cells and tissues, leading to disease or accelerated aging. What does this have to do with AGEs? Many AGEs act as potent *oxidants,* meaning that they generate free radicals, leading to increased or excessive oxidant stress.[2,3]

When Is Oxidant Stress "Normal"?

As just mentioned, a certain amount of oxidant stress is normal. Most living cells work like a factory and depend on fuel to set their motors in motion. Nothing happens—no functions are performed—without fuel (energy). The fuel for our body, of course, is the nutrients in our food. As the body burns nutrients, free radicals are exchanged extremely rapidly between the various departments in our cells, helping to execute important functions, such as generating the energy (such as ATP) that is required, for instance, for muscle contraction by the heart and skeletal muscles.

even to our genetic material, such as DNA. The newly glycated compound then goes through a series of transformations to ultimately form an *advanced glycation end product* (*AGE*). In essence, AGEs exist as modified proteins or lipids. As such, both their structure and their function in the body become altered, and they are no longer "normal."

Generally, oxidant stress is very well controlled by our own internal defense systems. A number of compounds in the body—called *antioxidants*—neutralize free radicals, preventing them from doing harm. Classic examples of antioxidant enzymes made by the body include catalase, superoxide dismutase, and glutathione peroxidase. Also, bacteria in the gut synthesize vitamins and other substances with antioxidant properties, such as vitamin B_{12}. A number of other important protective factors exist inside most cells—such as SIRT1 and AGER1—that help control the excess of oxidants as they perform multiple vital functions. (You'll learn more about SIRT1 and AGER1 on page 28.) And, of course, foods naturally contain many antioxidants, including vitamins C and E, alpha-lipoic acid, carotenoids, coenzyme Q10, curcumin, and phenolic compounds.

When Is Oxidant Stress Harmful?

Despite all of the antioxidants that the body can rely on to prevent tissue damage, these antioxidants can easily be used up or depleted—for instance, during an acute infection. This also happens when a large amount of AGEs comes pouring in as part of our modern diet.[3] AGEs from our food represent one of the largest sources of oxidants affecting the body. Once they react with cells and tissues in the body, AGEs are difficult to break down and remove. So they can persist for a long time, acting as oxidants that sop up antioxidants.

In an ill-fated twist, AGEs tend to form more easily and faster in the presence of too many oxidants, leading to a never-ending cycle of more AGEs, more oxidation, more AGEs, and so on. AGEs damage the body much like rust corrodes metal. And, as you will learn on page 27, when AGEs and oxidant stress increase, so does chronic inflammation—a condition that has been linked to all serious chronic conditions, from diabetes to cancer.

Proteins and lipids play countless vital roles in the body. For example, proteins are major components of every cell in the body's muscles, organs, bones, and blood vessels. They also function as enzymes, hormones, and antibodies. Lipids, too, are vital. For instance, they are a necessary component of the membranes that coat every cell. Proteins and lipids can coexist, for instance, in the lipoproteins that transport cholesterol throughout the body. So it is easy to see how the presence of too many altered proteins and lipids can spell trouble on many levels. AGEs are also known as *glycoxidants,* since they act as *oxidants.* (See the inset on pages 20 and 21.) And due to their often toxic properties, they are sometimes referred to as *glycotoxins.*

AGEs originate both inside the body (endogenously) from our own sugars and proteins or fats, and outside the body (exogenously) in the sugars, proteins, and fats present in our foods. Although not the subject of this book, it is worthy of mention that AGEs are also generated in large quantities in tobacco smoke, a fact that may explain many of the unhealthy effects of smoking.[1]

There are literally hundreds of different types of AGEs in the body and in the food supply.[4,5] Some are harmless—that is, they are inactive—so we won't worry about them. But others are potent oxidants that release free radicals and increase inflammation in the body. (See the inset on pages 20 and 21.) Once AGEs gather in quantity, they can damage every part of the body in ways that favor the development of chronic diseases and premature aging.[6,2] (See the list on page 44.) Since it is less important to know all of the chemical names of AGEs, and more important to know how to manage them, for simplicity's sake, we will refer to these substances simply as AGEs throughout this book.

AGES IN THE BODY

The body naturally produces a small amount of AGEs—known as *endogenous* or *native AGEs*—as a part of our normal metabolism. Since much of the body is composed of protein, fats, and carbohydrates, there is a steady supply of raw materials from which AGEs are born.

One of the reasons that AGEs managed to escape our attention for so long is that native AGEs tend to form very slowly, over weeks or months, and in small amounts. Moreover, our body is equipped with a number of systems to control, or degrade, them and flush them out in the urine. The kidneys are the unsung heroes in the AGE story, since they are the main route through which the body eliminates AGEs. So as long as the AGE load stays small, these substances can be handled quite easily. (See page 58 of Chapter 3 for more about AGEs and the kidneys.)

The classic example of a situation in which native AGEs get out of control is diabetes.[7] The formation of endogenous AGEs is markedly increased in diabetes because of the high levels of glucose (a form of sugar) present in the bloodstream. In fact, studies in people with diabetes were what provided the first clues about AGEs and their destructive nature. We now know that too many AGEs underlie many complications of diabetes, such as vascular disease, blindness, and kidney disease.

Although we continually produce some native AGEs *inside* the body, it is important to understand that most AGEs come from *outside* the body, through our diet. This is true because AGEs are generated much faster and in much greater quantity in our food whenever the three basic components—sugars, proteins, and fats—are mixed together in the presence of high-dry heat, which often happens during cooking.[8,9]

AGES IN OUR FOODS

For thousands of years, humans have been cooking food. Initially, this was done over a fire, and then via an array of tools and techniques that used some sort of heat source.

There is no question that at the moment our ancestors discovered fire, they took a decisive step toward their survival while securing our own place as the most successful mammals on Earth. Early on, man discovered that after a successful hunting or scavenging expedition, the scraps of leftover meat remained edible for a longer time if they were passed over fire or smoked. What humans didn't know was that this was due to the killing of bacteria that cause food to spoil. What else was imparted by the fire? That's right: AGEs! While cooking over fire helped preserve the food, it also generated large amounts of "tasty" AGEs. The combination of food preservation and a pleasant

AGEs Close Up and Personal

To get a close-up view of how AGEs form, try this simple experiment. Fill three-quarters of a small clear glass bottle with water. Add one egg white and a tablespoon of sugar, and mix them gently. Close the bottle tightly and let it sit at room temperature for a couple of weeks. The liquid will slowly go from colorless to yellow, gold, orange, and finally brown. The change in color registers the progress of the reactions between sugar and protein as AGEs are produced. This same process occurs inside the body when our own sugars and proteins interact. It also occurs in foods when we cook, although at a much faster rate than in the body. You can easily see its fast pace as you grill steak, roast chicken, or toast bread. That brown color and tempting aroma are due to the formation of AGEs!

flavor led us to develop a taste for AGEs, along with a preference for salt, sugar, and fat. As cooking habits and food preservation skills passed from generation to generation over thousands of years, they helped humans survive famine, migrate without fear of hunger, and spread across the continents. From an evolutionary perspective, there is no doubt that fire and cooking helped human development. However, in today's world, there is such an abundance of AGE-rich foods that these habits do much more harm than good.

While our ancestors long knew that cooking causes food to be more appetizing, it wasn't until the early 1900s that food chemists realized that the rich flavors and enticing aromas associated with cooking were actually due to AGEs, which first became known as *Maillard products*.[9] (See page 11 of Chapter 1 for more information.) In subsequent years, food manufacturers took this knowledge and developed new ways to optimize the levels of these compounds in food in order to make it more appealing and increase shelf life. Higher heat, longer cooking times, and drier conditions were found to drastically increase AGE formation. Different amino acids can produce different aromas and flavors. And certain sugars favor AGE formation more than others. Fructose, especially, increases the rate of glycation by more than ten-fold compared with glucose. Food chemists eventually figured out that there is endless room for different combinations of chemically produced flavors that imitate natural flavors. Many of these are chemically synthesized AGEs.

The food industry understands that AGEs are commercially valuable since they add delicious tastes and aromas to our foods, enticing us to eat more. Needless to say, food may sell better if it contains lots of AGEs. This is not an indictment of the entire food industry. It is hard to ignore the fact that dry-heat processing also made food more digestible and safer for storage.[10] It is only quite recently that we've begun to recognize the negative effects of foods with high levels of AGEs when over-consumed.[11,12] Moreover, not all industrially processed foods are high in AGEs. Plant-based products such as rolled oats, whole grain pasta, frozen vegetables, and canned beans are convenient, high in nutrients, and very appropriate for an AGE-less diet.

Commercially heat-processed foods can be a huge source of AGEs in the modern diet, but let's not forget that we also cook up many AGEs in our own kitchens. Anyone who has toasted bread or roasted meat has seen AGE formation in action. You cannot miss the changes in color and consistency, as the surface of bread or meat becomes first golden, then brown and crusty. In the case of meat, the surface becomes thick and caramel-like and, if you wait long enough or you brush it with a sweet glaze, it becomes dark or even black, with a crunchy texture. There is no doubt that AGEs are key to some of the more pleasant food experiences we have come to expect and enjoy.

HOW AGES CAUSE HARM

Once AGEs from food reach the body's tissues, they slowly pile up, especially since they resist breakdown by most normal enzymes. If you remember that in the background of AGEs there is always sugar, it is easy to visualize them as sticky substances that tightly adhere to tissues, much like Velcro! Eventually, this can affect organs all over the body, including the brain, heart, kidneys, bones, skin, and more.[8] Compare this to the unpleasant effects of a sanitation workers' strike. The situation may be tolerable at first, but eventually, the piles of garbage can bring an entire city to its knees because they disrupt so many normal activities. This is an apt comparison, because AGE buildup does not discriminate and can affect every part of the body. AGEs are linked to the most common diseases of the world today, including diabetes, cardiovascular disease, kidney disease, Alzheimer's, and many more. How exactly do AGEs cause harm? There are several distinct mechanisms, which are briefly described below. Understanding these mechanisms makes it easier to see how these substances can cause so many seemingly different diseases.

AGEs Provoke Inflammation

The body has a built-in mechanism to defend itself against threats such as bacteria, foreign substances, and even damaged cells and tissues that need to be repaired. This process is known as the *inflammatory response* and is part of our immune system. Most people already have a general idea of what acute inflammation is—the inflammation that occurs almost immediately in response to tissue injury, and quickly becomes severe. When you cut your finger, bang your knee, get a splinter under your skin, or get an insect bite, the event may be followed by pain, swelling, redness, or pus. When you get a viral or bacterial infection, you may have a fever. These are the typical symptoms of acute inflammation.

Inflammation is a vital protective machine meant to rid the body of harmful "irritants"—bacteria, viruses, damaged cells, and the like. When the body perceives a threat, the immune system employs an arsenal of white blood cells as "bodyguards" to keep us safe. These cells attack and destroy the offenders, and clean up the mess to get tissues ready for repair and renewal. To do all this, they generate a large excess of free radicals that coordinate an array of complex cellular processes that we have come to call inflammation. Symptoms of brief or acute inflammation recede as healing is completed. But if the body continues to be exposed to irritants, inflammation can become chronic or prolonged. It is now well accepted that chronic low-grade inflammation lurks beneath a host of health problems, including cardiovascular disease, obesity, diabetes, Alzheimer's, and what we generally view as conditions common in normal aging. And yet its origins have remained elusive.

Chronic inflammation depends on a sustained source of irritants or offenders. What can serve as such an abundant source of irritants in the absence of any obvious infection or trauma? AGEs, being fairly stable as oxidants, seem to be the perfect candidates. But native AGEs are sparse and not sufficient, since they are normally controlled by our defense systems. On the other hand, food AGEs, which can constantly flow into the body in an unregulated fashion, are a far more efficient source of oxidants—one that can drive and maintain chronic inflammation. Food AGEs are easily the best source of biological kindling to fuel chronic low-grade inflammation.

As AGEs begin to pile up in tissues, the immune system views them as invaders or irritants and mounts a defensive response. For example, immune cells such as macrophages have special receptors such as AGER1 (see page 29), that sense the presence of AGEs.[13,14] Then, like Pac-Men, they engulf them and set out to break them down. The remnants are then swept away in the blood, filtered out through the kidneys, and expelled in the urine. But if macrophages get filled with too many AGEs, they become exhausted and are then unable to keep up with any new AGEs that flood in with meals. The now frustrated macrophages recruit more immune cells, which then mount a stronger "inflammatory" immune response.[15,16]

Now you have a sense of how AGEs can be eliminated or, if not eliminated, how they can mount up in tissues. But how exactly do they damage the body's structures? Consider a case in which AGEs are stuck to connective tissue, such as that of our joints. As macrophages try to remove the AGEs, they must also bite off and break down pieces of the collagen strands to which AGES are welded, causing injury. (Think of this as collateral damage.) The more AGEs there are, the greater the damage. As inflammatory cells strive to rid AGEs from the body, they also spew out potent inflammatory proteins known as *cytokines*. These cytokines damage adjacent cells or structures and can increase the harm done by inflammation.

To make matters worse, if inflammation continues unabated, it leads to a vicious action-reaction cycle, which leads to more AGEs and more inflammation. In essence, AGEs can turn a normal *self-defense* into an abnormal *offense,* namely, chronic inflammation. After a while, tissues can become so bruised that organs begin to malfunction. This is one very common way in which AGEs can lead to chronic diseases—against a backdrop of persistent low-key inflammation.

This concept has been confirmed in studies of hundreds of people who, while considered healthy, actually had chronic systemic inflammation of which they were not aware. The extent of inflammation turned out to be proportional to the amount of AGEs in their diet.[17] Fortunately, we found that this type of inflammation can be quickly and effectively reduced by simply reducing the amount of AGEs consumed.[18] (See page 39 to learn more about this.)

AGEs Compromise Our Host Defenses

The body has an abundance of safety mechanisms that work to protect the well-being of our cells and tissues. These are collectively referred to as *host defenses* or *innate defenses*. One type of host defense is the immune system, which, among other things, orchestrates the inflammatory response just discussed and makes antibodies that fight foreign invaders such as bacteria and viruses. Another type of host defense is our native antioxidant system, which is able to neutralize and control oxidants, including AGEs. But AGEs can actually harm our host defenses—including some that have been rather newly recognized—and make them less effective. Two important host defenses that can be adversely affected by AGEs include SIRT1 and AGER1.[19]

SIRT1 belongs to a class of very important proteins known as *sirtuins*, which regulate many processes in the body. In humans, SIRT1 is a potent antioxidant and also affects numerous vital immune and metabolic functions, including, but not limited to, inflammation, insulin resistance, fat mobilization, and brain function.[20] All in all, it has been found to delay disease and extend lifespan in some insects and mammals. For these reasons, SIRT1 is often referred to as a "survival factor" or "anti-aging molecule." Needless to say, there has been a great deal of interest in finding ways to boost SIRT1. For instance, compounds (e.g., resveratrol) that are thought to mimic the actions of SIRT1 have been found in red wine, and small amounts have been found in vegetables, fruits, tea, and spices (polyphenols).

SIRT1 all but disappears in older adults and in people with chronic diseases such as diabetes. The reason for this decline in SIRT1 has long been a mystery—or it was, until we discovered that SIRT1 was depleted only in those people (or animals) who consistently consumed foods with high levels of AGEs, which bring with them high oxidant stress and a high inflammatory state. It would seem, then, that low levels of SIRT1 are not simply a random event caused by getting older or having a chronic disease. Rather, these levels may be due to long exposure to AGE-laden foods. In fact, SIRT1 is low even in young people if they consume a high-AGE diet.[21]

Found in most cells, especially macrophages, the "anti-AGE" receptor known as *AGER1* is the principal receptor that facilitates the removal of excess AGEs from the body. These receptors normally control AGEs by plucking them from the fluid around cells and pulling them into the cells, where they can then be destroyed. When levels of AGEs exceed the capacity of the body to detoxify them, they increase oxidant stress. As long as the levels of AGER1 are sufficient, this defensive factor helps maintain a normal oxidant balance, part of which is to support SIRT1. But like SIRT1, AGER1 seems to be depleted in people who have chronic diseases or are older. And just as with SIRT1, the depletion of AGER1 is linked to an AGE-rich diet.

The take-home message is that an AGE-rich diet depletes not only the classical antioxidants, such as SOD and glutathione; but also host defenses, such as SIRT1 and AGER1, discussed above; and many other protective factors, including PPAR and adiponectin, as well as glyoxalase I, an enzyme that degrades a very potent AGE called methylglyoxal. Although some of these newly discovered substances may not sound familiar to you, they are essential to your health. Just as important, all of these defenses can be rapidly restored to normal levels by following an AGE-less diet.

As you have now learned, the body has an abundance of defense mechanisms to protect it against threats from its environment. However, this capacity is not unlimited. And, unfortunately, we face increasing challenges from our environment, which has drastically changed over the last hundred years. We are now exposed to an unprecedented amount of toxins—in the air, in the water, and in our food. These changes are happening too fast for our defenses to adapt. As a result, the demands on our defenses may now exceed the body's considerable resources. AGE-rich foods, ingested in excess because we prefer them, make up the largest toxic exposure in today's environment. This makes our commitment to reducing food AGEs a most important way to both decrease this toxic burden and bolster the body's battered defenses.[8]

AGEs Make Our Tissues Stiff and Brittle

AGEs work like Velcro or glue to latch onto nearby proteins and form bridges between them. So, they "stick" molecules together that are not meant to be "stuck." The term we use for this formation of chemical bridges between proteins is *cross-linking*.[22]

To understand why this AGE property is so destructive, consider the vast network of connective tissue proteins that forms the backbone of most of our organs, including the blood vessels, heart, tendons, and even the lungs. We count on the collagen strands of connective tissue to be elastic, to stretch back and forth, or to glide freely over one another. This elasticity and flexibility is a real feat of engineering that allows us to fill our lungs with each breath of air, and to bend our joints from head to toe. Elasticity also allows us to pump blood from the heart through the blood vessels and ultimately reach every corner of the body.

When Velcro- or glue-like AGEs are inserted in this picture, the tissues become rigid. They can become immobile, harden, and distort countless little pieces of our body. These changes may take years to be felt, but as AGEs build up with time, they "weld" more and more proteins together, making blood vessels, joints, muscles, and tendons progressively thicker and inflexible. A common example of how this causes trouble is when stiff blood vessels that cannot dilate—so-called hardening of the arteries, or *arteriosclerosis*—lead to high blood pressure and heart disease. This triggers the recruitment of aggravated macrophages and local inflammation, as discussed earlier, causing further trouble.

The following is a list of the many ways in which AGEs cause damage in the body. Some of these harmful effects have been discussed in this chapter, and some have not, but will be discussed in Chapter 3. As you glance at the list, we hope that you also take time to consider that AGEs are abundant in some of your favorite foods.

Unlike any other contaminant or pollutant known to man in the recent past or present, food AGEs can simultaneously affect virtually every part of the body. Since these changes occur gradually and are neither felt nor visible to the naked eye, they mostly go undetected as they wreak havoc in the body.

The Many Ways Excess AGEs Can Be Harmful

❏ Since AGEs are oxidants, they generate an excess of free radicals, triggering oxidant stress—the root cause of inflammation, cellular injury, and cell death.

❏ Excess AGEs exhaust the body's native antioxidants and overwhelm innate defenses, making the body vulnerable to early aging.

❏ Excess AGEs fuel chronic, systemic inflammation—an underlying cause of all chronic diseases.

❏ Excess AGEs cross-link or "weld" proteins together, causing hardening of the arteries, stiff joints, cataracts, and wrinkled skin.

❏ Excess AGEs cause insulin resistance and promote the development of type 2 diabetes.

❏ Excess AGEs oxidize blood lipids,[23] which then get deposited inside our arteries and form "plaques" that plug blood vessels, leading to strokes, heart attacks, eye problems, kidney failure, and loss of limbs due to gangrene.

❏ Excess AGEs help retain AGE-fat, which is difficult to lose, all the while fueling inflammation. This is why AGE-fat is referred to as "bad" or "inflamed" fat.

❏ Excess AGEs get inside the brain, where they can damage brain cells, leading to loss of memory and other cognitive functions associated with Alzheimer's disease. AGEs also affect the nerves in the lower limbs and elsewhere.[24]

ARE AGES "ADDICTIVE"?

We eat far too many AGEs quite simply because AGEs are part of the taste, aroma, and appearance of foods that we have come to expect, enjoy, and, indeed, crave. Our busy lifestyles make it necessary for us to eat on the run, and we rely increasingly on restaurant or "grab-and-eat" meals. Many of these foods entice taste buds by being cooked until golden brown in the oven, in deep fat, or on the grill or skillet, with a crusty brown finish that intensifies the flavors. When we prepare food at home, our favorite recipes frequently use the very same techniques to increase AGEs and intensify our taste experience. And, of course, many of us also rely heavily on AGE-rich prepared foods that we purchase in the supermarket. Advertisers and food companies understand our preferences very well and add to the allure by making prepared foods inexpensive, readily available, and lavish in portion size.

A New Perspective on "Bad" Dietary Fats

For many years, there has been much discussion of "good" and "bad" dietary fats. Everyone agrees on the health hazards of hydrogenated oils and trans fats, but there is less agreement on saturated versus unsaturated fats. What gets totally overlooked is that dietary fat of all kinds—even the so called "good" fat—is easily oxidized by heat, and even by light or air. You are probably familiar with how easily butter becomes rancid as it oxidizes sitting out on the table. But few people realize that fat oxidation happens much faster when heat is applied, as in cooking.

As fat oxidizes, it generates free radicals that cause further oxidation of the fat, fueling the formation of AGEs on nearby fats and proteins, which are often mixed with some sugars or carbohydrates. This happens whenever you sear meat with oil in a hot skillet, bake a traditional cheese-topped pizza, or cook up a batch of fat-laden biscuits or croissants, to name a few examples. What if you don't sear your meat in a pool of oil, but instead cook it on the grill without any added fat? As many people know, there is still plenty of fat inside, and this fat can oxidize and help form AGEs. In fact, certain phospholipids, found on the surface or inside muscle cells, are especially potent AGE makers. But what few people realize is that muscle cells, like all cells, naturally contain small amounts of very reactive sugars that trigger super-rapid

We appear to have succumbed to a new lifestyle that includes constant overeating—and eating many of the wrong foods. AGEs seem to be in the driver's seat, spurring the appetite and urging us to reach for more food than is needed. It is almost as if eating AGEs causes us to crave more AGEs. While taste is a recognized factor in addiction, there is only limited evidence as of yet that AGEs, per se, are addictive. However, we are at an important crossroad. Research is looking at the peculiar "addictive" properties of processed foods and their effects on brain chemistry. The phenomenon of ceaseless eating and snacking suggest that there is something about our food that causes a craving which cannot be satisfied by foods such as fruits and vegetables, not even when sugar or salt are added to them. There is a growing consen-

AGE formation under heat. So even lean meats can form many AGEs when they are cooked with dry heat. This is why the method of cooking is so important when preparing any food, and especially when cooking meats.

There is no doubt that fats would be far less harmful if consumed in their natural state, before they are too oxidized and are still relatively low in AGEs, but we almost never eat them this way. For instance, nobody eats raw bacon or lard. Even the fats we think of as "uncooked," such as vegetable oils, have already undergone various processing steps that expose them to heat, light, and air—all of which trigger oxidation. Nuts and seeds undergo a drying process and may also be roasted. The effect of heating on fats is profound: Studies in our laboratory show a several-fold increase of oxidation products when vegetable oils are heated to typical cooking temperatures. Moreover, even "healthful" fats, such as omega-3s, may lose some of their good properties during cooking. This is due to the fact that the rapid oxidation of fats and free radicals released in the process of cooking basically robs them of their "good" properties.

The bottom line is that fats cooked at high temperatures tend to be highly concentrated sources of AGEs—which may be what originally gave some fats their bad name. More important, even "good fats" are vulnerable to AGEs. Chapter 6 provides tips for choosing the best fats and ways to minimize oxidation and AGE formation in these foods.

The Dark Side of Dark Sodas

Everyone knows that sweetened colas are "bad," since too much sugar can lead to obesity, diabetes, and vascular disease.[25] What is not realized is that what draws us to these drinks is not just the sweet taste of sugar, but also the taste of AGEs. Many consumers switch to sugar-free diet cola as a healthier substitute, since it provides a similar taste without the added sugar. Unfortunately, brown-colored diet sodas contain nearly the same amount of AGEs as their sugar-sweetened counterparts. The dark color and characteristic flavor of these beverages is due to AGEs that are made by caramelizing (dry heating) sugars. While these sodas are not exceptionally high in AGEs, they do contain common but very reactive precursor AGEs, such as methylglyoxal.[26,27] Once ingested, these pre-AGEs can generate additional AGEs when they mix with food proteins or fats. This interaction could be one reason why these sodas have such a damaging effect on the body. In fact, several current studies scientifically show that sugar-free diet drinks are associated with as much obesity as drinks that contain sugar. So in this respect, dark diet colas may not be much safer than sugar-sweetened varieties.

The bottom line is that all sweetened sodas, whether light or dark, contain far too much sugar and should be avoided for this reason alone. But if you drink soda, your best option is a clear or light-colored sugar-free soda, as this will be very low in AGEs. Even these should be limited, since they contain artificial sweeteners and other questionable ingredients.

sus that we have arrived at a point where our food has become dangerously "hyper-palatable," luring us into an "eating overdrive" and tipping the scales toward food addiction. AGEs, along with unhealthy doses of sugar, salt, fat, and artificial flavorings, contribute to this problem of overeating. Thus, in a never-ending cycle, AGEs help drive overeating, and overeating drives up AGE intake.

But even people who make a conscious effort to not overeat can unwittingly ingest far more AGEs than the body can safely handle. Our clinical studies show that AGE intake is often three to five times above the limit of safety in people who consider themselves very healthy. We have found that this is related to the *way* food is prepared, rather than to the *type* or *amount* of food consumed.

We can guess what you might be thinking: "I've already cut back on fat, sugar, and salt. Do I now have to give up foods just because they *taste good*?" Definitely not! Quite the opposite! You will find that an AGE-less diet resembles French and Mediterranean-style cuisines. These cuisines feature some of the finest food in the world. Just count the number of four-star restaurants in these categories! Did you ever imagine that the French paradox could be as much due to the savory stews, *en papillote* ("in parchment paper") cooking, and abundant fresh foods as it is to red wine?

You may also be wondering if it is possible to exchange old habits for new, healthier ones, especially when many available foods seem to be so addictive. In this day and age, with a fast food chain on every block and processed snack foods everywhere, it may seem impossible. But the evidence is unmistakable. Our studies—which involved direct experience with hundreds of people—demonstrated that an AGE-less diet can be easily adopted by everyone, especially since there is no need to feel food-deprived. Habits *can* be changed for the better. Consider how many people have given up smoking, how many have opted for leaner cooking methods and meatless meals, and how many people of all ages are now beginning to swap sugary sodas for water. Of course, it is much easier to replace unsafe eating habits with safer ones if the new habits are equally satisfying. You will see that eating the AGE-less way is both generous and rewarding. And because it focuses mainly on the way you cook, AGE-less principles can be applied to any type of diet in keeping with your personal preferences. Moreover, calories can be adjusted to allow for weight loss, weight gain, or weight maintenance, depending on your individual needs. (See Chapters 4 and 5.)

CONNECTING AGES IN THE BODY WITH FOOD AGES

Throughout the years that my team and other researchers performed the groundbreaking work described in Chapter 1, there was no data on the quantities of AGEs in each food, either in its raw state or after it had been cooked in various ways. It was impossible to even begin to speculate on the effects of AGEs in food without this basic knowledge. So we were the first to pick up the task of measuring AGE levels in common contemporary foods. We were also the first to publish a database listing the AGE content of hundreds of familiar foods, using one of the more common AGEs—and by now a universal AGE marker—CML (εN-carboxy-methyl-lysine).[28,29] Many of these foods have been listed in Chapter 4. A quick survey of this data will show you that the highest AGE levels are found in foods of animal origin, since these foods are richer in protein and fat, especially the type of fat that can be easily modified and form AGEs. In addition, these foods are very often cooked by broiling, grilling, roasting, or frying—in other words with high-dry heat, which is known to produce additional AGEs. Since animal products such as meat, butter, and cheese are very typical of our daily diet, it is easy to see how many of us can easily consume AGEs at levels that may be harmful, even toxic, even though we think our diets are healthful.

After creating a database, we still had to test our hypothesis that most people generally consume excessive, perhaps toxic amounts of AGEs. We then used our database to estimate the consumption of AGEs in healthy volunteers of different ages and ethnicities living in the New York City area. All of our subjects felt well, were nonsmokers, and were not aware of any health conditions. When we measured the AGE intake of these people, we found that it averaged 16,000 AGE kilounits per day, ranging from 12,000 to 20,000 AGE kilounits per day. This is more than twice what we have since determined to be a safe level. It was intriguing to see that blood levels of AGEs were proportional to the amount of AGEs consumed with food. We also discovered that levels of inflammatory markers in the blood were nearly double what is considered to be normal.[30,31] Moreover, blood levels of a prototypic inflammatory marker called TNFα (tumor necrosis factor alpha) also correlated with the amount of AGEs in the diet. In other words, those who consumed a high-AGE diet had chronic inflammation. Since chronic inflammation is linked to many health problems, such as diabetes, these people might have been at a higher risk for developing these conditions. So, there were good reasons to question whether, in fact, our volunteers were as healthy as they believed they were.

Testing for AGEs in the Human Body

Having long realized that AGEs are closely tied to chronic diseases and aging led us and others to propose that AGE levels be routinely measured to monitor health, just as blood pressure, blood sugar, and lipids such as cholesterol are monitored. For decades, scientists have been trying to nail down a practical, easily available method that measures those AGEs that cause disease. This has been challenging, in part because of the large number of chemical compounds that fall into the general category of AGEs. For this and other practical reasons, research studies are now carried out by using a few "representative" AGEs as markers, such as CML (εN-carboxy-methyl-lysine) or MG (methylglyoxal). These few AGEs are chosen because they are found in nearly all body components, as well as in foods. Many health problems have now been linked to abnormally high levels of these compounds, and in this respect, they serve as useful markers of disease. Currently, these AGE markers are tested by several methods.

Enzyme-Linked Immunosorbent Assay (ELISA)

This is by far the most widely used method and the one we and many other scientists employ. ELISAs use *antibodies*—proteins that are produced by the immune system to identify "foreign invaders" such as bacteria or viruses in order to target and then eliminate them. Taking advantage of this unique ability of antibodies, ELISAs work much like scanners to identify and count specific molecules. ELISAs are widely used in medicine and research to test levels of insulin, hormones, cancer, inflammatory markers, lipoproteins, enzymes, and more. In the case of AGEs, ELISAs measure certain AGE proteins or lipids, typically CML and MG.[32,33,34] The levels of these AGE compounds have been found to go hand-in-hand with inflammation and a number of conditions or disease processes, including insulin resistance, vascular disease, kidney disease, and mental decline. So they have been accepted as representing "harmful" AGEs.

Without a doubt, AGE-ELISAs will one day be available as routine blood tests at hospitals and doctors' offices. For now, testing for AGEs is done mostly in research settings. Under normal conditions, most of the AGEs circulating in the blood come from food, so testing for blood

AGEs is best done after an overnight fast. Based on thousands of tests in people of every age, race, and ethnicity, typical fasting levels of AGES (e.g., CML) fall into the range of 6 to 9 units of AGE per milliliter of serum (U/ml). One AGE unit (U) refers to one AGE modification or substance, such as CML, bound to a standard amount of protein or lipid. After a large meal, blood AGE levels may temporarily double to 15 U/ml. Patients with kidney disease or diabetes and overweight people with prediabetes or metabolic syndrome may have levels of up to 25 to 40 units per milliliter. It is important and encouraging to keep in mind that within two to four months after starting an AGE-less diet, blood AGE levels are significantly reduced and may even be restored to a normal level.

Chromatography-Mass Spectrometry Methods

Chromatography is a method of separating and analyzing mixtures of chemicals. Several types of chromatography are available, and they are often used in combination with a procedure known as mass spectrometry (MS), which is another means of chemical analysis. As technology is improving, these two tools of analytical chemistry are gaining popularity among food chemists.[35]

Chromatography-MS methods could, in theory, detect AGEs with a high level of accuracy. However, currently, this is possible only after the complete digestion and breakdown of proteins or peptides to their individual amino acids. This means that these methods can measure only "free" AGEs, which have not been shown to carry the toxic properties we have come to associate with protein- or fat-bound AGEs. Another problem is that these methods are not designed to work with lipids (fats), and therefore greatly underestimate the amount of AGEs present in tissues or food. For these reasons, chromatography-mass spectrometry techniques are not the best choice for clinical use.

Skin Autofluorescence

One of the oldest and simplest techniques, autofluorescence provides an estimate of AGEs that are deposited in the tissues by measuring these substances' natural emission of light through use of a simple reader on the forearm. This reading is used to estimate AGE accumulation in the body and the potential risk for AGE-related problems.[36]

At the moment, skin autofluorescence is of limited use in measuring AGEs. Although some AGEs have fluorescent properties, some—such as CML and MG—do not fluoresce, nor do they have color. This means that skin autofluorescence misses those AGEs with proven clinical importance, while at the same time picking up some harmless ones. Moreover, readings can be variable or unreliable in people with darker skin, after recent sun exposure, or in the presence of certain skin disorders and treatments. Skin autofluorescence is thought to be at least a useful extra tool in confirming the risk of serious cardiovascular or late kidney disease in white people,[36,37] although by itself, it is not yet ready to be used for either screening or monitoring early disease states.

An obvious and important question that surfaced at that point in our research was whether this heightened inflammation—and the risk for disease—could be minimized and, better yet, eliminated by reducing the consumption of AGEs found in foods. Half of the participants were asked to remain on their usual diet, and the other half was assigned an "AGE-less" diet for a period of four months. The AGE-less diet group was instructed to change *only* their cooking methods to favor stewing, braising, poaching, and steaming—all AGE-less cooking techniques—but not to change the type or amount of food they ate. Their calorie and nutrient intakes, therefore, would remain unchanged. The goal was to reduce food AGEs in this group by just one-half.

Both groups were tested for blood levels of AGEs and markers of inflammation[30,31] before and after the four-month period—and the results were impressive. Those who were instructed to reduce their intake of food AGEs by half showed a decrease in AGEs and inflammatory markers to normal blood levels in just a few months. It was clear that the experiment was successful. Dropping AGEs led to a decrease in risk for disease, at least for the test period. Again, remember that the participants' usual foods weren't replaced with different ones, nor were their usual caloric and nutrient intakes changed. The main change was in the ways in which they prepared meals in their own homes.

There were several other important take-home messages learned from these studies:

❏ A safe intake of food AGEs is below 8,000 AGE kilounits per day. At that level of AGE consumption, inflammatory markers do not exceed their normally low level.

❏ Many of us are under the impression that we are in good health. However, if we habitually follow the typical modern diet that is rich in AGEs, we are likely to consume at least twice as many AGEs as we should. Over a period of time, this is likely to increase our risk of developing inflammation-associated diseases such as diabetes, high blood pressure, kidney disease, Alzheimer's disease, and even cancer.

❏ It is completely possible for people with high blood levels of both AGEs and markers of inflammation to achieve a healthier state. Even if we are unable to cut down on the amount or type of food we eat, we can improve our odds for excellent health—within just a few weeks—by simply adjusting our cooking methods.

By reducing AGE intake through the use of different cooking methods, our participants essentially were able to reverse the path toward major disease that they were inadvertently following. The results of the initial studies have now been confirmed in subsequent trials in people with diabetes or kidney disease, as well as in overweight people with metabolic syndrome. It is clear that participants who applied themselves to the AGE-less program succeeded in securing better health. Importantly, this was done largely in their own homes and within a short period of time, with little effort and without extra expense.

In today's world, it is all too easy to find yourself on a high-AGE diet. This translates to a higher risk for debilitating disease and great personal expense, not to mention the larger societal cost. But it's just as easy to follow an AGE-*less* diet. Part Two of this book provides simple instructions and many delicious recipes that will help you become AGE-less.

CONCLUSION

The extensive experience and scientific evidence on dietary AGEs, which we briefly reviewed in this chapter, has been gathered over more than two decades. This evidence has led to nothing less than a completely new way of thinking about our health and health maintenance. We now know that AGEs provoke inflammation, undermine our body's innate defenses, and negatively modify our body proteins, fats, and DNA. A persistent AGE overload can affect every cell, organ, and system in the body, setting us up for many chronic degenerative diseases.

We also know that most AGEs in the body come from eating AGE-rich foods, and that even people who believe that they're eating a healthy low-calorie or low-fat diet can unwittingly ingest a large amount of AGEs. Worse yet, AGE overload can start at a young age. Today, we see many more children and adolescents with conditions such as obesity, high blood pressure, and prediabetes, all of which have been linked to an AGE-rich diet. That is the negative side of this issue.

On the positive side, since most AGEs enter the body through food, we now know that we can simply avoid them or at least sharply reduce them. It is never too late to start controlling AGEs, but the sooner you begin, the better the result. The AGE-less diet can keep AGEs at bay, reduce inflammation, and bolster the body's defenses against numerous diseases. We are confident that if you follow the AGE-less diet, your risk for chronic disease will be notably reduced. Moreover, if you have a chronic disease, considerable benefits may be derived from following this program. Chapter 3 takes a closer look at the many health problems that are linked to overexposure to AGEs, and the succeeding chapters will help you manage them effectively.

3.

_____

AGEs, Aging, and Chronic Disease

One of the great feats of human invention has to be the fact that we now live much longer than we did at any other time in history. For most of human history, *natural selection*—or the *survival of the fittest*—dictated how long people lived. Longevity depended on our ability to survive powerful forces of nature, including extreme weather conditions, predators, food shortages, and disease-causing microbes. Until the last millennium, the life span of *Homo sapiens,* the human species, averaged only about forty years. In contrast, survival in the modern world is shaped largely by industrial and scientific revolutions. Thanks to new drug discoveries, organ transplants, personalized medicine, and other feats of modern science, many people can expect to live at least twice as long as their ancestors. This gives a new meaning to getting old. However, since aging cannot be skipped altogether, the question becomes, *What can we do to "age well"?*

Among the most cited causes of early aging today are too many oxidants in the environment, diminished antioxidants, and inflammation. As you have learned, AGEs are a driver of the oxidation and inflammation that damage tissues and fuel chronic diseases associated with older age. AGEs also can diminish the body's natural antioxidant defenses, further tipping the balance toward oxidative stress and inflammation. In addition, AGEs can bind together, or *cross-link,* tissue proteins, which makes them less elastic and eventually stiff, with a tendency to tear. Over time, AGEs can cross-link proteins in all vital organs, causing hardening of the arteries, stiffer lungs, cataracts, inflexible joints, and much more. Once AGEs become lodged in tissues, there is no easy way to reverse this problem.

In the previous chapter, you learned how AGEs work on a molecular level to create havoc in the body. In this chapter, we will take a closer look at how the buildup of AGEs brings about a host of health problems and chronic diseases that were once associated only with aging, but are now also affecting much younger people. A complete list of these health problems would be very long. The following partial list includes only those health issues that will be discussed in the remainder of the chapter.

- Arthritis
- Cardiovascular disease
- Dementia
- Diabetes
- Intervertebral disc disease
- Kidney disease
- Maternal and infant health issues
- Muscle changes and muscle loss
- Obesity and overweight
- Osteoporosis (bone fragility)
- Skin damage
- Vision problems
- Wound healing problems

ARTHRITIS

Arthritis is a nearly universal complaint today—especially since the numbers of overweight, non-exercising people and those with chronic disease continue to increase. The word *arthritis* refers to joint inflammation and pain, and describes over a hundred different diseases and conditions that affect one or more of the tissue components that make up the joints. Some forms of arthritis involve the immune system and affect multiple organs of the body. Examples of this type of arthritis are rheumatoid arthritis, lupus, and gout.

All forms of arthritis, whether affecting isolated joints or multiple ones, generally cause joint pain and stiffness that is severe enough to impair the ability to perform everyday tasks. In fact, arthritis is the leading cause of disability in the United States. Experts frequently recommend that people with arthritis follow an "anti-inflammatory" diet. Unfortunately, most patients (and even their physicians) are still unaware that avoidance of dietary AGEs should be a key feature of any anti-inflammatory regimen. Let's take a look at two of the most common types of arthritis and the role that AGEs may have in their development.

■ OSTEOARTHRITIS

Osteoarthritis (OA)—the most common form of arthritis—is a chronic condition in which the cartilage that covers the ends of the bones and cushions the joints breaks down, causing bone loss and painful joints. It often affects weight-bearing joints, such as the spine, hips, and knees, although other joints can be affected as well.

OA has long been attributed simply to "wear and tear" of the joints or "old age." We now know it is much more complex than that. For instance, various genetic traits, obesity, injury, and overuse of the joints are linked to OA. AGEs also play a significant role. This is because cartilage, bone, and tendons are rich in connective tissues, such as collagen, that tend to have a low turnover rate, meaning that when injured, they are replaced very slowly. Moreover, due to their chemical structure, these tissues facilitate AGE formation. This leads to cross-linking, which, over time, causes tendons to become less elastic and more fragile. Additionally, AGEs activate immune cells, such as macrophages, causing prolonged inflammation, injury, and the eventual breakdown and loss of cartilage and adjacent bone.[1]

■ RHEUMATOID ARTHRITIS

Rheumatoid arthritis (RA) is an autoimmune disease in which a person's immune system attacks the *synovium*, which is the membranous pouch-like structure that surrounds the joints. RA is characterized by painful swollen joints, often leading to joint deformity and disability. This condition is associated with *systemic inflammation*, which means that inflammatory factors such as the potent cytokine *tumor necrosis factor alpha* (*TNFα*), are present in the blood at high levels. In fact, one of the most successful modern treatments for RA works by lowering TNFα levels using antibodies specific for this harmful protein. Excessive levels of such cytokines are often associated with problems in other organs, such as the kidneys and brain. So it's not surprising that patients with RA often experience symptoms in many organs.

AGEs have been found to exist inside the joint space and are also elevated in the blood of patients suffering from RA. Since these toxins can cause inflammation, there has been a suggestion that they play a role in RA.[2]

CARDIOVASCULAR DISEASE

The cardiovascular system, composed of the heart and blood vessels, moves blood throughout the body, and with it, the oxygen and nutrients that sustain life. *Cardiovascular disease* (*CVD*) refers to a variety of disorders that affect the heart and/or blood vessels. Common examples include coronary artery disease, heart failure, stroke, and peripheral arterial disease. In recent decades, death rates from CVD in the United States have declined, largely due to the availability of new medical treatments and a decrease in the number of people who smoke. But despite these gains, more people than ever are now living with disabilities due to CVD, and CVD still remains the most common cause of death in America today, accounting for more than half of all deaths in adults. As you'll see in the following discussions, AGEs are strongly associated with common heart and blood vessel problems.

■ DISEASES OF THE HEART AND BLOOD VESSELS

As we grow older, changes gradually take place in the heart and blood vessels. The normally supple and elastic walls of our blood vessels begin to stiffen. At the same time, fat, cholesterol, calcium, and other substances may begin to build up in the walls of the arteries, forming plaques that lead to *atherosclerosis*, which involves both hardening and narrowing of the arteries. As the arteries become less flexible and narrower, blood pressure rises and the flow of oxygen and nutrients to other parts of the body is restricted. Damage to the coronary artery, which supplies blood to the heart, is called *coronary artery disease* (*CAD*). Damage to the arteries that lead to other parts of the body—such as the arms and legs—is called *peripheral artery disease* (*PAD*). The heart, which is a muscle, can become enlarged and unable to pump sufficient blood to meet the needs of the body. This condition is known as *cardiac insufficiency* and can lead to *heart failure*.

What do AGEs have to do with these changes? Just about everything. It has been known for more than thirty years that oxidant stress and inflammation are linked to diseases of the heart and blood vessels. Studies have specifically shown that atherosclerosis—once thought to be mostly a lipid storage disease of the blood vessels—also involves an ongoing inflammatory response.[3] So it should not be surprising that by causing inflammation, AGEs may make things worse.

But how do AGEs cause inflammation in our blood vessels? As we learned in Chapter 2, our immune system sees AGEs as "foreign invaders" and responds accordingly. The process unfolds in the following way: As AGE-proteins and AGE-lipids pile up inside the cells of the blood vessel walls and overwhelm their defenses, the tissues become inflamed. They then send signals to the immune system, which responds by sending off cells called macrophages to deal with the damage. But problems arise when these macrophages become congested with AGEs. The overwhelmed macrophages respond by releasing potent inflammatory substances known as *cytokines*, some of which work as alarm signals to recruit even more inflammatory cells to help. A major downside of this is that these cytokines also damage normal cells—the very tissues they were sent to protect. If these newly recruited cells persist for a long time, they can spread the injury much as a wild fire spreads destruction.

Certain potent cytokines such as TNFα can also harm tissues by directly acting on cells. For instance, they can irritate platelets—the tiny cells that normally help blood to form clots—stimulating them to produce dangerous clots that can suddenly block the blood flow in an already narrowed vessel and cause a heart attack or a stroke.

AGEs can perpetuate CVD by a variety of other mechanisms, as well. The following list presents some of the different ways in which AGEs contribute to the development of cardiovascular disease.[4]

❏ AGEs promote inflammation in both vascular and immune cells.

❏ AGEs form cross-links that stiffen arteries and cause high blood pressure.

❏ AGEs reduce the activity of nitric oxide, which is a vital and potent vasodilator that widens blood vessels so they can fill up with more blood to deliver to tissues. When there is not enough nitric oxide in blood vessel walls, the result is increased blood vessel rigidity, higher blood pressure, and a higher risk of blood clots.

❏ AGEs cause small blood vessels (capillaries) to become leaky. Leaky blood vessels contribute to many problems, including edema (swelling of the tissues), eye and brain problems, metastasis of cancers, and more.

❏ AGEs cause blood clots that block blood vessels, leading to heart attack and stroke.

❏ AGEs accelerate calcification of the arteries—the deposition of calcium plaques that, over time, can narrow the arteries and reduce elasticity.

❏ AGEs oxidize LDL (bad) cholesterol, changing its structure so that it is harder to remove from the blood and more likely to end up entrapped in artery walls.

❏ AGEs oxidize HDL (good) cholesterol, changing its function and making it less protective.[5]

You now have a better idea of how AGEs can stir up inflammation and cause damage to the blood vessels. But two simple experiments illustrate the rapidity with which dietary AGEs can directly affect the cardiovascular system. The first was performed with healthy adults who were asked to drink just a single AGE-rich beverage made from a concentrated diet cola.[6] The second was conducted with diabetic patients who were given a single AGE-rich meal consisting of broiled chicken.[7] In both studies, the participants that ingested the AGE-rich foods showed a sharply reduced blood flow to the arm within less than half an hour, indicating a sudden dysfunction of the arteries. The faulty blood flow was associated with a sharp increase in markers of inflammation, signaling "injury" to the vessels. Fortunately, both abnormalities resolved after a few minutes, but these "challenging" tests demonstrated how rapidly changes can be provoked by AGEs. When people habitually consume AGE-rich meals, the resulting vascular injury may no longer be reversible.

Having these results in mind, we examined both "normal" and diabetic subjects over a few weeks. But now, the participants were given either a diet with the usual amount of AGEs or a similar diet prepared the AGE-less way. After consuming the AGE-rich diet, the blood flow tests again indicated vascular dysfunction, but after the AGE-less diet, they remained normal.[7] While these studies must be confirmed by larger and longer clinical trials, we believe that by cutting back on dietary AGEs, it is possible to reduce the risk for cardiovascular disease. Furthermore, even when CVD is present, it may be possible to postpone a heart attack or stroke.

■ STROKE

A *stroke* occurs when the blood flow to an area of the brain is interrupted or severely reduced, depriving the brain of oxygen and causing brain cells to begin to die. This can result in loss of memory and cognition, or in loss of muscle control, causing an inability to walk, stand, move, or speak. These events often take the form of an *ischemic stroke*, which occurs when a blood vessel carrying blood to the brain is blocked by a clot, or a *hemorrhagic stroke*, which happens when a weakened blood vessel ruptures.

AGEs can easily find their way into the brain's blood vessels or cells, causing a localized inflammation. We now know that this inflammation can remain "silent" for long periods of time, while AGEs slowly—in the ways listed on page 48—cause arteries to and within the brain to close down and eventually get blocked. This is the most common cause of stroke. Moreover, as we discovered from working with laboratory mice, after a stroke, brain damage can be more extensive and serious if the affected brain tissue already contains too many AGEs.[8] Studies show that AGEs can spell double trouble for the brain. First, they wear down or injure brain arteries and make them susceptible to blockage, just as they do in vessels of other organs. Second, they can make brain arteries leakier, enabling AGEs to escape the vessels and gain entry to the brain cells themselves, where they cause injury. If too many AGEs have been deposited in the brain over a long period of time, this may have already caused a depletion of the brain's protective defenses and can reduce the brain's chances of recovery from an event such as a stroke.

Although definitive human trials on stroke remain to be done, these initial animal study results make logical sense, especially when tied to what studies in humans have revealed about AGEs and the brain. When AGE deposits build up in the brain, they cause inflammation and aging, just as they do elsewhere in the body. It is no longer far-fetched to see AGEs as a cause not only of cardiovascular disease, but also of dementia.[9]

DEMENTIA

One of our worst fears as we grow older is *dementia,* a chronic disorder marked by problems with memory, the ability to concentrate, a sense of connection, and learning. This fear is not unfounded, since the risk of dementia rises exponentially with age, doubling about every five years after age sixty.

There are many causes of dementia. For instance, it can arise due to a lack of vitamins or micronutrients or from an infection or a reaction to medications. This type of dementia may be reversible by correcting the underlying problem. It can also occur after an event such as a stroke, which can cause immediate and profound symptoms. But most often, dementia develops over many years with the gradual erosion of cognitive function caused either by Alzheimer's disease or by *vascular dementia,* which is brought about by impaired blood flow to the brain. Alarmingly, the prevalence of dementia is growing worldwide, and preventive measures and effective treatments are lagging behind.

Cognitive decline is more common in people with diabetes, heart disease, high blood pressure, and kidney disease—the same diseases that have surged in the last fifty to seventy years. What underlies this uncanny coincidence? Scientists have considered everything, from genetic causes and altered gut bacteria to a loss of natural antioxidants, too much stress, and new environmental toxins. But there is one point of agreement: All forms of dementia stem from chronic inflammation and oxidant stress. Does that sound familiar?

The earliest clue that AGEs might be involved in cognitive decline was found more than one hundred years ago. Researchers noticed that brain cells accumulated a kind of yellow-brown pigment named *lipofuscin*. This fatty pigment—which was also found in the heart, eyes, and kidneys—was identified as a mix of oxidized lipids and proteins generally thought to be cellular debris. It seemed reasonable to suspect that lipofuscin also contained lots of AGE-lipids. Since the brain is extremely rich in lipids, it was a matter of time before we and others found that brain lipofuscin-like material contained AGE-lipids, that levels of AGEs in the brain increase with age, and that this can coincide with a disturbance of brain function.

The most common form of dementia is *Alzheimer's disease* (*AD*). This slowly progressing disorder is characterized by the loss of brain cells, by the loss of connections between brain cells, and by an abundance of two abnormal structures—plaque-like deposits call *amyloid plaques* and *neurofibrillary tangles,* which are twisted protein threads (think of a mass of tangled hair). These hallmarks of Alzheimer's are especially common in those areas of the brain that command memory. A typical early symptom is difficulty in recalling specific recent events, but brain changes may begin long before any symptoms appear. Although in some cases, a family history of this disease or certain genetic traits are recognized as risk factors, there is no agreed-upon cause nor any effective treatment.

How are AGEs linked to Alzheimer's? While the brain is an exceptionally well-protected area, over the years, it can become like an old fortress with crumbling walls. By causing brain vessels to become leaky, AGEs can damage the protective barrier that insulates the brain from the rest of the body. This, in turn, allows these harmful compounds to get inside the brain. Once behind the brain barrier, AGEs bond with proteins specific to the brain, such as beta-amyloid or tau protein, resulting in the formation of amyloid plaques and neurofibrillary tangles. Both of these structures are thought to be quite injurious to the human brain, and there is convincing experimental evidence that AGEs can instigate or accelerate their formation. [10]

The first compelling evidence that supported a direct relationship between the AGEs present in food and AD came from a highly publicized study that our group did on mice.[11] We discovered that when mice were fed the standard AGE-rich type of mouse diet until old age—in this case, a year and a half—not only did they get an excess of AGEs stashed in their brain, but they developed dramatic brain changes that closely resembled those seen in Alzheimer's disease, including amyloid deposits, inflammation, and loss of memory. Importantly, this was associated with decreased coordination and motor skills, just as it is in humans. In contrast, mice fed AGE-less food had much lower levels of AGEs in their brains and only minimal amyloid deposits and inflammation. The truly remarkable finding was that the very old mice fed the AGE-less diet did not develop any cognitive or motor decline.

Also intriguing was the fact that SIRT1, a potent anti-inflammatory protein and a key factor in brain function as well as metabolism (see page 28), remained perfectly normal with an AGE-less diet. This was important, because it had long been known that SIRT1 is suppressed in AD and in aging in general. Also, AGER1, the AGE receptor that helps clear AGEs (see page 29), remained normal, as did other protective factors. These studies highlighted how harmful an AGE-rich diet can be to the brain. More important, they demonstrated that a low-AGE diet can "protect" against Alzheimer's disease—at least in mice. The question was whether these findings would pertain to humans, as well.

To begin sorting this out, we studied older people who were living independently in the New York City area. At the time, these people were free of dementia and conditions that are associated with dementia, such as diabetes and insulin resistance. After testing their memory, we instructed them to keep an AGE-food diary by listing their food intake and, especially, keeping notes on cooking methods. We collected their notes at the clinic, where they were followed for five years. As we had seen before, the levels of AGEs and inflammatory markers in the blood were a direct reflection of the amount of AGEs consumed with food. But the most telling new finding was that in people who were habitual consumers of AGE-rich foods, *and only in them*, memory had gotten significantly worse. These people belonged to a single group that had both the highest levels of AGEs and inflammation and the lowest levels of protective SIRT1 and AGER1.[11,12] The finding that older but still healthy individuals who simply share a preference for high-AGE foods can suffer a measureable loss of memory in just five years was eye-opening. This was the first clear indication that AGEs are toxic to the human brain, a sobering finding.

As remarkable as these study results were, there is no question that more clinical studies need to be performed to determine whether the AGE-less diet will prevent or—just as important—*restore* memory loss in humans. Given how slowly this disease develops, such trials may require decades to complete. However, there are already many good reasons to reduce the consumption of AGEs as a preventive measure against dementia. As a society, we currently have no effective protection against the debilitating and costly effects of Alzheimer's disease and other types of cognitive impairment. Reducing dietary AGEs is simple, cost-effective, and has no down-sides, making it just what the doctor ordered.

DIABETES

Diabetes is a condition in which the level of blood glucose is abnormally high. It is among the most common chronic diseases of the developed world, and it is the leading cause of cardiovascular disease (CVD), kidney disease, blindness, loss of limbs, dementia, and reduced life span. Nearly 30 million people in the United States have diabetes, and the number of newly diagnosed cases is expected to double every ten years. In addition, 86 million adults have *prediabetes*, a condition in which blood sugar is higher than normal, but is not high enough to be classified as diabetes. All in all, about 50 percent of the United States adult population has either diabetes or prediabetes.

One of the main jobs of insulin, the hormone produced by the beta-cells (β-cells) of the pancreatic islets, is to enable glucose to pass into the body's cells, where it can be converted into energy. Diabetes develops when the pancreas does not make enough insulin (*type 1 diabetes*) or the body is not able to use the insulin properly (*type 2 diabetes*), causing glucose to accumulate in the blood. Type 2 diabetes is the most common form of the disease, accounting for about 90 percent of all cases.

Insulin resistance, a condition in which the cells respond poorly or not at all to insulin, usually precedes type 2 diabetes. In an attempt to overcome the problem, the pancreatic islets work overtime to produce more insulin. As long as the pancreas can produce enough insulin to surmount the insulin resistance, blood glucose levels stay in the normal range. But eventually, the pancreas may become exhausted, unable to produce the large amounts of insulin needed. This is when glucose builds up in the blood, leading first to prediabetes and then to diabetes. Insulin resistance can also be linked to a cluster of dysfunctional changes known as *metabolic syndrome,* which increases the risk for diabetes, dementia, and cardiovascular disease, and is linked to many other health problems. (For more information about metabolic syndrome, see page 64.)

As we have discussed, AGEs form from reactions between sugars and proteins or fats. Since people with diabetes have high blood sugar levels, they have the "fuel" to make more AGEs. The hemoglobin A1C test, which is used to monitor average blood sugar levels in people with diabetes, actually measures "glycated" hemoglobin—a precursor of AGEs, or *pre-AGE.* Based on the knowledge that AGEs form from sugars and proteins, it would seem logical to conclude that blood sugar is the primary source of the increased AGE levels seen in diabetes. However, this is only partly true. While all diabetics who have high blood sugar will likely have high A1C levels, not all of them have high AGEs. And many patients with nearly normal A1C can have high levels of AGEs. While high blood sugar can cause more AGEs to form within the body, we now know that much of the AGEs that are found in circulation—even in people with diabetes—come from foods.[13] Something else to consider is that the kidneys, which help excrete AGEs from the body, have a direct effect on the level of circulating AGEs. For instance, diabetics who have high blood sugar may not have high blood AGE levels because their kidneys are still healthy enough to excrete these substances. (For more about kidneys, see page 58.)

For decades, scientists have searched for ways to prevent the devastating complications of diabetes. Since one of the most obvious features of diabetes is high blood sugar, it seemed logical that if you implemented "tight" or "intensive" control to maintain blood sugar levels as close to normal as possible, you would successfully prevent these problems from developing. This turned out to be an overly simplistic view. A number of large studies have looked at the control of blood sugar, and their results have been very inconsistent. Indeed, current evidence suggests that diabetic complications are more related to the presence of AGEs than to high blood sugar. A large body of research has shown that AGEs are involved in and even drive the most devastating complications of diabetes, such as cardiovascular, brain, and kidney disease. Interestingly, there is evidence that in the relative absence of AGEs, these complications are slowed down or do not develop despite the presence of high blood sugar or A1C levels in diabetics—even after a period of fifty or more years. [14]

In addition to driving the complications of diabetes, a high-AGE diet may precipitate or hasten the development of diabetes itself. What is the evidence? For one, data in mice show that a high-AGE diet can induce both type 1 and type 2 diabetes.[15] Also, epidemiological studies on human twins who were followed since childhood showed that those who ended up developing type 1 diabetes were those who had high blood levels of AGEs. These high levels were present long before they became diabetic, pointing to a source of AGEs other than the body's own sugar.[16] These studies were repeated and confirmed in a larger group of "non-twin" children. [17] Taken together, the studies nail down the environment as the major source of AGEs and place them squarely in the category of major risk factors for the development of diabetes.

The following list shows the various ways in which AGEs are believed to contribute to diabetes:

❏ AGEs in food increase appetite and promote obesity, a major risk factor for type 2 diabetes.

❏ AGEs increase oxidant stress and inflammation, two factors that precede both type 1 and type 2 diabetes.

❑ AGEs have toxic effects on insulin-producing β-cells of the pancreas, causing a decrease in insulin production and leading to type 1 diabetes and the late stages of type 2 diabetes.

❑ AGEs affect how our tissues—our fat cells, muscles, and liver—respond to insulin, leading to insulin resistance.

❑ AGEs can modify the insulin molecule, which can cause it to lose its function.

The studies discussed earlier raised many interesting questions. What could cause the higher AGE levels in healthy people who go on to develop diabetes? Could food AGEs be the problem? It would be unethical and impractical to expose healthy people to high-AGE diets for the many years needed to develop diabetes just to prove this point. Rather, we discovered something equally convincing: People who habitually favored a high-AGE diet were likely to display prediabetes or insulin resistance.[18] Even more to the point, we turned the question around by asking if people who already had diabetes could become more healthy. And, indeed, we found that just four months of the AGE-less diet substantially reversed a lingering insulin resistance in patients with type 2 diabetes.[19] These findings were strengthened by a larger and longer study of one hundred obese patients with prediabetes.[20] We found that over a period of a year, the AGE-less diet was able to nearly normalize insulin resistance, which if left untreated, could have led to diabetes and its many complications. Moreover, the AGE-less diet brought about this remarkable result without requiring a reduction in calories. (To read more about this study, see page 69.)

Despite the significant progress that had been made, we searched for stronger proof that these benefits of the AGE-less diet were precisely due to reducing the amount of food AGEs entering the body, and not to some unforeseen effect of the diet. Luckily, we were able to directly address this question soon after. By coincidence, we had found a drug that, although it was not absorbed in the gut, could bind with food AGEs, preventing the toxic substances from being absorbed into the blood and instead causing them to be eliminated in the stool. The drug, sevelamer, had a long history of use in people with kidney disease, where it binds to excess phosphate in the gastrointestinal tract and carries it out of the body, essentially doing part of the job that the kidneys normally carry out.

It was a risky expedition, but we went on to study sevelamer in two controlled trials in patients with type 2 diabetes who also had diabetic kidney disease. [21] During the trials, the patients continued their usual diet and medical care. The only change was that they took the drug three times per day with meals. We could hardly believe the results. The AGEs in the blood were successfully reduced by sevelamer by at least as much as they would have been reduced by the AGE-less diet. And, as with the AGE-less diet, this was accompanied by a significant reduction in markers of inflammation and a near normalization of antioxidant and anti-inflammatory factors—also called host defenses—including AGER1, SIRT1, and others. Now, we had the proof: *Toxic quantities of AGEs most certainly do come from our food, regardless of the presence of diabetes.*

To our surprise, many of these patients also had shown a significant improvement in hemoglobin A1C. This was an interesting discovery since these patients, despite being under excellent medical care, still had elevated A1C. In fact, these patients were all receiving multiple "anti-diabetic" drugs and were being carefully followed by one of the premier diabetes groups in New York. In addition, they were following a diet prescribed by the American Diabetes Association, and a dietician experienced in diabetes care was seeing them. In other words, they were receiving "optimal" care. Yet reducing the absorption of food AGEs could bring blood glucose under even better control. Our findings offered definitive evidence that food AGEs must be avoided, especially by diabetics.

INTERVERTEBRAL DISC DISEASE

Back pain due to chronic stress to the spine, or *intervertebral disc disease,* is a near universal problem. Not only older people but also overweight and diabetic individuals very often suffer from back pain, and medical science has not offered a way to prevent the problem. Because of the role AGEs plays in tissue breakdown, we often wondered if there was a connection between the deterioration of discs and AGEs.

To find out, we set up another study: After mice were fed either an AGE-rich or AGE-less diet for their entire life (almost two years), we found that the AGE-rich diet led to distinct degenerative changes in the spine and the intervertebral discs, similar to those seen in human diabetes, old age, and obesity. By comparison, the spines and discs of mice exposed to the AGE-less diet had remained healthy.[1] This well-controlled study made a fairly strong case for the fact that the chronic ingestion of AGEs in our food contributes to changes in the spine and intervertebral discs. Clinical trials will hopefully shed more light on this subject soon.

KIDNEY DISEASE

Most people don't give much thought to their kidneys. These bean-shaped organs—located against the back muscles, just below the rib cage—are each about the size of your fist. Although they tend to silently go about their business, the kidneys are truly hardworking, versatile, and adaptive organs. Their best-known job is filtering toxic waste products from the blood and forming urine to remove this waste from the body. But they also perform several other heavy-duty jobs. Our kidneys help maintain the crucial balance between salt and water in the body. They produce or control many hormones that help regulate the heart, control blood pressure, produce red blood cells, and control normal bone growth. And importantly, the kidneys are the only organs that can expel excessive amounts of toxic food-derived AGEs. Such vital functions explain their enormous blood flow, energy requirements, and impressive reserve capacity. Even if one of our two kidneys is removed, the remaining kidney can still easily cope with day-to-day needs.

But, as you have learned, AGEs are good at gumming up the works. These substances are "sticky" and can adhere to the tissues of all organs. They accumulate along our huge network of blood vessels, significantly reducing their ability to get the blood to where it is needed. This greatly affects the kidneys. Although the kidneys are small, they have a lot of blood vessels, and every minute, they are exposed to about 20 percent of the body's total blood volume. Over time, the accumulation of AGEs in the kidneys progressively undermines many of their vital functions. Cells in the blood vessels and other parts of the kidneys are injured, and the organs begin to get scarred and shrivel up, greatly reducing their ability to excrete AGEs.

There is something else to consider: We have calculated that the amount of AGEs that pour into the body each day with food may exceed the capacity of the kidneys to flush them out by at least two- to three-fold.[22,23] Imagine, then, all the AGEs that cannot be cleared from the body and end up in our tissues, day after day, month after month, year after year.

This situation gets even worse if the kidneys are not working perfectly. Remember that the kidneys are the body's main exit for AGEs. So when kidney function declines, in essence shutting down this exit, AGE levels rise in the blood, flooding all the tissues of the body. This sets the stage for greater damage to not only the kidneys themselves, but all other organs, as well. This may be why kidney disease is linked to diabetes, heart disease, cancer, Alzheimer's, and aging. High levels of AGEs in the blood are an excellent predictor of reduced renal function in older adults. In fact, patients with kidney failure have AGE levels that are five to seven and even ten times above the normal level.[24]

■ DIABETES, AGEs, AND THE KIDNEYS

Diabetes—today, an epidemic—is the most common cause of reduced kidney function, or *chronic kidney disease*. This means that the reality of kidney disease looms over more people now than it has at any other time in history. Every person with diabetes is potentially at risk. As we have learned, people with diabetes have abnormally high levels of both sugar and AGEs in their blood. This raises the question of whether food AGEs are more or less harmful to the kidneys than high blood sugar itself.

From animal studies, we know that blocking the formation of AGEs inside cells with special anti-AGE drugs protects the kidneys from the effects of diabetes, even though hyperglycemia is still present. The drugs used in some of these studies are at the stage of clinical trials or on the way to becoming available for clinical use. But are new drugs the only answer to controlling AGEs, or is another approach available?

To find out, we studied mice that were genetically diabetic, and as a result, were prone to kidney disease. The mice were fed either regular mouse chow, which is made into pellets using a dry-heat process, or an AGE-less diet, which was specially prepared without excess heat. All the mice were fed the same amount of food in terms of nutrients. In just a few months, it was clear that the AGE-less diet had almost completely protected these diabetic mice from kidney disease, even though they remained diabetic.[13]

Two points are worth noting. First, the AGE-less diet worked despite persistently elevated blood sugar levels. This meant that high blood sugar was not the main problem. Second, despite the fact that these mice had defective genes that could make them susceptible to kidney disease, kidney disease did not develop when they were fed the AGE-less diet. Therefore "bad" genes did not cause the kidney disease, although they certainly raised the odds. But exposure to a "bad" trigger—a high-AGE diet—did create problems. In other words, genes may matter to an extent, but a trigger matters a lot: No trigger, no trouble. In short, diabetic kidney disease may have less to do with high blood sugar and a great deal more to do with high AGEs, most of which come from food.

Of course, the important question is, do these findings in mice apply to people? As discussed on page 57, we have published two clinical trials in patients with kidney disease and diabetes, using the drug sevelamer, which prevented food AGEs from being absorbed into the body. The drug quickly and effectively lowered AGE levels in the blood of our patients, just as occurs with an AGE-less diet. Better yet, there were improvements in both inflammation and albuminuria (protein loss in the urine) and a recovery of lost defenses such as antioxidant and anti-inflammatory factors SIRT1 and AGER1, proving that reducing food AGEs can be beneficial for kidney disease.[25]

The patients participated in the trial for only six months, but we saw changes which suggested that kidney disease might be arrested. A concern here is that while this drug worked very well, it may be many years before it is approved for this use. Also, drugs often interact with other drugs and have serious side effects, and they certainly cost money. So the AGE-less diet is still the best option. No doubt, a combination of a drug and the AGE-less diet could be more effective than either alone in many cases of diabetic kidney disease.

More and larger trials are likely to spring from these innovative studies. Until that time, the important and practical message is that lowering the consumption of AGE-rich foods may provide protection against the development or progression of kidney disease in diabetes, without compromising either nutrition or the enjoyment of eating.

■ AGING AND THE KIDNEYS

Conditions such as high blood pressure and diabetes are well-known risk factors for kidney disease, especially as people get older. However, most healthy people can also show a decline in kidney function with age. After age forty, it is estimated that kidney function declines in about a third of the healthy population. This raises important questions, since the cause of this decline is unknown. Could it be somehow linked to the AGE-associated general inflammation of older age?[26]

To investigate whether AGEs might be a trigger for aging-related kidney decline, we took young healthy laboratory mice and fed them either an AGE-less diet or regular mouse chow until they were very old. Both groups of mice were fed the same amount of food. We found that mice fed the AGE-rich diet developed kidney changes that were consistent with their old age, such as shrinking and scarring of kidney tissues, a decline in kidney function, and a shortened life span. In contrast, the AGE-less mice did not develop kidney changes and had a stronger and more youthful heart and blood vessels.[27] No wonder, then, that these mice lived a larger part of their lives in good health than did their littermates, who were fed the usual AGE-rich food.

As always, the next question was whether humans would derive similar benefits from an AGE-less diet. While it has not been possible to control the diet of humans for a lifetime while tracking their health, we did learn a great deal from one of our studies of patients with advanced kidney disease.[28] The participants were maintained on a nutritionally complete diet, but with about half the usual amount of AGEs. After just one month, blood AGE levels were decreased by half, and this was accompanied by a similar improvement in markers of inflammation. Since these participants had significant kidney disease, usually intractable to treatment, even these results were remarkably rapid and signalled a clear improvement in the patients' overall condition. The study was much too short for a major improvement in kidney function to materialize. However, the AGEs excreted in the patients' urine doubled during the study, indicating a substantial recovery in one of the main functions of the kidneys, the removal of toxic substances. Improved AGE clearance was indeed responsible for the reduced inflammatory state in these people.

An important message here is that staying away from AGE-laden foods can mean improved kidney health. The earlier this message becomes integrated into the overall care of people with kidney disease, the better their quality of life is likely to be. The more general message is that protecting your kidneys from a heavy AGE load may be a way of keeping your entire body younger and healthier. In the long run, this is a worthwhile investment.

MATERNAL AND INFANT HEALTH ISSUES

It is common knowledge that women should avoid smoking and alcohol during pregnancy, because of the potential harm posed by these substances to the unborn baby. Due to concerns that excess AGEs may predispose infants and children to diabetes or other health problems, it appears that limiting dietary AGEs should be added to this list. Since AGEs are able to cross the placenta and transfer from the mother's blood to the developing fetus, avoidance of dietary AGEs should start during pregnancy.

Along these lines, we can offer the following intriguing fact: Blood AGE levels in newborn infants can closely correlate with those in their mother's blood, and soon after, with levels of AGEs found in infant formulas. Breast milk has the lowest level of AGEs compared with commercial infant formulas, which can contain over one hundred times more AGEs. Alarmingly, infants with higher circulating AGEs can show a tendency for insulin resistance. This, if persistent, could precondition them to an early onset of diseases such as diabetes, obesity, or high blood pressure.[29] These findings were supported by studies conducted in newborn mice that were followed well into adulthood.

One study was conducted in mice that were genetically prone to type 1 diabetes, and the other, in mice prone to type 2 diabetes. The results of both of these studies were striking. Compared with pups fed the standard dry-heat-processed mouse chow, those who got the AGE-less diet had a significantly lower incidence of type 1 diabetes or a marked delay in the onset of age-related type 2 diabetes, which became lower with each successive generation.[15]

The above information leads us to believe that an AGE-rich diet during pregnancy, infancy, and childhood may overwhelm immune defenses and lead to many diseases later in life. There is increasing evidence that allergies, asthma, diabetes, and autoimmune diseases such as rheumatoid arthritis and inflammatory bowel disease are all occurring at an earlier age than in previous generations. It is not yet completely clear what role AGEs play, but data from both animal and clinical studies suggest that this merits further investigation.

MUSCLE CHANGES AND MUSCLE LOSS

As we get older, we are likely to experience any number of muscle changes, including a loss of muscle strength and function or loss of muscle mass, known as *sarcopenia*. Another common aging-related problem is muscle stiffness and loss of flexibility. These changes can greatly impair balance, gait, and the ability to perform the routine tasks of daily living. Sarcopenia is a real problem, leading to frailty in old age and increasing the risk of falls and fractures. But that's not all. Loss of muscle causes a decline in basal metabolic rate, making it easier to gain unwanted pounds. It also increases insulin resistance, making it easier to develop diabetes and cardiovascular disease. Muscle mass typically starts to decline sometime in the thirties, but the loss accelerates later in life. Sarcopenia is most severe in people who are sedentary, but the fact that it also occurs in physically active people indicates that other factors are involved.

AGEs are likely to be a causative factor in muscle loss and weakness. As we get older, most adults are likely to develop more cross-linked collagen, in part because of an excessive amount of AGEs being "stuck" between the muscle bands, as well as in the tendons and the sheaths that contain each muscle. This probably plays a significant role in overall muscle stiffness. AGE-induced injury of muscle cells can likewise cause a loss in muscle cells, leading to loss of muscle mass.[30] An interesting connection between AGEs and muscle dysfunction is the finding that older adults with the highest blood levels of AGEs have weaker "grip" strength [31] and slower walking speed compared with those with lower AGE levels.

OBESITY AND OVERWEIGHT

Obesity or overweight affects the majority of adults and a growing number of children in modern society. Let's take a look at why this is such a serious problem.

Too much fat in the body has long been known to be the easiest way to make our body resistant or even unresponsive to insulin. First discussed on page 54, insulin resistance can be a huge problem because insulin is what makes it possible for cells to take in glucose and convert it into energy.

Strange though it seems, the more we eat and the fatter we get, the more resistant our cells become to insulin, a state known as *insulin resistance.* In other words, our cells starve despite having an excess of glucose in the blood. This sends frantic signals to the pancreatic islets, calling for more insulin in an effort to get sugar into our cells. But more insulin does not always solve the problem. When the blockade persists, unused glucose accumulates in the blood, leading to the diagnosis of type 2 diabetes and all of its complications. Eventually, the β-cells that produce ever more insulin can get fatigued and stop working altogether. This can lead to insulin-dependent, or type 1, diabetes.

As we already learned, long before diabetes develops, insulin resistance can be linked to a cluster of dysfunctional changes known as *metabolic syndrome.* Like diabetes, this syndrome often goes unrecognized because there are no obvious symptoms. There are however, some classic signs: Excess abdominal fat, high blood triglycerides, low HDL "good" cholesterol, high blood pressure, and high blood sugar. Metabolic syndrome now affects about 35 percent of all adults in the United States and half of adults over age sixty. It is also prevalent in Europe and is rapidly spreading to the rest of the world. Another important point: It used to be the rule for metabolic syndrome to affect middle-aged and older adults. Now, this condition is increasingly common among people in their twenties and thirties, and even adolescents and children.

Obesity, insulin resistance, and metabolic syndrome are all connected—and a state of high oxidant stress, and thus inflammation, ties them all together. What does this have to do with AGEs? As you know by now, AGEs are key players in oxidant stress and inflammation. But they also act in other ways. For instance, AGEs attack the tiny bridges that insulin uses to transport glucose inside the cells, causing a breakdown in the ability of cells to metabolize glucose. To add insult to injury, food AGEs, by enticing you to overeat, fight your weight-loss efforts every step of the way and favor the deposition of body fat, especially belly fat, which notoriously exacerbates insulin resistance.

■ AGEs, WEIGHT, AND BODY FAT

Many different nutritional plans have been offered for weight loss, and while a number are effective in the short term, most fail to keep off the lost weight for long periods of time. A 2014 *meta-analysis*—a statistical method that combines the results from multiple similar studies—illustrates the reality of weight-loss diets. One year of dieting produced an average weight loss of about sixteen pounds, and the results were similar for both low-carbohydrate and low-fat diets. While everyone knows someone who has lost a much larger amount of weight on a "diet," over the long term, few people are successful at losing weight and keeping it off.

A clue often misplaced here is the concept of *caloric balance*—that is, every time you eat more calories than you burn for energy, the excess calories are deposited in the body as fat and, therefore, extra weight. If you keep eating more than you utilize, the amount of fat keeps accumulating. Where do food AGEs fit into this equation? By way of adding flavor, aroma, and color to most foods, AGEs quite simply drive us to over-consume calories. So just like unhealthy doses of sugar, salt, fat, and artificial flavorings, AGEs make the modern food supply dangerously hyper-palatable, which entices us into overeating and possibly even to food addiction.

Although it is true that maintenance of weight requires caloric balance, it seems that some foods, such as those that are rich in AGEs, may have a more profound effect on fat accumulation than others. An experiment we performed in mice illustrates this point very well.[32] We fed normal healthy mice a high-fat diet, which is designed to lead to the development of obesity and diabetes. However, half of the mice had their food prepared by exposing it to dry heat to increase AGE content, and the other half had the same fatty food prepared the AGE-less way, with low heat and moisture. So both groups consumed the same amount of fat and calories, the only difference being the AGE content of the diet. After six months, the high-AGE diet group accumulated twice as much visceral (deep belly) fat as the mice on the low-AGE diet, and their plasma insulin levels increased by several times above their own baseline. In other words, they became insulin resistant. However, insulin levels remained normal in the mice on the AGE-less diet.

This phenomenon was confirmed in subsequent, far longer studies in which several generations of mice were fed high-AGE or AGE-less standard mouse diets. In these studies, we found something even more intriguing: With each successive generation, the mice on the high-AGE diet not only accumulated more abdominal fat than mice on the low-AGE diet, but also became fatter much earlier in life. The high-AGE mice also had more AGEs in their fat tissue. To dig further into this, we put the fat tissue under a microscope, where we found fat cells surrounded by many inflammatory cells (macrophages), all full of cytokines, indicating that this fat was of an especially inflammatory nature.[15]

How might AGEs favor the accumulation of this damaging type of body fat? One process is related to those all-important protective mechanisms, or host defenses, first discussed on page 28. We learned that AGEs can cause a serious deficiency in such vital mechanisms as SIRT1, PPARγ, glyoxalase I, and antioxidants.[33] These "protectors" normally keep a lid on inflammation and also help nutrients to be properly metabolized. SIRT1 is crucial for moving fatty acids from visceral fat out to the liver to be metabolized.[34] If there is no SIRT1, then the movement of fatty acids, including AGE-fat, can slow down, causing fat to get "stuck" in fat stores. This is clearly evident as "belly fat," which can be extremely difficult—even impossible—to eliminate. Worse yet, AGE-belly fat is dangerous precisely because, as we saw, it spews inflammatory cytokines into the bloodstream, enabling the cytokines to reach and harm other organs, including the heart, kidneys, and brain.

■ DO AGEs INFLUENCE FAT GENES?

If your parents are overweight, and their parents for generations before have been overweight, does that mean you will inevitably be overweight, no matter what you eat? Do we inherit "fat" genes? Scientists have tirelessly grappled with the question of whether obesity has a genetic component. While the data is still not clear, it appears that there are genes that *predispose* some people to becoming fat, given the right environmental conditions. In other words, genes load the gun, but environment pulls the trigger. In this case, AGEs could be one of the triggers.

For instance, a 2015 study compared the body mass index of participants in the Framingham Heart Study—a large ongoing study of people in Framingham, Massachusetts, now following its third generation of participants. Curiously, they found that people with high levels of the obesity-associated FTO gene who were born after 1942 were more likely to become obese than those who were born earlier. [35]

The authors suggested that this increase in fatness must be due to something that changed in the environment after the 1940s. That "something" could be a factor in the diet that activated this gene and led to obesity. Food AGEs could be such a factor, since they became more prominent following the transformation of our food industry that followed World War II. New technologies allowed mass-produced, heat-processed foods with an extended shelf life to become part of the everyday diet. It is possible that these food AGEs could "trigger" obesity genes, just as they trigger genes controlling inflammation and insulin resistance, as we have already learned. While there is no firm evidence of a direct link, the more we learn about how AGEs are formed in foods and how they influence our eating behavior, the easier it is to see the connection. Food AGEs will fight your efforts to lose weight every step of the way by enticing you to eat far more than you can "burn," and then, to add insult to injury, by facilitating the deposition of "bad" AGE-fat, especially around your belly.

■ THE "HEALTHY" AND "UNHEALTHY" OBESITY PARADOX

It is well established that obesity is a major risk factor for health problems such as insulin resistance, diabetes, and cardiovascular disease. With the rising tide of obesity, the situation is very likely to get worse. But it is also confusing: Although many obese individuals develop diabetes or heart disease, others remain healthy, with no signs of metabolic dysfunction for many years. It is as if not all fat is bad.

To clarify this issue, we carried out a study that compared overweight or obese people who were "healthy" with others who were "unhealthy," because they had one or more conditions of metabolic syndrome, such as high blood pressure, high triglycerides, low HDL cholesterol, or elevated blood sugar.[33] We found that obese people who had high serum AGEs (two to three times the normal level) were sure to have insulin resistance and inflammation as well as several conditions of metabolic syndrome, but those obese who had lower or normal serum AGEs had none of these signs. When we reviewed their nutritional history, we found that unhealthy obese people routinely consumed at least 50 percent more food AGEs than did healthy obese people. The unhealthy obese, in other words, turned out to be devout consumers of AGE-rich foods, preferring their foods grilled, broiled, and roasted.

Type 2 diabetes is a well-known and frequent outcome of metabolic syndrome. As explained earlier in the chapter (see page 54), before full-fledged diabetes develops, people often go through a stage called prediabetes, in which insulin levels are high and blood sugar is elevated, but not enough to be classified as diabetes. Intrigued by the findings that "unhealthy" obese people with metabolic syndrome share a taste for exceedingly high-AGE food, we went on to test whether reducing dietary AGEs—but not calories—would reverse or stall prediabetes. Obese individuals with prediabetes were divided into two groups. Half were offered an AGE-less diet, which contained no more than 8,000 to 10,000 kilounits per day of AGES, instead of their usual 25,000 to 40,000 kilounits per day. Importantly, they were asked not to change the quantity of calories and nutrients they normally ate, but only to switch to AGE-less food preparation methods. The other half remained on their usual high-AGE diet. We closely followed them for twelve months, making sure that there was no lowering of calories, fat, or other nutrients in their diets.

One year later, the results were nothing less than spectacular. There was a marked improvement in levels of insulin and other markers of insulin resistance in people on the AGE-less diet. In fact, insulin levels had nearly returned to normal levels. An unexpected surprise was weight loss averaging seven to ten pounds in those on the AGE-less diet. This change, although small, was unexpected, since the diet did not involve calorie restriction. Some participants happily reported that they shed pounds more easily while on the AGE-less diet than on other regimens, even though that was not the point of the study. No less striking was the improvement in protective (host defense) mechanisms—such as SIRT1 and related antioxidant players—together with an equal improvement in the overall inflammatory state, matching in magnitude the decrease in blood AGE levels.[20]

We cannot overemphasize the crucial fact that no reduction in calorie intake was required to achieve the near reversal of insulin resistance and inflammation, and the profound recovery of lost host defenses seen in these obese patients. This showed that an excessive intake of calories, often in the form of fatty foods in general, are not to be blamed alone. What matters is "bad" fat gathering inside the abdomen and spewing inflammatory factors, as already learned from well-controlled lifelong mouse studies.[36] That kind of fat can come from a diet rich in AGEs. In other words, it is found in our favorite Western diet, which is heavy on animal products, especially red meat; and rich in fats, which are broiled, fried, or otherwise exposed to high-dry heat, and are all too easily oxidized or transformed by the body into AGE-fat.

At the same time, we cannot ignore the modest loss of weight that occurred during the study, and that if kept up, could amount to slow but sustainable progress. The participants, although they still were overweight or even obese, exited our project in a much-improved state

A Debate on Diet and Longevity— Low Calories Versus Low AGEs

Over the last fifty years or so, scientists have tried to sort out the effects of particular nutrients and other dietary factors on the rate of aging. The results have been rather unreliable, with one exception—*calorie reduction* or *calorie restriction* (*CR*). Across a wide spectrum of animal species, drastically reducing calorie consumption (by 25 percent or more) has been found to unequivocally delay the effects of aging, leading to fewer chronic diseases and a significantly longer life span.

Why would drastically cutting calories improve health outcomes? Aging is accompanied by increased free radical production, harmful changes to the DNA, and inflammation. These effects should now be familiar to you—*they are identical to those caused by AGEs.* Calorie restriction, it turns out, lowers free radical production, prevents unwanted DNA changes, and tamps down inflammation and its harmful effects. One of the significant effects of calorie restriction also turns out to also be an increase in SIRT1, the "survival factor" first discussed in Chapter 2. (See page 28.) SIRT1 helps mitigate most of the effects of aging—although, as we already learned, it decreases with age as well as with diabetes and Alzheimer's disease.

Reasoning that ingesting less food also means ingesting fewer AGEs, we wondered if the anti-aging benefits of CR were due to cutting down on calories, cutting down on AGEs, or perhaps both. To answer this question, we divided a group of mice into two groups and fed each a specific diet for life. Both groups were fed exactly the same amount of calories, but one group got only half the amount of AGEs as the other. As the mice got older, only those on the AGE-less diet showed benefits. Compared to mice on the "normal" diet, mice on the AGE-less regimen kept a healthier and more youthful heart and kidneys, maintained greater levels of physical activity, remained leaner, and were more resistant to the development of diabetes. The mice on the AGE-less diet also lived, on average, about 13 percent longer than those on the "normal" diet.[27] This is equal to no less than twenty years of human life, so it is no small benefit.

One conclusion from these studies was that when fewer food AGEs enter the body, both oxidative damage and inflammation decrease.

This outcome spells "success" not only for a longer life span, but also for a better *health span,* the length of time when one is generally free of serious disease. In other words, reduced exposure to food AGEs could explain the benefits of CR. This, again, is not trivial. Calorie restriction seemed to hold promise, enough for it to have many followers. But is it really an effective anti-aging diet?

Since a calorie restriction diet requires long-term adherence to a very strict, hunger-inducing regimen, its general utility remains doubtful. The long-term safety of CR is another issue, since it may be difficult to get enough essential nutrients on a diet that is low in calories. For obvious reasons, a quest for new drugs that can imitate the effects of calorie restriction has been gaining in popularity. A famous example is *resveratrol,* a compound found in relatively large amounts in grapes. In animal studies, resveratrol has been found to mimic some of the protective anti-inflammatory actions of SIRT1. However, the story did not pan out as well when it came to humans, and the jury is still out on many new types of SIRT1-like drugs.

Our own research took a different, perhaps deeper look at the question of what causes a deficiency in SIRT1. It turns out that a decrease of this key substance in older age is not simply due to getting older. Rather, it is the excessive burden of oxidants such as AGEs— for the most part, stemming from a lifetime of exposure to AGE-rich foods—that uses up and depletes SIRT1 and our other protective resources. Weaker defenses leave the door to inflammation open, allowing it to surge.[15]

As you learned in the discussion of dementia, the AGE-less diet enables SIRT1 levels to remain normal, just as a CR diet does. (See page 52.) Over and above these effects, however, is the fact that with the AGE-less diet, there is no need to drastically reduce calories or constantly feel hungry! Plus, the AGE-less diet has the ultimate advantage of being nutritionally healthy and completely safe.

It may be some time before these issues are sorted out. Perhaps a combination of drugs (not yet available), calorie restriction (neither practical nor safe for all), and an AGE-less diet (which is already available, practical, and healthy) may be useful in some instances. But why make life complicated? When it comes to aging, AGE-less eating seems to be the key to improved healthspan and longevity.

of health. A critical new ground seemed to have been conquered. Now, we know that it is no longer necessary to feel hungry for long stretches of time, which is a great problem when people follow most diet plans. We also know that excessive body fat or even obesity doesn't have to be automatically equated with the unhealthy and risk-fraught metabolic syndrome. Our year-long study revealed that the vicious cycle of high AGEs, bad fat, inflammation, and insulin resistance can be broken. Equally important, the entire range of risky events was reversed within less than a year. Neither medications nor other nutritional interventions had been able to achieve these goals. A take-home message is that these changes can be easily implemented by most people in their daily lives, without medical attention and the associated costs.

OSTEOPOROSIS

Osteoporosis, which literally means *porous bones*, is a disease in which bones lose density and become fragile. Approximately one in two women and up to one in four men age fifty and older will break a bone due to osteoporosis. Bone mineral density (BMD) tests are used to assess the risk of osteoporosis. These tests measure how much calcium and other types of minerals are in an area of bone such as the hip or spine.

Another common cause of bone fragility and fracture that many people are not aware of is type 2 diabetes. Unlike osteoporosis, bone fragility associated with type 2 diabetes is not caused by low bone mineral density. In fact, people with type 2 diabetes often have normal or even high bone density. Rather, the bone fragility seen in type 2 diabetes is due to deterioration of bone *quality,* largely related to damage to the collagen matrix that provides elasticity and support to bone.

AGEs are a major cause of the bone fragility seen in both osteoporosis and diabetes. High levels of AGEs may explain why older people or those with diabetes are at a greater risk for fractures, even though they may have normal bone mineral density.[37] The accumulation of AGEs in the collagen matrix of bones makes bones more susceptible to fracture. AGEs can also trigger oxidant stress and inflammation in bone cells, which, over the long term, weaken and damage bones.[38]

Another way in which AGEs may impact bone health is through their effect on the kidneys. The kidneys play a major role in bone health because they control bone mineral content and AGE removal (excretion). Healthy kidneys balance calcium and phosphorus levels in the blood. They also activate vitamin D, which the body needs to absorb dietary calcium. Since excessive AGEs can cause kidney injury in a number of ways (see page 58), they may cause bone disease.

SKIN DAMAGE

The skin is the body's largest organ, though we may not think of it that way. Beyond just protecting us from outside elements, the skin provides a barrier against harmful microbes, gives us the ability to feel, and manufactures vitamin D. Further, its blood vessels help regulate our body temperature, while its sweat glands cool the body off and rid it of toxins. But when the skin is damaged by overexposure to the sun or, as we will see, by AGE accumulation, it can have a negative effect on both our health and our appearance.

■ WRINKLES AND SAGGING SKIN

The skin is one of the best mirrors of our health and age. This is not surprising, since skin is in constant and direct contact with the environment. Just being exposed to sun, to air, and to air's pollutants makes skin vulnerable to irritation, trauma, and disease. It is a well-known fact that most common skin problems are due to inflammation, often referred to as *dermatitis*. Sunburn, a good example, is caused by ultraviolet light that causes skin cells to produce lots of free radicals, which trigger our familiar oxidative damage. Even low amounts of sun exposure on a repeated basis and the attendant oxidative damage can make skin wrinkled and inelastic. Over time, AGEs can have similar effects on the skin.

Just as AGEs are deposited in other tissues, they are deposited in the skin, affecting both its structure and its function. AGEs preferably bind to proteins such as collagen, a constituent of connective tissue, which, as we learned on page 45, has a low turnover rate and therefore does not get replaced very often. They construct cross-links between collagen molecules, causing the skin to become less elastic and leading to sagging and loss of radiance. The formation of cross-links is exacerbated in the presence of diabetes, and together with inflammation, it leads to delayed or abnormal wound healing.[39] Of course, wrinkling inevitably occurs as people grow older, but it may commence at an early age if there is an overexposure to harmful elements such as sun; smoking (which is another source of AGEs);[40] and, of course, the AGEs in foods. Because the restriction of AGEs has been found to improve wound healing in diabetic mice,[39] it seems likely that an AGE-less diet can offer similar benefits in human beings.

■ CELLULITE

Another way that AGEs may affect the appearance of the skin is by accumulating in the fatty layer that lies just beneath the skin, known as *subcutaneous fat*. This AGE-laden fatty tissue tends to expand rapidly and often looks lumpy. The lumps, also known as *cellulite*, are extremely common in women, occurring in up to 98 percent of them, and are influenced by age, obesity, and—to some extent—heredity. Cellulite is notoriously difficult to "melt away," even with drastic dieting. In addition, new research shows that this AGE-fat may not be harmless. AGE-fat accumulates not only loosely between connective tissue strands but also inside fat cells that, like the skin's own macrophages, can spew inflammatory cytokines, eventually causing harm to skin cells and skin components. This can lead to localized skin atrophy (decline) and unsightly sagging due to loss of youthful elasticity. AGE-fat is almost impossible to lose, which may be the main reason why these areas of cellulite are notoriously resistant to even drastic diets.

The lower the AGE burden, the less AGE-fat is formed, and the easier it is for your body to lose fat and repair damaged skin. This means that over time, your skin will remain more youthful. And, of course, minimizing oxidative damage from the sun should also be part of any sensible skin care program. (For more information about

AGEs and skin health, see the discussion of wound healing on page 76.)

VISION PROBLEMS

In many ways, vision is the most valued of our senses. In order for us to see clearly, light must pass through the lenses of our eyes to reach the retina in the back of the eyes. The lenses are made of translucent proteins that allow light to pass through without diffraction (bending of the light waves) so we may enjoy perfectly sharp images. In children and young people, the lenses are crystal clear. It is for this reason that major lens proteins were named *crystallins.* The lenses of young people are also elastic and adjust their shape as needed to sharpen the focus on close-up or far-away objects. Unfortunately, age and/or health problems such as diabetes can greatly affect our vision. And AGEs appear to play a part in the development of common aging-related vision problems.

■ CATARACTS

With age, the lenses of the eyes can become progressively cloudy or opaque, causing a decrease in vision. This condition is known as *cataracts.* Affected patients often experience this problem as "curtains of white water falling" in front of their eyes. The lens also gradually becomes stiff and inelastic. This is one reason that over time, we lose the ability to focus and we require new glasses. As you may guess, the trouble begins with AGEs, which cross-link the crystallins together, disrupting the clear crystal-like organization of these proteins and causing both stiffness and cloudiness. Eventually, a solid opaque or brown mass of proteins cross-linked by AGEs occupies the whole lens. Unless the lens is removed, blindness can result.

The involvement of AGEs in cataracts has been known for many years. Long ago, we demonstrated that when young laboratory mice were injected with AGEs, they developed cataracts identical to those of older or diabetic animals. But when these mice also received an AGE inhibitor, cataracts did not develop, nor did heart and kidney problems due to aging. [41] It is now well established that cataracts are far more common when AGE levels are high, such as in diabetes and aging, as well as with chronic smoking, another source of AGEs.[40]

■ AGE-RELATED MACULAR DEGENERATION (AMD)

Another feared eye disease is *age-related macular degeneration (AMD)*—the deterioration of the central portion of the *retina,* the part of the eye that records the images we see and sends them to the brain via the optic nerve. AMD is the most common cause of blindness in the elderly, and people affected with this condition have both inflammation and AGE deposits in their damaged retina.[42] Experiments in animals suggest that AGEs could be a cause of this condition, but no clinical trials have been done to prove this point in humans.

In view of the strong evidence linking AGEs to cataracts and the potential role of AGEs in AMD, the AGE-less diet might offer a safe way to help keep our vision crystal clear. Even more broadly, protecting eye health by addressing the source of the problem could not only save millions of dollars in medical expenses, but also prevent the suffering of those who have little recourse but to lose their sight.

WOUND HEALING PROBLEMS

After an injury, the ideal scenario is rapid healing without scars or redness—just smooth, elastic skin, like that of children. But this is not the reality for many people. As we get older, simple wounds tend to heal more slowly and may leave scars that are bigger or darker. Many people also suffer from *chronic wounds,* which fail to heal within a reasonable length of time. While all types of wounds have the potential to become chronic, chronic wounds can be categorized as *venous ulcers,* which generally occur in the legs due to improper function of the veins; *diabetic ulcers,* which are due to vascular damage and can appear as sores in multiple stages on the feet of people with diabetes; and *pressure ulcers (bedsores),* which are injuries to the skin and underlying tissues that most often develop in people who are confined to bed for long periods of time. Most often, wounds due to trauma heal within days, but advancing age, obesity, diabetes, and blood vessel disease increase the likelihood that wound healing will be impaired.

Once a wound occurs, an orchestrated process is set into motion to repair the damage. The first order of business is to stop the bleeding by constricting blood vessels and forming a clot. Next comes the familiar inflammation. This is initially a protective immune response—which features redness, heat, swelling, pain, and loss of function—that targets invading microbes and cleans up cellular debris in the wound area. As inflammation subsides, the proliferation of new cells begins, helped by a new network of blood vessels. Finally, the wound closes up as tissue grows and matures over the wound surface.

Many factors, including general health status, stress, medications, nutrition, and more, can affect the healing process. The proper oxygen level, for instance, is critical to wound healing. Oxygen induces the development of new blood vessels, increases the growth of new tissues, and promotes wound contraction. One reason why people who have diabetes, are obese, are older, or smoke take longer to heal is that they often have poor tissue oxygenation (hypoxia) related to poor blood flow or blood vessel disease. Blood vessel damage caused by AGEs (see page 46) is undoubtedly a factor in poor wound healing.

On a more direct level, AGEs accumulate in the skin, just as they do in other tissues, and are known to get in the way of the healing process. From studies in animals, we know that an AGE-rich diet and, by extension, a high body AGE burden make it harder for wounds to heal in a timely manner and more likely for them to become infected or form unseemly scars. AGEs affect various components involved in wound healing by prolonging inflammation or by impairing collagen synthesis and wound closure. An AGE-less diet[40] and anti-AGE agents have been found to speed the healing process in animal studies, but further studies are needed to learn more about the mechanisms through which AGEs impair wound healing in humans.

The entire body depends on a constant state of repair and renewal, and our cells are constantly being replaced by new ones. The skin is a perfect example of this extraordinary process, and it is clear that an excess of AGEs can adversely affect it in many ways.

CONCLUSION

The acronym AGEs was originally coined to remind us that these substances are linked to aging. Over the past several decades, volumes of scientific data have expanded and strengthened the case against AGEs. It has become clear that AGEs are a major factor that underlies not only the aging process in general, but also numerous specific problems that are associated with older age. The list includes some of the most common and costly conditions, such as Alzheimer's disease and other types of dementia, diabetes, heart and kidney disease, arthritis, and much more. It is critical to remember that the effects of AGEs are systemic and affect all tissues and organs in our body. We must also remember that abundant amounts of AGEs are hidden in our daily food. No other single nutrient, environmental contaminant, or pollutant can boast the same pervasiveness as AGEs.

In these first three chapters, we have reviewed what AGEs are, how we have come to rely on a secure and steady supply of foods overloaded with AGEs (the standard Western diet), and what health consequences have been earned as a result. It is clear that AGEs are at the very heart of the early aging process and chronic disease.

We are used to caring for our health by taking simple preventive measures. For instance, we protect our teeth by avoiding sugary foods and brushing and flossing regularly. We eat vegetables and fruits for important nutrients, and we exercise to keep our body in shape. We perform these acts to prevent the very diseases discussed in this chapter. However, our lifestyle is also in many ways indulgent, and one of those indulgences—a diet rich in AGEs, a root cause of disease and accelerated aging—has been largely overlooked. The AGE-less diet offers an important solution and a safe way to ward off these problems. The remaining chapters present and reinforce the principles of AGE-less meal planning and help you put these principles into practice.

4.

The AGE-Less Diet

Our research has taken us on a long and exciting journey. First, we discovered AGEs in the body and linked them to faster aging and chronic diseases. Next, we found that the main source of AGEs in the body was actually the foods that we consume daily. We learned that the amount of AGEs found in food can markedly differ depending the on the way the food is cooked. And, initially in studies using mice, we confirmed that food AGEs had profound negative health effects. This meant that the large amount of AGEs coming from our food could be the major driver of chronic diseases such as diabetes, Alzheimer's, osteoporosis, and even cancer. Just as important, we learned that lowering the intake of AGEs in animals could slow down or prevent the development of every single one of these conditions. The AGE-less diet clearly enabled the animals to live longer and healthier lives.

By comparison, the next step seemed easy enough. We had to determine if what we had learned in animals also applied to humans. But even before we could get to that, we hit a huge roadblock because no one had ever measured AGE levels in human foods before. There wasn't even a known way to address this problem. To move forward, our only choice was to take on this new task, however daunting. Ten years and hundreds of thousands of tests later, we created the first database listing AGE levels in hundreds of commonly consumed foods.[1] This information formed the basis for the AGE-less diet used in our clinical (human) trials. These trials have shown that reducing the intake of AGEs not only lowers levels of AGEs in the human body, but also markedly reduces inflammation and turns the disease clock back in those who have health issues. (See Chapter 3.) Therefore, our chance for a long and healthy life could well depend on how many AGEs we consume with food every day.

This chapter describes what we learned about AGE levels in foods and explains how to lower your daily AGE intake to safe levels. You will learn which foods add the most AGEs to your diet, which foods are naturally low in AGEs, and how you can keep AGEs out of your meals through proper cooking techniques. It comes down to knowledge of three basic principles, which can be applied whether eating at home or at a restaurant. You will also learn about potential AGE therapies—drugs that may be able to lower AGE levels in the body. But, as you will discover, the easiest and most effective way you can preserve your well-being *right now* is by following a diet that limits AGEs through the wise selection of foods and meal-preparation methods.

UNMASKING FOOD AGES

By the time we began testing for AGEs in foods, the process by which they are formed (the Maillard reaction) had been studied by food scientists for decades.[2] (See Chapter 2.) It was well known that higher heat, longer cooking times, and dry (low in water) conditions drastically increased this reaction in foods. It was also known that the addition of sugar or fat to foods and higher pH (alkalinity) increased the speed of this chemical reaction.

Anyone who cooks has witnessed the Maillard reaction in their own kitchen. For instance, chicken that is roasted, broiled, or grilled—all classic "dry-heat" cooking methods—develops a crusty golden-brown exterior. This is a key sign of certain kinds of AGEs. Deep-frying is another type of dry-heat cooking, and as such, it also produces the familiar AGE-rich crusty brown finish. To think of deep-frying as dry heat may seem counterintuitive unless you keep in mind that water and oil do not mix, and in fact, repel each other. So there is no water in a

Measuring Food AGEs

In the inset on page 37, we explained the three methods currently in use to measure AGE levels in the human body as a means of monitoring health. Although the autofluorescence method of estimating AGEs is not appropriate for testing foods, the other two methods discussed in that earlier inset—ELISA and chromatography-mass spectrometry—*are* used to assess food AGE levels.

By now, you may be aware that a large number of different chemical compounds fall into the general category of AGEs, and no method measures all of them. For practical reasons, research is carried out using selected or "representative" AGEs that serve as markers of AGE consumption.

Enzyme-Linked Immunosorbent Assay (ELISA)

This is the method we have employed in our many studies. As described in Chapter 2, ELISA uses antibodies to capture and quantify certain AGE-proteins or lipids.[3-5] One of the better-studied AGEs is a stable compound known as $^{\varepsilon}$N-carboxy-methyl-lysine (CML). This is one of the AGEs that we typically measure in foods and use as representative of AGE content. CML belongs to those AGEs that do not have a brown color. However, it is associated with markers of disease in healthy people and is elevated in obese people and in patients with diabetes, vascular disease, kidney disease, and dementia. This lends credibility to its use as a marker for AGEs in foods and also serves to remind us that even when a brown color is not present in foods, harmful AGEs may be there in substantial amounts.

AGE-ELISAs measure some of the most common AGE substances that are bound together with proteins or fats. Among these are the forms of "harmful" AGEs as they exist in our tissues, blood, and urine, as well as in foods. This test allows scientists to track the passage of AGEs from ingested foods to the blood or tissues, and to assess their impact on our health.

Food AGEs measured by ELISA are expressed in *kilounits* (kU), or thousands of units (*kilo* means *thousand*). One kilounit (kU) refers to one thousand AGE units in a standard amount of protein or lipid. Comparing kilounits per standard amount or serving of food puts the AGE content of various foods into context. The more kilounits there are, the more AGEs the food contains.

Chromatography-Mass Spectrometry Methods

As discussed in Chapter 2 (see page 38), these methods measure only "free" AGEs,[6] not the AGEs that are bound to proteins and fats. "Free" AGEs have not been demonstrated to have the toxic effects we have come to associate with protein- or fat-bound AGEs. Therefore, these methods may measure wholly different substances that may not be the best choice for determining those food AGEs that have been connected with disease.

Another major problem with chromatography-MS methods is that they do not measure lipid (fat)-associated AGEs. The glycation and oxidation (glycoxidation) of fat is a major source of AGEs. Thus, chromatography-MS methods can grossly underestimate the amount of AGEs present in most foods, especially in fatty foods such as butter, cheese, oils, and meats. This is a critical problem, since these foods have been found to bring about many modern diseases.

What to Believe About the AGE Content of Foods

There clearly is controversy among scientists regarding the AGE content of foods based on different methodologies, such as chromatography versus ELISA, and the use of certain AGEs as markers of total AGE content. None of this is unusual nor should it be alarming, given that this is a new field with much active research in progress. Despite any areas of disagreement, over the past several decades, researchers have gained a great deal of knowledge on the subject and have agreed on several basic principles:

❏ Cooking with lower temperatures and more moisture minimizes AGE formation in foods.

❏ Dehydration increases AGEs. Dehydration occurs, for example, when water is removed from milk to make powdered milk, when moisture is lost from meats during roasting or grilling, and when grain products are baked or heat-processed until they are dry and crisp.

❏ Fruits, vegetables, and legumes have a negligible AGE content.

As mentioned earlier, a major difference between the ELISA and chromatography methods has to do with the amount of AGEs found in high-fat foods. Chromatography-based methods do not measure lipid-AGEs, and therefore underestimate the AGE content of fatty foods such as meats, cheeses, butter, and oils. While there is still room for improvement, our ELISA methods for testing food AGEs offer estimates of both protein-AGEs and lipid-AGEs, and these results form the basis for the AGE-less diet that we have validated in both human and animal studies. Our data highlights the very important concepts that animal foods high in protein and fat are AGE-rich, and that care must be taken when choosing and preparing these foods. In addition, fats and oils—even vegetable oils—can be AGE-rich and should be selected carefully and used in accordance with the principles outlined in this book.

We have come a long way in testing for AGEs both in the body and in foods. There are ongoing efforts to arrive at a practical and universally available clinical AGE test. These are mostly matters of fine-tuning. In the meantime, we need to remain mindful of the undisputed facts: First, AGEs in food are—and have been for a very long time—a major threat to our physical and mental health. Second, we can do a lot about it.

deep-fat fryer, but there is plenty of heat and AGE formation. This absence of water is, in effect, dry heat. On the other hand, chicken that is either poached or steamed—classic "moist-heat" cooking methods—does not develop the brown finish characteristic of many types of AGEs.

More evidence of AGE formation can be seen in baked goods. Those made with lots of sugar develop a dark brown crust, while sugar-free versions remain much lighter in color. Baked goods leavened with baking soda (which is alkaline) develop a darker crust than those leavened with baking powder (which is acidic). As we began our task of measuring food AGEs, we thought that variables such as these might be important factors. But whether other factors were involved, or certain foods or food groups would prove to be higher in AGEs than others, remained to be seen, since none had been measured as of yet.

Once we began measuring AGEs in foods, a fascinating pattern began to emerge: The items most heavily laden with AGEs were among the most popular foods in the United States, and many of them were prepared using dry-heat methods, such as grilling, baking, roasting, and frying. The list of AGE-rich foods included steaks, fried chicken, bacon, pizza, cheeses, and butter. Foods high in protein and fat, especially those of animal origin, were clearly among those that had the highest amounts of AGEs. The higher the heat and the longer the cooking time, the more AGEs in the food. A surprise was that foods such as oils and cheeses, which don't have the classic "browned" appearance of roasted or grilled foods, could also deliver large amounts of AGEs. This may be unexpected, but it is due to the fact that many AGE compounds lack the typical gold-brown color. In fact, CML—the compound we use as representative of AGE content when measuring food AGEs (see the inset on page 81)—is colorless. This is why even when a food is not brown, we cannot assume that it is low in AGEs.

As we continued to test a wide variety of foods, looking at variables such as cooking time, cooking method, fat and sugar content, and pH, we were able to come up with three basic principles for planning the AGE-less diet.

THE THREE PRINCIPLES OF THE AGE-LESS DIET

Your transition to eating the AGE-less way must begin with an understanding of three basic principles. These principles will enable you to keep dietary AGEs to a reasonable level that your body can safely handle and eliminate so that these substances do not accumulate and overwhelm the body's defenses, leading to inflammation and chronic disease. The principles are:

1. Learn which foods are lowest in AGEs.

2. Choose cooking methods that prevent the formation of AGEs.

3. Use ingredients that deter the formation of AGEs.

The three principles of the AGE-less diet, which are discussed in detail on the pages that follow, are based on over ten years of testing, observations, and clinical trials.

Principle 1. Learn Which Foods are Lowest in AGEs

After analyzing hundreds of different foods, one thing that has become perfectly clear is that foods rich in protein and fat (particularly of animal origin) tend to be highest in AGEs. However, it is vitally important to understand that the AGE content of foods ultimately depends on how they are *cooked or processed*, as discussed on page 91. This means that a food with a low AGE content can become AGE-rich through use of the wrong cooking method! With this in mind, let's start by looking at the three food groups that are consistently highest in AGEs: *meats, cheeses,* and *fats*. After that, we'll review vegetables, fruits, and other foods that provide a relatively low level of AGEs.

Meats and Meat Alternatives

Meat typically adds more AGEs to the diet than any other food group. Beef tends to have the highest levels of AGEs, followed by poultry and pork. Fish has more moderate AGE levels, while eggs and legumes (dried beans, peas, and lentils)—which can be eaten in place of meat—rank lowest on the AGE scale. Of course, it all depends on how the food is cooked. For instance, grilled chicken can have more AGEs than stewed beef. (See Table 4.1 on page 86.)

When choosing meats, leaner is better, but even lean red meats and skinless chicken can contain high levels of AGEs when cooked with high-dry heat. This is because lean muscle cells naturally contain small amounts of reactive fats and sugars, which rapidly accelerate AGE formation in the presence of dry heat.

Several strategies can help you avoid getting too many AGEs from meats. First and foremost, switch from dry-heat to moist-heat cooking methods, as described in the section that starts on page 91. This is especially important for people who prefer a high-meat diet, which has the potential to greatly exceed a safe limit of AGEs. As you will learn on page 93, marinating uncooked foods in an acidic liquid (lemon juice, vinegar, or wine) can also help deter AGE formation, especially in meats that are grilled or broiled. Another smart strategy is to favor more fish and vegetarian choices over meat proteins. Still another way to cut back on dietary AGEs is to rearrange your meal plate to reduce

Table 4.1 AGE Content of Selected Meat and Meat Substitutes

Food	AGEs per Serving
Beef steak, grilled (3 ounces)	6,700 kU
Beef steak, stewed (3 ounces)	2,200 kU
Chicken, skinless, grilled (3 ounces)	4,400 kU
Chicken, skinless, poached (3 ounces)	800 kU
Egg, fried (1 large)	1,200 kU
Egg, poached (1 large)	30 kU
Kidney beans (3 ounces)	190 kU
Pork ribs, roasted (3 ounces)	3,985 kU
Pork tenderloin, braised (3 ounces)	1,000 kU
Salmon, broiled (3 ounces)	3,400 kU
Salmon, poached (3 ounces)	1,550 kU
Soy burger (2 ounces)	60 kU

the portion of meat and increase the portions of vegetables, fruits, and whole grains. Besides being naturally much lower in AGEs, plant foods contain phytonutrients that may help combat some of the damaging effects of AGEs. Of course, combining all of these strategies is the best scenario for keeping dietary AGEs to a minimum.

Cheeses

Cheeses are another big contributor to our AGE load. Why are cheeses so AGE-rich? After all, they are neither cooked nor browned. A variety of factors may be involved, including dehydration, since the removal of liquid whey is an early step in the cheese-making process, and dehydration is known to drive AGE formation in foods. Also, heat is typically applied through pasteurization and various processing steps. This, too, powers AGE formation. In addition, many cheeses undergo long holding or "aging" times. This is done in caves, cellars, or chilling units, where the temperature ranges from about 50°F to 55°F. Glycation continues to occur even at these cool temperatures, although at a slower rate, which causes the accumulation of AGEs over the long term. So the longer a cheese is aged, the more AGEs it will contain.

The bottom line is that those cheeses which are lower in fat, are less processed, and have shorter aging times tend to be lowest in AGEs. For example, cheddar cheese made with 2-percent milk has about half as many AGEs as cheddar cheese made from whole milk (4-percent milk), and about 70-percent less AGEs than processed American cheese. (See Table 4.2.)

Table 4.2   AGE Content of Selected Cheeses

Food	AGEs per Serving
Cheddar cheese (2% milk) (1 ounce)	740 kU
Cheddar cheese (whole milk) (1 ounce)	1,660 kU
Cottage cheese (whole milk) ($^1/_2$ cup)	1,600 kU
Parmesan cheese (2 tablespoons)	2,500 kU
Processed American cheese (1 ounce)	2,600 kU

Fats and Fat Sources

While many fats are now lauded for their nutritional attributes, such as omega-3 fatty acids, until now, little thought has been given to their AGE content. Fats and oils, especially animal-based fats such as butter, are rich in AGEs. Factors that may be involved include exposure to heat in combination with exposure to air and the dry conditions present during extraction, purification, and other procedures that take place during processing. For instance, conventionally processed vegetable oils may be exposed to temperatures of 400°F or higher during refining. Even oils that are "cold-pressed" may be exposed to warm temperatures, simply as a result of the friction created during pressing or grinding. Also, the longer oils sit on the shelf, especially once they are opened and exposed to air, heat, and light, the more AGEs are formed. Storing oils in the refrigerator has been found to help slow oxidation and AGE formation.

Whole or minimally processed foods such as raw nuts and seeds, avocados, and extra-virgin olive oil are the preferred sources of fat for the AGE-less diet. Of these foods, nuts tend to be highest in AGEs, and if eaten in large quantities, they can add many AGEs to the diet. This is likely due to the fact that most nuts are subjected to a drying process (to produce a crisp texture and extend shelf life) before being sold for consumption. And, of course, many nuts are roasted, which can double their AGE content compared with raw nuts.

With that caveat, including nuts as part of a healthy diet is supported by numerous scientific studies. People who eat an ounce of nuts per day have a lower risk for health problems such as cardiovascular disease and diabetes. These benefits may be related to nutrients such as fiber, folate, magnesium, and potassium, as well as nuts' minimal effect on blood sugar compared with the foods they may replace in the diet.

Foods such as raw nuts and seeds, avocados, and extra-virgin olive oil can add wonderful taste as well as important nutrients to the diet. The key is to enjoy these foods in moderation in order to keep AGEs in check. Something else to remember is that foods which are high in fat are calorie-dense, so moderation can also help you maintain a healthy weight.

Table 4.3 AGE Content of Selected Fats and Fat Sources

Food	AGEs per Serving
Almonds, raw (1 ounce)	1,600 kU
Avocados (1 ounce)	470 kU
Butter (1 tablespoon)	1,890 kU
Olive oil (1 tablespoon)	450 kU
Pumpkin seeds, raw (1 ounce)	560 kU
Sunflower seeds, raw (1 ounce)	750 kU
Sunflower seeds, roasted (1 ounce)	1,400 kU

Vegetables and Fruits

If animal-derived foods contribute the most AGEs to the diet, which foods are lowest in AGEs? Plant foods—which include vegetables, fruits, and grains—consistently contain lower amounts of AGEs than animal foods.

Vegetables and fruits are naturally low in AGEs owing to their relatively low content of protein and fat and their high content of water. The high amounts of antioxidants and vitamins in vegetables and fruits may also diminish AGE formation in these foods. Freezing, canning, or juicing does not appreciably raise the AGE content. Drying—used to turn grapes into raisins, for instance—raises AGE levels. However, the amount of AGEs in dried fruit is very small compared with AGE levels in meats, cheeses, and fats. Moreover, both starchy vegetables (such as corn and potatoes) and non-starchy vegetables (such as green beans and carrots) are low in AGEs. Of course, loading up on too many starchy foods should be avoided since they can raise blood sugar levels.

Grilling, broiling, or roasting can raise the AGE content of fruits and vegetables ten-fold, but even when prepared this way, they have just a small fraction of the AGEs found in grilled or broiled meats. Obviously, deep-frying vegetables, drenching them with butter or oil, or making fruits into rich desserts adds many AGEs. (See Table. 4.4.)

Table 4.4 AGE Content of Selected Vegetables and Fruits

Food	AGEs per Serving
Apples, baked (3^1/$_2$ ounces)	45 kU
Apples, raw (3^1/$_2$ ounces)	15 kU
French-fried potatoes (3 ounces)	1,000 kU
Peppers and mushrooms, grilled (3 ounces)	260 kU
Plums, dried (1 ounces)	50 kU
Sweet potatoes, baked (3^1/$_2$ ounces)	70 kU
Tomatoes, raw (3^1/$_2$ ounces)	20 kU

Grains

Like vegetables and fruits, grains are naturally low in AGEs, and when they are boiled or steamed—as in brown rice, bulgur wheat, or oatmeal—the AGE level remains low. Problems occur when grains are turned into foods such as crackers, chips, and cookies, which are processed with dry heat through baking, frying, or other techniques. For instance, many popular snack foods and breakfast cereals undergo a mechanical extrusion process that uses high-temperature low-moisture conditions to produce appealingly crisp chips, puffs, curls, or other bits of crunchy "food."

Many processed grain foods also contain added ingredients such as butter, oil, cheese, eggs, and sugar, which increase AGEs during dry-heat processing. For example, biscuits have more than ten times as many AGEs as low-fat breads, rolls, and bagels. And cheese-flavored corn chips may have twenty times more AGEs than steamed or boiled corn. Since these foods are also high in carbohydrates, they can contribute to higher blood sugar levels in the body. Table 4.5 shows that as moisture is lost and sugar and fat are added, the AGE content of grain-based foods rises.

Table 4.5 AGE Content of Selected Grain Products

Food	AGEs per Serving
Biscotti (1 ounce)	970 kU
Biscuit (1 ounce)	400 kU
Bread (1 ounce)	25 kU
Bread, toasted (1 ounce)	50 kU
Cracker, graham (1 ounce)	370 kU
Cracker, toasted wheat (1 ounce)	275 kU
Crisp rice cereal (1 ounce)	600 kU
Oatmeal, cooked ($^3/_4$ cup)	25 kU
Rice, cooked ($^1/_2$ cup)	10 kU

Milk and Yogurt

As discussed on page 86, cheeses tend to be very high in AGEs. This is likely due to their low moisture content, exposure to heat during processing, and long aging times. On the other hand, dairy foods with high water content such as milk and yogurt are low in AGEs, and this is true for both low-fat and whole milk products. Milk products that should be avoided include evaporated and dried milks and hot cocoa made from a dehydrated mix. These are subjected to dehydration and extra heat processing, which can increase AGE levels far beyond those present in regular milk and yogurt. (See Table 4.6.) Dairy products that are high in sugar should also be avoided.

Table 4.6   AGE Content of Selected Milk Products

Food	AGEs per Serving
Hot chocolate, from packet (1 cup)	660
Ice cream, vanilla (1 cup)	85
Milk, nonfat (1 cup)	2
Milk, whole (1 cup)	12
Yogurt, vanilla (1 cup)	10

Principle 2. Choose Cooking Methods That Prevent the Formation of AGEs

While most foods naturally contain some AGEs, it is the way they are prepared that ultimately determines their AGE content. (See Table 4.7.) The concept is simple: The main cause for the increase of AGEs in food is high-dry heat, such as baking or roasting foods in an oven or cooking foods on a grill. Any kind of cooking that uses a lot of heat, chars the outside, and dries out the food causes a dramatic rise in toxic AGEs. Therefore, the use of cooking methods such as searing, grilling, broiling, roasting, and frying should be minimized. What about foods that are "breaded" prior to frying—are they any better? No. The breading not only adds more calories but also soaks up a lot of fat, and when the food is dry-heated, it produces large amounts of AGEs.

It is also important to remember that the amount of AGEs present in a food has little to do with calories. For instance, the longer a steak is broiled or grilled, the more AGEs it contains! The formation of new AGEs happens despite the fact that the calories in the meat stay the same. Many people who believe they are eating a "healthy" low-calorie meal such as grilled chicken are surprised to discover that this meal can be very high in AGEs. This is because food AGEs are directly tied to cooking method.

So what are the best ways to deter the formation of AGEs during cooking? Moist-heat cooking methods such as poaching, steaming, stewing, and braising are ideal. These simple low-fuss techniques are very much in tune with the needs of busy people. Table 4.7 illustrates how the AGE content of chicken varies depending on the cooking method used. For safety reasons, foods like meats and poultry must be cooked to certain minimum temperatures, and poaching, steaming, stewing, and braising can accomplish that while causing far fewer AGEs to form than dry-heat methods. Chapter 7 provides more details about AGE-less cooking, and you will find many delicious ways to use these cooking techniques in the recipe section of this book, which begins on page 175.

Table 4.7 Effect of Cooking Method on AGE Content of Chicken

Chicken	AGEs per Serving
Raw (3 ounces)	400–700 kU
Poached, braised, stewed, steamed (3 ounces)	600–1,000 kU
Microwaved (3 ounces)	1,300–1,500 kU
Roasted, broiled, grilled (3 ounces)	4,000–6,000 kU
Deep-fried, oven-fried fast food chicken nuggets (3 ounces)	7,000–9,000 kU

Principle 3. Use Ingredients That Deter the Formation of AGEs

As you have seen, moisture is a powerful deterrent of AGE formation. Another AGE deterrent that you should know about is acid. Far fewer AGEs are formed in an acidic environment such as lemon juice, wine, vinegar, and tomato juice. These ingredients can be used in marinades and cooking liquids to help inhibit AGE formation. For example, you can incorporate some lemon or wine in poaching liquids and include some wine or tomatoes in soups and stews. This will both add flavor and discourage AGE formation during cooking.

Marinating meats for even a couple of hours prior to grilling or roasting meat may reduce AGE formation by about 50 percent. Of course, the degree to which the marinade will deter AGEs will partly depend on the thickness of the meat and the amount of acidic liquid around it. In Chapter 7, you will find some helpful guidelines for marinating food to reduce AGEs.

PUTTING IT ALL TOGETHER

Now that you understand the basic principles of the AGE-less diet, you can use them to make your daily food choices. Table 4.8 provides a general guide to foods according to AGE content. You can easily see how foods high in animal protein and fat and cooked with high-dry heat dominate the high-AGE categories. On the other hand, plant foods and foods cooked with moist heat dominate the lower-AGE categories. The remaining chapters of this book offer a wealth of practical tips for shopping, cooking, and dining out the AGE-less way.

HOW DOES YOUR DIET STACK UP?

By using the food AGE counts that have been presented throughout this chapter, you can compare your diet with the AGE-less diet. Use the data provided in this chapter's food tables to estimate your typical AGE intake and to also get ideas for substitutions that will help you eat the AGE-less way. You will note that the biggest reductions in AGEs come from paying attention to foods in the meat and

Table 4.8   AGE Categories for Selected Foods*

Very Low (<100 kU/serv)	Low (100–500 kU/serv)	Medium (501–1000 kU/serv)
Bread (low-fat varieties)	Avocado	Cheese (reduced-fat)
Eggs (poached, scrambled, or boiled)	Fruits (dried, roasted, or grilled)	Chicken (poached, steamed, stewed, or braised)
Fruits (fresh)	Legumes (cooked or canned)	Chocolate, dark
Grains (boiled or steamed)	Olive oil	Fish (poached or steamed)
Milk	Olives	Sunflower and pumpkin seeds (raw)
Soy milk	Pasta	Tofu (raw)
Vegetables (fresh or steamed)	Soy veggie burgers	Tuna or salmon (canned)
Yogurt	Vegetables (roasted or grilled)	

*AGE content is based on standard serving sizes. For instance, the serving size for meats is 3 ounces; cheese, 1 ounce; butter, 1 tablespoon, etc. So if you eat larger servings, you get more AGEs.

fat groups. For instance, stewing or braising meat instead of grilling or roasting can reduce AGEs in meats by at least two-thirds. Replacing butter with olive oil results in similar savings. Substituting lower-AGE foods such as legumes, eggs, and seafood for meats is still another way to reduce AGE intake.

As discussed in Chapter 2, when we used our database to analyze food records from a large group of healthy people in the New York City area, we estimated their average dietary AGE intake to be approximately 16,000 AGE kU per day. Based on subsequent studies in both animals and humans, we believe that reducing this amount by at least half is vital to health and longevity, which is why we suggest aiming for an upper limit of 5,000 to 8,000 AGEs kU per day.

From the data presented, it is easy to see how people who eat a diet rich in grilled or roasted meats, fats, and highly processed foods could easily achieve an intake in excess of 20,000 kU AGE per day, while the intake of some obese individuals can exceed 40,000 kU per day.[7] Although we provide these numbers for your information, we

High (1001–3000 kU/serv)	Very High (3001–5000 kU/serv)	Highest (>5000 kU/serv)
Beef or pork (stewed or braised)	Chicken (skinless broiled, grilled, or roasted)	Bacon (fried)
Butter	Fish (breaded and fried)	Beef (roasted, grilled, or broiled, well done)
Cheese (full-fat and processed varieties)	Pork chops (pan-fried)	Chicken with skin (broiled, grilled, or roasted)
Fish (grilled, broiled, or baked)	Single cheeseburger (fast food)	Chicken (fried or fast food nuggets)
French fries	Toasted cheese sandwich	Double cheeseburger (fast food)
Nuts and seeds (raw)	Tofu (broiled or sautéed)	Fish sandwich (fast food)
Sweets (donuts, pies, cakes, pastries, etc.)	Turkey (roasted)	Hot dog
		Pizza
		Sausage

caution against getting caught up in counting AGEs. A better and far easier way to AGE-proof your diet is to simply follow the basic principles outlined in this chapter along with the practical information found in the remaining chapters of this book. This will automatically curtail your AGE intake to recommended levels.

POTENTIAL ANTI-AGE THERAPIES

Over the years, as we studied the detrimental effects of AGEs, it was natural to consider the use of pharmaceuticals to initially lower the AGE levels in patients. Before we end this chapter, it is important to discuss the use of potential anti-AGE therapies.

There are several drugs that can neutralize AGEs and their actions. More than thirty years ago, in the journal *Science,* our research group at the Rockefeller University reported on the first drug that could bind and inhibit the negative actions of AGEs: aminoguanidine.[8] This exciting finding was confirmed and expanded in many subsequent animal studies in our laboratory and those of others. The drug became an instant star as a potential new "fountain of youth." Several more anti-AGE agents were produced that protected the heart and kidneys in laboratory animals.[9–12] Unfortunately, most of these drugs got only as far as animal testing. A few short-term studies were conducted in humans, some of them promising,[13] but large clinical trials that can answer questions about safety and efficacy are still many years away. Table 4.9 lists some drugs and nutrients under investigation as anti-AGE therapies.

Table 4.9 Potential Anti-AGE Therapies

AGE Inhibitors
● Aminoguanadine-HCL
● Benfotiamine (a fat-soluble form of thiamine)
● Pyridoxamine (a natural form of vitamin B[6])
● Thiamine-PP (thiamine pyrophosphate, the active form of the B vitamin thiamine)
AGE Breakers
● ALT-711 (alagebrium)
● PTB (phenacylthiazolium bromide)
Molecules That Sweep Up AGEs in the Blood
● Anti-AGE antibodies
● Lysozyme
● sRAGE (soluble RAGE)
Antioxidants and Radical Scavengers
● Alpha-lipoic acid
● Vitamin E

In addition to the investigational drugs and nutrients listed in the table, some medications that are currently in use appear to have anti-AGE effects. These include metformin, which is chemically similar to aminoguanidine, and is used in the treatment of diabetes; and ACE (angiotensin converting enzyme) inhibitors, which are used to treat high blood pressure, kidney disease, and heart failure.[14] Another drug of interest is sevelamer, which is used in the treatment of bone disease in patients with advanced or end-stage kidney disease.[15] This medication was recently shown to bind food AGEs in the gut and reduce their absorption. (See the earlier discussion on page 56.) The anti-AGE effects of these drugs may explain some of their benefits.

The search is also on for natural compounds to thwart AGEs, and many plant foods, including spices, have been found to have anti-AGE properties. This is an active area of research, especially with regard to a class of phytonutrients known as flavonoids. Some flavonoids are potent antioxidants, others activate enzymes that neutralize AGEs, and still others act as scavengers, trapping AGEs or AGE precursors.[16,17] Some foods of interest for their anti-AGE phytonutrients include:

- Culinary herbs and spices, including allspice, capers, cinnamon, cloves, garlic, marjoram, parsley, sage, rosemary, tarragon, thyme, and turmeric.

- Fruits and vegetables, including apples, chili peppers, cranberries, cruciferous vegetables (such as broccoli, Brussels sprouts, cauliflower, and cabbage), red grapes, mangos, mangosteen, pomegranates, strawberries, and tomatoes.

- Beverages such as green tea, black tea, and maté (a tea made from the South American yerba maté plant).

A diet rich in plant foods has been proven time and again to help prevent heart disease, cancer, diabetes, and many other health problems. The ability of these foods to help neutralize AGE damage is a likely reason for these effects, not to mention that plant foods are naturally low in AGEs. So now you have another compelling reason to build your diet around vegetables, fruits, legumes, and whole grains.

CONCLUSION

Over the years, we have seen time and time again how the modern Western diet—high in red and processed meats, cheeses, sweets, fast food, and junk food—is tied to many health problems. Certainly these foods have plenty of "bad stuff" to offer, such as saturated or trans fats, excess sodium, high glycemic load, low nutritional value, and an abundance of calories. But what most people don't realize is that these foods are also loaded with AGEs. And, as we have learned, AGEs instigate the underlying processes that put us directly in harm's way. No other single food, nutrient, contaminant, or pollutant shows the same pervasiveness and clear health risk as AGEs.

You can dramatically lower your AGE intake both by smart food selection and by changing the way you cook. Preparing AGE-less foods can be easy, cost-effective, and delicious. There is no need to purchase exotic and expensive ingredients. Overall, moving away from the typical Western diet toward a diet focused more on vegetables, fruits, and whole grains, with lean meats and fish prepared the AGE-less way, will not only reduce your AGE intake, but also allow you to meet all of your nutritional needs while you enjoy tasty meals.

The search is on for drugs or supplements that can thwart AGE formation or diminish the damage caused by AGEs, but large clinical trials that can answer questions about safety and efficacy are many years away. The real question is, who can afford to wait? The same question is raised for many chronic conditions. A number of drugs exist for the treatment of heart disease, high blood pressure, and diabetes, but they come into play too late in the game and are not always effective. They would likely be far more helpful, or even unnecessary, if combined with a strategy that deals with the root cause of the condition. Following an AGE-less diet may well be the best way to take a big chunk of AGEs right off the top. Why waste this opportunity?

5.

Applying the AGE-Less Way to Different Diets

Perhaps the best thing about eating the AGE-less way is that there is no need to go on a highly restrictive diet or eliminate entire food groups. Nor is there a need to drastically reduce calories. This is because we can dramatically lower our daily intake of AGEs just by modifying our food choices and using the right meal-preparation techniques. The AGE-less diet has many similarities with the Mediterranean diet, which has been proven time and again to be among the most healthful dietary patterns in the world. However, any eating plan that features more vegetables, fruits, whole grains, seafood, and legumes—with less meat, sweets, and refined grains—is a good start to eating the AGE-less way.

With that said, AGE-less principles can be applied to *any* type of diet—from low-carb to low-fat, from omnivore to vegetarian, and everything in between. In this chapter we will be focusing on five of the most popular diet philosophies: low-carbohydrate diets, low-fat diets, the Mediterranean diet, the Paleolithic diet, and the vegetarian diet. You will see how simple it is to integrate the basic AGE-less principles into these diets to make them even more healthful. If your particular diet is not among these five, the practical information provided here will guide you in converting the diet you favor into a better food plan, the AGE-less way.

LOW-CARBOHYDRATE DIETS

As the name implies, a low-carbohydrate—or low-carb—diet limits carbohydrate-rich foods and emphasizes foods high in protein and fat. There are many types of low-carb diets, each with varying restrictions on the types and amounts of foods that are allowed. Some low-carbohydrate diets drastically restrict carbs at the beginning of the diet and then gradually liberalize the amount of carbs that are allowed. Popular examples of low-carb diets include the Atkins and South Beach diets.

Low-carb diets have attracted the interest of both consumers and the medical community as a means of treating obesity, diabetes, cardiovascular disease, and other problems. But unless these diets are prudently planned to limit AGEs, over the long term, they may actually contribute to the same health problems they are meant to prevent. The reason for this is simple: The foods that form the basis of the low-carb diet—foods that are high in protein and fat—tend to be the highest in AGEs, especially when they are cooked or processed with dry heat. A low-carb diet:

- Emphasizes high-protein foods such as meat, poultry, seafood, eggs, cheese, and nuts.

- Allows non-starchy vegetables such as asparagus, broccoli, cauliflower, and lettuce.

- Limits or excludes starchy vegetables (such as potatoes, corn, and peas), legumes, fruits, grains, and sweets.

- Includes various amounts of fats, such as butter, oil, and cream.

Extreme low-carb diets that feature piles of grilled or roasted meat, cheese, and fat; limited vegetables; and few or no fruits are guaranteed to deliver an overload of AGEs. Low-carb dieters who snack on large quantities of nuts and seeds (especially if they are roasted) can also unwittingly add many AGEs to their diet. Furthermore, many AGEs can slip into the diet with low-carb baked goods and desserts made with ingredients like nut meals or nut flours (finely ground nuts), butter, cream, and cream cheese.

Fortunately, there are also a variety of reduced-carb diets that emphasize lean protein foods such as fish and chicken, generous amounts of vegetables, and other "good carbohydrates" such as fresh fruits and whole grains. These are much easier to work with when it comes to keeping AGEs in check. Examples of reduced-carbohydrate diets include the Zone diet; the later phases of the South Beach diet; and the OmniHeart diet, a reduced-carb version of the DASH diet.[1] (To learn more about the DASH diet, see the discussion of low-fat diets on page 102.)

Because low-carb diets feature so many foods with a high potential to be AGE-rich, it is imperative to apply AGE-less principles to meal planning and preparation. Table 5.1 shows AGE counts for some foods typically included on low-carb diets, and also demonstrates how cooking methods and the selection of low- or high-fat options can impact the AGE content of some foods.

Table 5.1 AGE Content of Selected Foods

Food	AGEs per Serving
Beef steak, grilled (3 ounces)	6,700 kU
Beef, stewed (3 ounces)	2,200 kU
Chicken, grilled (3 ounces)	4,400 kU
Chicken, poached (3 ounces)	800 kU
Salmon, broiled (3 ounces)	3,400 kU
Salmon, poached (3 ounces)	1,550 kU
Egg, fried (1 large)	1,200 kU
Egg, poached (1 large)	30 kU
Cheddar cheese (whole milk) (1 ounce)	1,660 kU
Cheddar cheese (2% milk) (1 ounce)	740 kU
Butter (1 tablespoon)	1,890 kU
Olive oil (1 tablespoon)	450 kU
Cashews, roasted (1 ounce)	2,900 kU
Cashews, raw (1 ounce)	2,000 kU

AGE-Less Modifications for Low-Carb Diets

While many people find that reducing carbs helps them manage their weight, control diabetes, or deal with other health problems, you have learned that low-carb diets can easily deliver an overload of AGEs. The following strategies can be used to minimize AGEs in low-carb diets.

- Use AGE-less cooking methods such as steaming, poaching, and stewing.

- Favor foods that are lower in AGEs. Choose lean meats and lower-fat cheeses, eat nuts and seeds in their raw state, and use olive oil instead of butter.

- Enjoy generous portions of fresh vegetables with meals.

LOW-FAT DIETS

A low-fat diet limits fat and emphasizes foods high in carbohydrates. These diets have long been recommended for weight loss and preventing heart disease. Many athletes also enjoy a low-fat diet, since they need carbohydrate-rich foods to fuel their vigorous physical activities. However, these diets can lead to a number of health problems unless prudently planned (more on this later).

The most evidence-based low-fat diet is the DASH diet, which stands for Dietary Approaches to Stop Hypertension. The DASH diet is based on research sponsored by the National Heart, Lung, and Blood Institute (NHLBI) and has been shown to be associated with lower blood pressure, improved blood cholesterol levels, and a reduced risk of cardiovascular disease. The DASH diet:

- Emphasizes vegetables, fruits, and whole grains.

- Includes low-fat dairy products, fish, poultry, legumes, nuts, and seeds.

- Limits sodium and foods high in saturated fat, such as fatty meats, full-fat dairy products, and tropical oils such as coconut and palm oils.

- Limits sweets and sugary beverages.

The DASH diet is a smart low-fat diet pattern because it empha-sizes "good carbs" such as vegetables, fruits, and whole grains. Be aware, however, that low-fat diets can also be high in sugar, white flour, and other processed carbs. This can actually worsen health by raising insulin and sugar levels, which can adversely affect blood cholesterol and triglycerides, among other things.[2]

What about AGEs? While limiting fats can certainly help curb AGE intake, many people following low-fat diets get an abundance of AGEs from foods such as grilled, roasted, or oven-fried chicken. Another pitfall is heat-processed grain foods such as low-fat crackers and cookies, which not only raise AGEs but also increase sugar intake.

AGE-Less Modifications for Low-Fat Diets

A well-planned low-fat diet helps many people manage their weight, improve their health, and fuel their active lifestyle. The following strategies can assist you in minimizing the AGEs in a low-fat diet while making sure that your meals are rich in health-promoting nutrients.

- Favor whole natural foods—that is, foods that are compatible with the DASH diet pattern, such as fruits, vegetables, and whole grains.

- Eat nuts and seeds raw rather than roasted or toasted.

- Prepare meats using AGE-less cooking methods such as steaming, poaching, and stewing.

THE MEDITERRANEAN DIET

The "traditional" Mediterranean diet is based on the food traditions of Crete, Greece around the middle of the twentieth century, and it is very similar to the AGE-less diet. The Mediterranean eating plan:

- Features a high proportion of vegetables, fruits, whole grains, and legumes.

- Includes small to moderate portions of animal foods, with fish and poultry served much more often than red meat.

- Uses olive oil as the principal fat, instead of butter or margarine.

- Includes the regular consumption of nuts and seeds.

- Uses liberal amounts of herbs and spices.

- Recommends a moderate consumption of wine.

- Encourages fresh fruit for dessert.

The "Best" Diet—An Ongoing Debate

While there are many diets proposed to optimize health, few have undergone rigorous controlled clinical trials. This point was emphasized recently in a report by a committee of scientists who were tasked with reviewing the literature and preparing evidence-based recommendations for updating the Dietary Guidelines for Americans, the nation's go-to source for nutrition advice.

Several important and unexpected recommendations were included in the report. First, dietary cholesterol was no longer considered a "nutrient of concern," as the group could find no strong evidence that dietary cholesterol raises blood cholesterol levels. Second, the report did not specify an upper limit of total fat consumption. What was the reason for this surprising decision? The committee concluded that the common practice of reducing total fat by replacing fat with refined carbohydrates does not lower the risk of cardiovascular disease. Instead of this strategy, more emphasis should be placed on simply consuming less *saturated* fat.

The committee recommended a greater focus on choosing healthful foods, including more vegetables, fruits, whole grains, seafood, legumes, and low-fat dairy products to prevent obesity. Specifically, people should consume less meat, less sugar-sweetened foods and beverages, and less refined grains. Moreover, the group stressed that "consumption of 'low-fat' or 'nonfat' products with high amounts of refined grains and added sugars should be discouraged."[3]

These statements are in remarkable contrast with countless earlier guidelines presented over the last several decades. At the same time, they are strikingly consistent with the AGE-less diet. However, the AGE-less diet introduces new and very critical recommendations regarding cooking methods.

The Mediterranean diet is supported by over fifty years of strong scientific evidence. People in the modern world who adhere closely to this traditional dietary pattern have been found to have lower rates of heart disease, diabetes, and dementia, and higher life expectancy.[4,5] A likely reason for the benefits of this cuisine is, of course, an abundance of nutrient-rich foods. But the Mediterranean diet also contains far fewer AGE-rich fast foods, junk foods, sweets, desserts, and red and processed meats compared with Western diets. In addition, many Mediterranean foods are cooked the AGE-less way. For instance, soups, stews, and braised and poached meats and fish are all prominently featured in this food plan. A recent controlled clinical trial from Spain has shown that some of the benefits of the Mediterranean diet may be explained by a lower content of AGEs.[4]

AGE-Less Modifications for the Mediterranean Diet

The Mediterranean diet is renowned for both its fine cuisine and its many health benefits. Following the basic principles of the Mediterranean diet is a very good start to eating the AGE-less way. The tweaks presented below can make it even better:

- Use AGE-less cooking methods, such as steaming, poaching, and stewing.

- Choose lean meats and reduced-fat cheeses.

- Eat nuts and seeds raw rather than roasted or toasted.

THE PALEOLITHIC DIET

The modern dietary regimen known as the Paleolithic diet—also referred to as the Paleo diet, caveman diet, and hunter-gatherer diet—is based on the premise that modern humans are genetically adapted to the diet of their Paleolithic ancestors. Therefore, the ideal diet is one that resembles the ancestral diet of wild plants and animals that humans consumed during the Paleolithic Period.

The Paleo diet has gained interest from both consumers and the scientific community due to claims that it prevents the chronic health conditions that plague us today—problems such as obesity, diabetes, cardiovascular disease, and brain disease. However, it is important to remember that the average lifespan of people in the Paleolithic Period was quite short. So one reason that cavemen might have died less often from chronic diseases may be that they did not live long enough to develop them.

The actual composition and best modern interpretation of the real Paleolithic diet remains an ongoing debate. However, a typical "contemporary" version of the Paleolithic diet:

- Emphasizes meat, seafood, eggs, vegetables, and fruits as dietary staples.

- Encourages grass-fed meats and wild-caught or wild-gathered foods whenever possible.

- Includes nuts, seeds, and some oils, such as olive, walnut, coconut, and flaxseed.

- Excludes grains, legumes, dairy products, salt, refined sugar, and processed foods.

The biggest potential sources of AGEs in the Paleo diet are meats, nuts, and oils. Some Paleo followers eat some or all of their animal foods raw—as in steak tartare, sashimi, and ceviche. This certainly reduces AGEs, but keep in mind that people who eat raw animal foods risk exposure to foodborne pathogens such as listeria, salmonella, and *E. coli*, as well as parasites that may be in raw fish or meats.

AGE-Less Modifications for the Paleo Diet

A well-planned Paleo diet can be nutrient-dense, and many people have lost weight and improved their health by eating this way. However, as with low-carb diets, a Paleo diet has the potential of being high in roasted or grilled meats, nuts, and oils, all of which deliver very high amounts of AGEs. To minimize AGEs, you can do the following:

- Choose lean organic meats and cook them using AGE-less methods, such as steaming, poaching, and stewing.

- Eat nuts and seeds raw rather than roasted or toasted.

- Use oils lightly.

VEGETARIAN DIETS

Vegetarian diets are plant-based eating plans that include a range of variations. As a whole, study after study has shown vegetarian diets to be among the healthiest in the world. These diets are associated with a lower risk of many health problems, including high blood pressure, heart disease, type 2 diabetes, obesity, and some types of cancer.[6] One reason for these benefits is that plant foods are rich in fiber, antioxidants, and other important nutrients. Many people who follow vegetarian diets also choose organic foods and avoid processed snack foods and sweets. Finally, plant foods are naturally low in AGEs, so a plant-based diet can limit AGE intake. However, as with all dietary patterns, the devil is in the details. Let's take a look at some of the variations of the vegetarian diet.

■ RAW VEGETARIAN DIETS

This plant-based diet centers on the philosophy that all foods should be eaten in their uncooked form. While cooking is not allowed, many people prepare elaborate meals using blenders, food processors, juicers, and dehydrators. People often lose weight on this diet, since many raw foods are high in fiber and low in calories. The diet also better preserves many vitamins and phytonutrients that are diminished by cooking.

Something to keep in mind is that a diet comprised only of plant foods requires supplementation with vitamin B_{12}, which is found primarily in animal foods. Typically, a raw vegetarian diet:

- Features abundant raw fruits, vegetables, nuts, seeds, sprouted grains and legumes, and fresh herbs.

- Includes varying amounts of sweeteners such as raw agave and evaporated cane juice.

- Includes varying amounts of cold-pressed vegetable oils.

- Excludes foods that are heated above a certain temperature, usually 118°F.

- In most cases, excludes all animal foods, although some people may consume foods such as raw (unpasteurized) milk or cheese or even raw fish, such as sashimi or ceviche.

It may be logical to assume that AGEs are not a problem in a raw vegetarian diet since there are no cooked foods and typically no animal products. However, this is not always true. For instance, nuts are eaten in abundance by many followers of this diet, and ounce for ounce, raw nuts such as almonds, walnuts, and cashews are on par with grilled or roasted chicken with regard to AGE content. (See Table 5.1.) Vegetable oils, even if cold-pressed, are another potential source of AGEs in the raw vegetarian diet. Cold-pressed oils are less processed than conventional oils, but they may still be exposed to temperatures of up to 120°F during extraction. Exposure to these temperatures plus contact with air and light can trigger oxidation and the accumulation of AGEs.

Dehydrators are popular kitchen appliances for raw foodists, and herein lies another way that AGEs can sneak into the diet. Remember that dehydration, or removal of water, drives AGE formation. This is most pronounced in foods that are high in protein and fat, such as nuts and seeds. Nuts and seeds are often ground, mixed with other ingredients, and then dehydrated for hours to make crispy treats like crackers, chips, and cookies deemed suitable for the raw diet. These foods can be a rich source of AGEs, negating many of the health benefits of a raw vegetarian diet.

AGE-Less Modifications for Raw Vegetarian Diets

Many people enjoy a raw vegetarian diet, and many others would benefit by including more fresh, raw foods in their diet. However, there are a few pitfalls to watch out for when you want to keep AGEs in check. Guidelines for raw foods include the following:

- Eat nuts and seeds in their raw state and in reasonable portions.

- Avoid using dehydrators on high-protein, high-fat foods like nuts and seeds, which are most vulnerable to AGE formation.

- Use oils sparingly.

■ VEGAN DIETS

A vegan diet is one that excludes all animal foods. However, unlike the raw vegetarian diet, heat-treated and cooked foods are allowed. The basic vegan diet:

- Includes a high proportion of raw or cooked fruits, vegetables, whole grains, legumes, tofu, nuts, and seeds.

- Features varying amounts of vegetable oils and sweeteners such as maple syrup, brown rice syrup, and sugar.

- Excludes all animal foods, including dairy and eggs.

Like any diet that eliminates all animal foods, a vegan diet often does not supply enough vitamin B_{12}. While some vegan foods are fortified with this nutrient, supplementation may still be necessary.

Like a raw vegetarian diet, vegan diets may seem ideal for AGE-less eating. However, AGEs can sneak in with foods such as nuts (especially if roasted), oils, and grilled or broiled tofu. People who eat large amounts of these foods may consume more AGEs than they realize.

AGE-Less Modifications for Vegan Diets

Vegan diets can be extremely beneficial because they eliminate meats, cheese, and other high-fat, high-AGE foods. To further reduce the intake of dietary AGEs, guidelines for this type of eating plan include the following:

- Eat nuts and seeds in their raw state and in reasonable portions.

- Use oils sparingly.

- Serve tofu raw or cooked the AGE-less way—steamed or simmered in a soup.

■ LACTO-OVO VEGETARIAN DIETS

Lacto-ovo vegetarians eat a plant-based diet that also includes milk products and eggs. Variations include lacto-vegetarians, who eat dairy foods but no eggs; and ovo-vegetarians, who eat eggs but no dairy foods. Basically, this diet:

- Emphasizes raw or cooked fruits, vegetables, whole grains, legumes, nuts, and seeds.

- Includes eggs and dairy foods such as milk, yogurt, and cheese.

- Features varying amounts of fat, including oils and butter.

- Features varying amounts of sweeteners such as honey, maple syrup, and sugar.

- Excludes meat, poultry, and seafood.

The major sources of AGEs in the lacto-ovo vegetarian diet are cheeses (especially those that are high-fat and aged), butter and cream, nuts, oils, and fried eggs. Compared with people who follow vegan and raw vegetarian eating plans, people on a lacto-ovo vegetarian diet also have a greater variety of processed snack foods and rich desserts to choose from. And as you know, these options can add many AGEs to the diet.

AGE-Less Modifications for Lacto-Ovo Vegetarian Diets

Even though a lacto-ovo vegetarian diet eliminates meat, poultry, and seafood, as you just learned, it does supply foods that can contribute AGEs to the diet. To minimize AGEs when following a lacto-ovo food plan, use these guidelines:

- Choose lower-fat cheeses.

- Cook eggs using AGE-less methods—by poaching, boiling, or scrambling rather than frying.

- Serve tofu raw or cooked the AGE-less way—steamed or simmered in a soup.

- Substitute olive oil for butter.

- Eat nuts and seeds in their raw state and in reasonable portions.

- Limit sweets and processed snack foods.

■ FLEXITARIAN DIETS

Flexitarian is a combination of two words—*flexible* and *vegetarian.* Flexitarians follow a mostly vegetarian diet but occasionally eat fish, poultry, or meat. The flexitarian diet:

- Emphasizes raw or cooked fruits, vegetables, whole grains, legumes, nuts, and seeds.

- Includes eggs and dairy foods such as milk, yogurt, and cheese.

- Features varying amounts of fat, including oils and butter.

- Features varying amounts of sweeteners such as honey, maple syrup, and sugar.

- Occasionally includes meat, poultry, and seafood.

    Potential sources of AGEs in the flexitarian diet include meats, poultry, or seafood, especially when grilled or roasted; nuts, especially when roasted; high-fat cheeses; butter and cream; processed snack foods; and sweets.

AGE-Less Modifications for Flexitarian Diets

Of the various types of vegetarian diets, flexitarian eating plans have the greatest potential to offer high levels of AGEs. To minimize these substances, follow these guidelines:

- Choose lower-fat cheeses.

- Cook eggs using AGE-less methods—by poaching, boiling, or scrambling rather than frying.

- Substitute olive oil for butter.

- Eat nuts and seeds in their raw state and in reasonable portions.

- Limit sweets and processed snack foods.

- Cook meat, poultry, and seafood using AGE-less methods, such as steaming, poaching, and stewing.

- Serve tofu raw or cooked the AGE-less way—steamed or simmered in a soup.

CONCLUSION

Each person is unique in his or her food preferences. Different diet philosophies work for different people, and a wide variety of dietary patterns—from vegetarian, to Mediterranean, to Paleo—have been found to confer individual health benefits. This chapter has shown that AGE-less principles can be applied to any diet, allowing you to follow the plan that appeals to you. But it is important to re-emphasize that any "healthy" diet can become unhealthy by simply "turning up the dial" and cooking food at higher temperatures and with less moisture. Conversely, the unhealthy effects of many diets can be avoided by turning the heat down.

The following chapters will further guide you in putting AGE-less principles into practice, whether selecting foods in the grocery store, preparing foods in your own kitchen, or eating away from home. You will find that it can be both easy and delicious to eat the AGE-less way at any time and any place.

6.

Stocking the
AGE-Less Pantry

Now that you understand the basics of eating the AGE-less way and how to apply the AGE-less way to different diets, it's time to consider the ins and outs of grocery shopping. As you shop for food, keep in mind that the AGE content of the Western diet has increased vastly in the past fifty years due to our ever-increasing reliance on processed foods. Processing refers to all the ways that food is altered from its natural state, whether for safety reasons, for convenience, or to increase palatability. Processed foods are often exposed to heating and/or dehydration, and both treatments increase the reactions between sugars, proteins, and fats that create AGEs. However it's important to point out that not all processed foods are unhealthy or high in AGEs. This is particularly true of plant-based foods such as rolled oats, whole grain pasta, brown rice, frozen vegetables, canned beans, milk, and yogurt, to name a few examples. These foods are convenient, high in nutrition, and very appropriate for an AGE-less diet.

This chapter highlights foods that can fit into an AGE-less eating plan, offers smart substitutions for high-AGE foods and ingredients, and provides additional tips for selecting and preparing foods. You will find that AGE-less food can be tasty, easy to prepare, and economical. By keeping your pantry, refrigerator, and freezer stocked with the right foods, you will always have the makings of a healthful and delicious meal or snack on hand.

MEATS, POULTRY, AND SEAFOOD

It bears repeating that animal protein, especially red meat, is the biggest contributor of AGEs to many people's diets. The good news is that simply using moist-heat cooking methods markedly limits the creation of further AGEs. An additional benefit can be obtained by marinating with acidic liquids such as lemon juice, vinegar, and wine, since acid inhibits AGE formation in foods. (See the discussions on pages 93 and 286.) Here are some guidelines for choosing foods that are compatible with the AGE-less diet.

Beef. When choosing any kind of meat, keep in mind that a higher fat content means more AGEs, so choose lean cuts and cook them the AGE-less way. Many cuts of beef can be braised (as in pot roast), simmered (as in soup), or stewed. The leanest cuts have "loin" or "round" in the name. Examples include eye of round, top round, and sirloin. You can also tell a lot just by looking at meat. Fatty steaks and roasts have more "marbling" or intramuscular fat, which shows up as white streaks throughout the meat. They also tend to have a thick layer of fat on the outside, but unlike marbling, this external fat can be easily trimmed away. As for ground beef, look for meat that is at least 93-percent lean. A good visual guide is that the leaner the ground meat, the darker the color will be. Purchase organic, grass-fed beef as often as possible. (See the inset on page 121.)

Chicken and Turkey. Chicken is lower in AGEs than beef and it is well suited for AGE-less cooking methods such as stewing, poaching, braising, and steaming. Various cuts of turkey are also good choices for braising, stewing, or making soups. As with beef, a higher fat content means more AGEs. For instance, roasted chicken skin, which is very fatty, has more than twice as many AGEs as roasted skinless chicken meat. When purchasing ground chicken or turkey, look for meat that is at least 93-percent lean. Fresh chicken and turkey Italian-type sausages are also available. (Again, look for products that are at least 93-percent lean.) These are a better choice than greasy pork and beef sausages. Choose poultry that is organic and pasture-raised as much as possible. (See the inset on page 121.)

Lamb. Although classified as a red meat, lamb appears to be lower in AGEs than beef. This may be because it comes from younger animals. Like other meats, lamb should be stewed or braised rather than roasted, grilled, broiled, or fried. Purchase organic, grass-fed lamb as much as possible.

Pork. Once again, higher fat means more AGEs. In fact, fried bacon, a favorite American food, is the most AGE-rich food item in the American diet. However, lean cuts of pork are similar to chicken in AGE content. Lean cuts have the word "loin" in the name—such as tenderloin and sirloin. As with beef, a visual inspection can reveal a lot about fat content in pork. Leaner pork has less marbling and external fat. To minimize AGEs, pork should be cooked with moist heat as in a pot roast or stew. Choose pork that is organic and pasture-raised as much as possible. (See the inset that begins on page 121 to learn more about organic pasture-raised meats.)

Seafood (fresh and frozen). Seafood, including fish and shellfish, is lower in AGEs than meat and poultry, so consider substituting seafood for meat often. Fatty fish such as salmon, especially when it is farm-raised, has more AGEs than lean fish like cod and flounder. Even so, salmon has about half the AGEs of a similarly cooked serving of beef. In addition, salmon is an excellent source of healthful omega-3 fats. Low-AGE cooking methods such as poaching, steaming, and cooking en papillote (steaming in foil or parchment packets) are ideal for seafood. (See Chapter 7 for more details about cooking methods.) When choosing seafood, important issues include safety in regard to both mercury and other environmental contaminants, and sustainability in regard to overfishing. The inset on page 118 will help you make the best choices.

Seafood (canned). Canned seafood, such as tuna, salmon, crab, clams, sardines, and herring, are convenient lower-AGE foods to keep in your cupboard. To minimize AGEs, choose seafood that is packed in water, rather than oil. In the case of sardines, those canned in a low-fat sauce such as tomato or mustard sauce would also be a good choice.

AGE-Less Tips for Cooking
or Replacing Meats, Poultry, and Seafood

❑ **Limit portions of animal protein to a quarter of the plate.** Then fill the remainder of the plate with plant foods. Enjoy more salads, soups, and stews that combine moderate portions of meat with generous portions of vegetables.

❑ **Replace some meals of meat and poultry with seafood or vegetarian alternatives.** In general, seafood is much lower in AGEs than other animal proteins. Vegetarian alternatives such as legumes are even lower than seafood.

❑ **Whenever possible, use AGE-less cooking methods, such as steaming, poaching, and stewing.** When recipes call for intense browning with high heat and lots of oil or fat—all of which contributes to AGE formation—lightly brown the meat in a ceramic or nonstick skillet using medium heat and nonstick cooking spray or a small amount of oil.

❑ **Use chopped mushrooms as a ground meat "extender."** Swap the desired amount of ground meat for an equal weight of mushrooms. For instance, replace 8 ounces of ground meat with 8 ounces (about 3 cups) of chopped fresh mushrooms. Both white button and baby portabella mushrooms work well. Replace up to half of the ground meat in recipes such as tacos and a quarter to a third of the meat in meatballs, burgers, and meatloaf.

❑ **Instead of sausage, add sausage flavor to foods with herbs and spices.** A bit of fennel seed and dried Italian seasoning will lend Italian sausage flavor to a pasta dish or casserole. Sage and a pinch of red pepper suggest pork sausage flavor.

❑ **Keep flavorful cooking liquids on hand.** Because of the importance of simmering, poaching, and stewing in AGE-less cooking, you'll want to stock your pantry with cartons of fat-free and low-fat chicken, beef, and/or vegetable broth. Broth made from bouillon is also an acceptable choice.

Table 6.1   AGE Content of Selected Meats, Poultry & Seafood*

Food	Portion Size	100 kU or less — Very Low	100–500 kU — Low	501–1000 kU — Medium	1001–3000 kU — High	3001–5000 kU — Very High	5000–12,000 kU — Highest
BEEF							
Grilled, broiled, or roasted, well done	3 ounces						▓
Grilled steak, rare	3 ounces			▓			
Raw	3 ounces			▓			
Stewed	3 ounces				▓		
CHICKEN							
Deep-fried							▓
Grilled, broiled, or roasted (skinless)	3 ounces					▓	
Grilled, broiled, or roasted (with skin)	3 ounces						▓
Poached or steamed	3 ounces			▓			
LAMB							
Leg, braised	3 ounces			▓			
Leg, broiled	3 ounces				▓		
PORK							
Bacon, fried	2 slices						▓
Pork chop, pan fried	3 ounces					▓	
Pork Italian sausage, grilled	3 ounces					▓	
Pork tenderloin, braised	3 ounces			▓			
SEAFOOD							
Flounder, steamed	3 ounces		▓				
Salmon, broiled	3 ounces					▓	
Salmon, poached or steamed	3 ounces			▓	▓		
Tuna, canned in oil	3 ounces				▓		
Tuna, canned in water	3 ounces	▓					

*Note that in the case of some foods, such as poached salmon, two boxes—"Medium" and "High," for instance—have been marked. This indicates that the food is on the "borderline" of two categories, and therefore belongs in both categories.

Safe and Sustainable Seafood

Seafood is a highly recommended part of the AGE-less diet. It is much lower in AGEs than meat and poultry and provides omega-3 fatty acids, which the standard diet lacks in sufficient amounts. However, care must be taken to choose those varieties that are lowest in environmental contaminants. This is especially important for women who are pregnant or who might become pregnant, for nursing mothers, and for young children.

Sustainability is another huge concern, as many species are being overfished to the point where their numbers have become dangerously low. Groups such as FishWatch, the Monterey Bay Aquarium Seafood Watch, and the National Resources Defense Council offer advice for choosing the safest seafood and most sustainable varieties. (See the Organizations and Websites section.) The National Resources Defense Council compiled the information presented in Table 6.2 based on both mercury content and sustainability. Choose low-mercury seafood most often, and eat moderate-mercury seafood six times or less a month and high-mercury seafood three times or less per month. Seafood that is high in mercury should be avoided entirely. Keep in mind that this information may change periodically, so it is important to check it on a regular basis.

Table 6.2 Mercury Levels in Seafood

LOWEST IN MERCURY

Anchovies	Herring	Sardine
Butterfish	Mackerel (Atlantic chub)	Scallop*
Catfish		Shad (American)
Clam	Mullet	Shrimp*
Crab (domestic)	Oyster	Sole (Pacific)
Crawfish/Crayfish	Perch (ocean)	Squid (calamari)
Croaker (Atlantic)	Plaice	Tilapia
Flounder*	Pollock	Trout (freshwater)
Haddock (Atlantic)*	Salmon (canned)†	Whitefish
Hake	Salmon (fresh)†	Whiting

MODERATE IN MERCURY		
Bass (Striped, Black)	Jacksmelt	Skate*
Carp	(Silverside)	Snapper*
Cod (Alaskan)*	Lobster	Tuna (canned
Croaker (White Pacific)	Mahi Mahi	chunk light)
	Monkfish*	Tuna (skipjack)*
Halibut (Atlantic)*	Perch (freshwater)	Weakfish (sea trout)
Halibut (Pacific)	Sablefish	

HIGH IN MERCURY		
Bluefish	Mackerel (Spanish, Gulf)	Tuna (canned Albacore)
Grouper*		
	Sea Bass (Chilean)*	Tuna (Yellowfin)*

HIGHEST IN MERCURY		
Mackerel (King)	Shark*	Tilefish*
Marlin*	Swordfish*	Tuna (Bigeye, Ahi)*
Orange Roughy*		

* These fish are perilously low in numbers or are caught using environmentally destructive methods.
† Farmed salmon may contain PCBs, which are toxic chemicals with serious health effects.

MEAT SUBSTITUTES

Many plant foods are rich in protein and make tasty and budget-friendly alternatives to meat. For instance, one cup of cooked dried beans provides 14 to 16 grams of protein, which is about what you get in 2 to 3 ounces of meat, poultry, or seafood. Since plant foods are much lower in AGEs than animal foods, an easy way to trim AGEs from your diet is to enjoy these foods as often as possible.

Dried Beans, Peas, and Lentils. Also known as legumes, dried beans, peas, and lentils are the seeds of pod-bearing plants that are allowed to fully mature and dry on the vine before being harvested. Legumes are a staple in many delicious cuisines throughout the world. Middle

Eastern hummus, Latin American black beans and rice, and Mediterranean white bean cassoulet are just a few examples of popular legume-based dishes.

In addition to being low in AGEs, legumes are inexpensive, supernutritious, and highly versatile. Enjoy them in soups, casseroles, dips, salads, spreads, and more. Legumes are also a low-glycemic index food, meaning they have minimal impact on blood sugar levels despite their relatively high carbohydrate content. Look for organic canned beans, or cook them from dried.

Edamame. Edamame is another name for fresh green soybeans. These beans have a light nutty flavor and are packed with fiber and other nutrients. They can be purchased fresh or frozen, either shelled or in the pods.

Although they are a type of legume, unlike dried legumes, edamame beans can be boiled or steamed, and are ready to eat in just a few minutes. Many people enjoy edamame in the pods as a snack, although the pod itself is not edible. Shelled edamame is delicious in salads, casseroles, soups, pilafs, dips, and many other dishes.

Tofu. Also known as bean curd, tofu is made from soymilk in a process similar to cheese making. It has a mild taste and absorbs the flavors of the other ingredients in your recipe, making it adaptable to a variety of dishes.

Tofu can be used in soups, sauces, dips, smoothies, and more. To minimize AGEs, serve tofu raw, steamed, or simmered in a soup. When grilled or broiled, tofu's AGE content can rival that of grilled chicken.

Vegetarian Meat Alternatives. A variety of meat alternatives—including bacon, burgers, sausages, and burger-style crumbles for use in chili and tacos—can be found in the freezer case of most supermarkets. These are typically made from a combination of soy, vegetables, whole grains, and seasonings, and are much lower in AGEs than their animal-based counterparts. A caveat is that for added protein and a chewy texture, many of these products contain wheat gluten, which some people must strictly avoid. In addition, some are high in sodium, so you'll want to balance them out with lower-sodium choices in the rest of your meal.

AGE-Less Tips for Using Meat Substitutes

❑ **Keep your AGEs in check by replacing meat, poultry, and seafood with plant-based meat alternatives as often as possible.**

❑ **To keep AGE formation low, eat tofu raw, steamed, or simmered in a soup.** Avoid broiling and grilling your tofu.

❑ **Enjoy nuts and seeds in moderation.** These foods are a good source of protein, with 4 to 7 grams per quarter-cup serving, but they are much higher in AGEs than foods like dried beans, peas, and lentils. Since nuts contain more fat than protein, they are discussed in the section on fats and oils, which begins on page 134.

Table 6.3 AGE Content of Selected Meat Substitutes*

Food	Portion Size	100 kU or less Very Low	100–500 kU Low	501–1000 kU Medium	1001–3000 kU High	3001–5000 kU Very High	5000–12,000 kU Highest
Kidney beans, canned	½ cup		■				
Tofu, boiled	3 ounces			■			
Tofu, broiled	3 ounces					■	
Tofu, raw	3 ounces		■	■			
Vegetarian bacon	2 strips		■				
Veggie burger	3 ounces	■					

*Note that in the case of some foods, such as raw tofu, two boxes—"Low" and "Medium," for instance—have been marked. This indicates that the food is on the "borderline" of two categories, and therefore belongs in both categories.

The Benefits of Going Organic

There is no difference between the AGE levels of organic vegetables and fruits and those of produce that's grown conventionally. However, by choosing organic products, you will reduce your exposure to other toxins, such as the synthetic pesticides, herbicides, and fungicides usually used on crops. Organic producers must use natural processes and materials, and their farming practices must maintain soil and water quality and conserve the ecosystem. Organic foods must also be free of genetically modified organisms, or GMOs. In the United States, the National Organic Program regulates standards for producing and labeling organic foods. Complete guidelines can be found at the USDA National Organic Program website. (See page 304 of the Organizations and Websites section.)

Of course, organic food often costs more. To maximize food dollars, it pays to know which foods are highest and lowest in pesticides and other agricultural chemicals. This can help you decide when you want to buy organic produce and when you can economize by opting for conventional produce. The Environmental Working Group (EWG) (see page 303) maintains lists of the "Dirty Dozen Plus," which are more likely to contain pesticides, and the "Clean Fifteen," which are less likely to contain these harmful chemicals. These lists are updated from time to time, so it is important to review them regularly.

The EWG's Dirty Dozen Plus

- Apples
- Celery
- Cherry tomatoes
- Cucumbers
- Grapes
- Hot peppers
- Kale/collard greens
- Nectarines
- Peaches
- Potatoes
- Snap peas
- Spinach
- Strawberries
- Sweet bell peppers

The EWGs Clean Fifteen

- Asparagus
- Avocados
- Cabbage
- Cantaloupe
- Cauliflower
- Eggplant
- Frozen sweet peas
- Grapefruit
- Kiwi
- Mangos
- Onions
- Papayas
- Pineapples
- Sweet corn
- Sweet potatoes

What about animal foods such as meat, poultry, eggs, and milk? USDA organic regulations require that animals are fed 100-percent organic food, and do not receive growth-promoting antibiotics or hormones. These animals are also supposed to be raised in living conditions that accommodate their natural behaviors, like the need to graze on pasture. However, this guideline is currently vague, and some producers adopt higher standards than others. It pays to check with producers to determine the criteria they're using. A number of farmers and producers have websites that offer this type of information.

Many people assume that organic meat comes from exclusively grass-fed or pasture-raised animals, but this is not necessarily true. For instance, many organically raised animals start out grass-fed and then are "fattened up" on a diet of dried corn and other grains; foods such as soy, peanut, or sunflower meal (residue that is left after vegetable oils are extracted); and molasses. Why does this matter? There is little doubt that these feeding practices drive the raw meat's AGE content up significantly. Grass-fed and pasture-raised meats are not only lower in AGEs, but also leaner and lower in calories than grain-fed meat, and they contain a healthier balance of essential fatty acids. (Grass-fed meat contains more omega-3s and fewer omega-6s.) So when it comes to animal foods, the ideal option is to use meat that is both organic *and* grass-fed or pasture-raised as much as possible. When used correctly, both terms mean that animals were raised outdoors on a range or pasture where they could roam and forage.

Note that the term *grass-fed* typically refers to beef (and dairy foods), lamb, goats, and bison, whose natural diet is grass. *Pasture-raised* typically refers to pigs and chickens (and eggs), whose natural diet includes a variety of plants, insects, and animals. However, only the term "grass-fed" has a legal definition. The USDA defines grass-fed as meaning a diet solely of grass and other forage since the time of weaning. Pasture-raised is currently not a regulated term, so it pays to check with producers to see what criteria they're using. Many farmers and producers have websites that offer this information.

Of course, a big concern for many people is that organic grass-fed and pasture-raised meats cost more. One way to offset the cost is by consuming smaller meat portions—for instance, have a bowl of beef and barley soup instead of a steak. You can also use legumes to make many delicious and creative meatless meals. The recipe section of this book offers plenty of ideas. These strategies will trim your food budget *and* your AGEs.

EGGS

A good source of high-quality low-AGE protein, eggs are perfect for a quick meal at any time of the day. In the past, eggs were often viewed as unhealthy due to their high cholesterol content. However, cholesterol in foods has not been found to have a major effect on blood cholesterol levels in most people. The latest consensus is that eating one egg a day is not a problem. A caveat is that people who have diabetes or high LDL "bad" cholesterol may be more vulnerable to the effects of cholesterol-rich foods. Therefore, health care professionals may advise this group to eat fewer yolks and more egg whites, which are cholesterol-free.

Fresh Whole Eggs. Enjoy whole eggs poached, boiled, steam-basted, scrambled, or in omelets. The yolks are higher in AGEs than the whites, but the AGE content of whole eggs is still much lower than that of meat. Choose organic pasture-raised eggs as much as possible.

Liquid Egg Whites. These are typically 100-percent egg whites, with no additives or preservatives. Liquid egg whites are sold in cartons next to whole eggs in grocery stores. Enjoy them scrambled or in omelets.

Egg Substitutes. Fat-free egg substitutes, such as Egg Beaters, are made from egg whites with added colors such as beta-carotene so they look like beaten whole eggs. Egg substitutes may also contain added seasonings, vitamins and minerals, and other ingredients. These products can be scrambled or used in omelets as you would whole eggs.

AGE-Less Tips for Cooking With Eggs

❏ **Use eggs as a high-nutrient, low-AGE source of protein.** Speak to your health care provider about which egg products—whole eggs, egg whites, or egg substitutes—are best for you.

❏ **Cook your eggs using AGE-less methods.** To keep AGE formation at the lowest possible level, poach or scramble your eggs. Hard-boiling is also good. Avoid frying, as this raises AGE levels.

Table 6.4 AGE Content of Selected Eggs and Egg Substitutes

Food	Portion Size	100 kU or less — Very Low	100–500 kU — Low	501–1000 kU — Medium	1001–3000 kU — High	3001–5000 kU — Very High	5000–12,000 kU — Highest
Egg, fried	1 large				■		
Egg, poached	1 large	■					
Egg, scrambled or omelet	1 large	■					
Egg substitute, scrambled	¼ cup	■					
Egg white, hard boiled	1 large	■					
Egg yolk, hard boiled	1 large		■				

DAIRY FOODS AND SUBSTITUTES

Dairy foods are rich in high-quality protein and calcium. Many dairy foods can be enjoyed on the AGE-less diet. For those who choose to avoid these products, a number of vegan options are suitable for AGE-less eating. Choose from among the following dairy foods and nondairy alternatives:

Cheese. Care must be taken when choosing and cooking with cheeses, since many contain very high levels of AGEs. Hard, aged cheeses such as Parmesan are among the highest in AGEs. Fortunately, they are very flavorful, so a little bit can go a long way, allowing you to use just a light sprinkling to add flavor. "Light" cheeses, such as those made from 2-percent milk, are lower in AGEs than full-fat cheeses, so choose these products most often. Avoid processed cheeses such as American, which undergo additional heating steps during production that can add AGEs. Above all, add cheeses to food at the end of the cooking period so that AGE formation is minimized.

Milk. Nonfat, low-fat, and even whole milk are low in AGEs. Cream, on the other hand is high in AGEs. Instead of cream, use whole milk in coffee, tea, and recipes to add flavor and body.

Nondairy Milk. Most soy milk, almond milk, and other plant-based milks are good low-AGE options. The majority of these products are low in fat and fortified with calcium and other nutrients. They are sold in cartons alongside the dairy milk in most grocery stores. Choose plain, unsweetened versions instead of those with added sugars. Full-fat coconut milk on the other hand, which is often sold in cans, is much higher in AGEs due to its exceptionally high fat content (about 40 grams per cup). If you like coconut milk, choose the lower-fat versions (with about 5 grams of fat per cup), which are typically sold in cartons near soy and nut milks.

Yogurt. Choose plain yogurt or flavored versions that have little or no added sugar. Even better, start with plain yogurt and add your own fruit and just a teaspoon or two of sweetener. For everyday use, choose nonfat or low-fat products, as lower fat means lower AGE levels. Save the higher-fat versions for occasional use in recipes that require a creamier texture.

Greek-Style Yogurt. Authentic Greek yogurt is yogurt that has been strained to remove part of the whey (liquid). This creates a creamy, thick texture similar to that of sour cream. Avoid imposters that are thickened with cornstarch and contain added ingredients such as dry milk powder, which may increase the AGE content. Greek yogurt is delicious served with fresh fruit and a sprinkling of nuts or seeds. It also makes a healthy alternative to sour cream.

AGE-Less Tips for Using Dairy Foods and Dairy Alternatives

❑ **Choose lower-fat cheeses, as they tend to have lower AGE levels.**

❑ **Avoid cheeses with labels like "processed cheese," "prepared cheese product," or "cheese food."** These foods have undergone additional heating, melting, and processing steps compared with "natural" cheeses, and all of this processing raises the AGE content.

❑ **If cheese is to be melted (as in a pizza or casserole), add it only during the last minute or two of cooking.** Then be sure to cook the cheese just long enough for it to melt. Do not brown it or place it under a broiler, since this blast of heat will cause an explosion of AGEs.

❏ **For a low-AGE alternative to cheese, try crumbling a bit of firm raw tofu over salads.**

Table 6.5   AGE Content of Selected Dairy Foods

Food	Portion Size	100 kU or less Very Low	100–500 kU Low	501–1000 kU Medium	1001–3000 kU High	3001–5000 kU Very High	5000–12,000 kU Highest
CHEESE							
American	1 ounce					▓	
Brie	1 ounce					▓	
Cheddar, full-fat	1 ounce					▓	
Cheddar, 2% milk	1 ounce			▓			
Cottage cheese (1% fat)	½ cup			▓			
Feta	1 ounce				▓		
Mozzarella, reduced-fat	1 ounce			▓			
Parmesan	2 tablespoons					▓	
MILK AND CREAM							
Cream, heavy	2 tablespoons			▓			
Nonfat, reduced-fat, and whole	1 cup	▓					
NONDAIRY MILK							
Coconut milk (full-fat)	1 cup			▓			
Soy milk	1 cup	▓					
YOGURT							
Plain (whole milk)	1 cup	▓					
Vanilla (whole milk)	1 cup	▓					

VEGETABLES

Since plant foods are naturally low in AGEs, eating plenty of produce is key to the AGE-less diet. As a bonus, plant foods provide an abundance of disease-fighting, anti-aging nutrients.

Choose a rainbow of colors every day to ensure a good assortment of phytonutrients, many of which give veggies their vibrant colors. Also choose organic vegetables whenever you can. Organic methods do not affect AGE content, but they do reduce your exposure to other toxins, such as the pesticides, herbicides, and fungicides often used on crops. (See the inset on page 121.)

Fresh Vegetables. As often as possible, feature abundant fresh vegetables in your meals and snacks. For the best quality and price, purchase veggies in season and look for locally grown options from venues such as farmers markets and U-pick farms.

Frozen Vegetables. Vegetables that are grown for the purpose of freezing are picked at the peak of ripeness and quickly frozen to maintain quality. As a result, frozen vegetables may actually be more nutritious than fresh produce that has been sitting in the store or in the refrigerator for too long. Choose plain frozen vegetables instead of those packaged in sauce, as the sauces may add ingredients such as fat, salt, sugar, and artificial flavors and colors.

Canned Vegetables. Canning does not appreciably raise AGE content, so a variety of canned foods can be included in the AGE-less diet. Canned dried beans and tomatoes are handy staples to keep in your pantry. Jarred marinara sauce, artichoke hearts, roasted red peppers, and olives are other convenient foods to keep on hand. Look for organic lower-sodium varieties.

AGE-Less Tips for Using Vegetables

❏ **Enjoy abundant portions of vegetables.** Veggies are low in AGEs, provide a bounty of nutrients, and may prevent AGEs from damaging your body.

❏ **Keep the amount of AGEs low in vegetables by going easy on**

added fats. A good tip is to add just a tablespoon of flavorful extra-virgin olive oil to a pan of vegetables instead of drenching your dish with oil, butter, or cheese sauce. Keep in mind that a bit of healthy fat such as olive oil not only adds flavor, but also increases the absorption of nutrients such as vitamin E, lycopene, and beta-carotene.

❏ **Be aware that roasted, broiled, and grilled vegetables *can* be enjoyed as part of the AGE-less diet.** Vegetables prepared this way have more AGEs than raw or steamed vegetables, but the amount of AGEs in these dishes is very small compared with the amount in roasted and grilled meats.

❏ **For meaty taste and texture, grill or roast portabella mushrooms to enjoy in sandwiches and salads.** You will be surprised by how "meaty" they taste.

Table 6.6 AGE Content of Selected Vegetables

Food	Portion Size	100 kU or less / Very Low	100–500 kU / Low	501–1000 kU / Medium	1001–3000 kU / High	3001–5000 kU / Very High	5000–12,000 kU / Highest
Carrots, canned	1/2 cup	▓					
Cucumber	1/2 cup	▓					
Eggplant, grilled	3.5 ounces		▓				
Eggplant, raw	3 ounces	▓					
Tomato, raw	3.5 ounces	▓					
Tomato sauce, canned	1/2 cup	▓					
Vegetable juice	1 cup	▓					

FRUITS

Like vegetables, fruits are naturally low in AGEs, so it makes sense to include them as a regular part of your diet. Be sure to choose a variety of colorful fruits to ensure you are getting a wide array of AGE-fighting nutrients, and whenever possible, purchase fruit that is organic, locally grown, and in-season. It's tastier, more nutritious, contains fewer pesticides, and is better for the environment, too.

Fresh Fruits. Fresh fruit is the best way to satisfy a sweet tooth, so enjoy it daily in meals and snacks. When fruit is at its best, it has a vibrant sweet taste that requires no added sugar. Sadly, much of the fruit in grocery stores has been picked under-ripe, shipped long distances, and stored for months, and it's mealy and tasteless. For the best quality and flavor, purchase fruit in season, ideally from local farmers markets or U-pick farms.

Frozen Fruits. Fruits grown for the purposes of freezing are picked at their peak of ripeness and quickly frozen to preserve quality. For that reason, frozen fruit may be more nutritious than "fresh" fruit that has been sitting for too long. Frozen fruits are convenient to keep on hand for smoothies. Choose a product that has been frozen without any added sugar or syrup.

Canned Fruits. Canning does not appreciably increase AGE content, so canned fruits can be included in an AGE-less diet. To reduce your intake of added sugars, choose fruits packed in juice rather than sugary syrup.

Dried Fruits. Dried fruit has had the majority of its water removed, either through sun drying or through the use of dehydrators. Although drying does raise AGE content, dried fruits are still very low in AGEs when compared with meats, cheeses, and fats. Keep in mind that because dried fruit is so concentrated, 3 to 4 tablespoons has about the same amount of calories as a whole cup of fresh fruit. The best advice is to eat fresh and frozen fruit most often and to enjoy dried fruit in moderation.

AGE-Less Tips for Using Fruits

❏ **Whenever possible, satisfy your sweet tooth with whole fresh fruit.** It's low in AGEs and high in nutrients and fiber.

❏ **Remember that roasted, grilled, baked, or broiled fruit *can* be enjoyed on an AGE-less diet.** A caramelized baked apple has more AGEs than raw or poached fruit, but it's still much lower in AGEs than meat cooked with these methods.

❏ **Get in the habit of having a small dish of fruit for dessert or as a snack instead of cakes, pies, cookies, and other concentrated sweets.** This not only keeps AGEs down but also helps control blood sugar levels.

Table 6.7 AGE Content of Selected Fruits

Food	Portion Size	100 kU or less Very Low	100– 500 kU Low	501– 1000 kU Medium	1001– 3000 kU High	3001– 5000 kU Very High	5000– 12,000 kU Highest
Apple, baked	3.5 ounces						
Apple, raw	3.5 ounces						
Banana	3.5 ounces						
Cantaloupe	3.5 ounces						
Dried plums	1 ounce						
Raisins	1 ounce						

GRAIN PRODUCTS

A variety of breads, cereals, and grains may be enjoyed on the AGE-less diet. The key is to choose *minimally processed whole grains.* This will boost your intake of AGE-fighting nutrients and antioxidants, which are concentrated in the grain's bran and germ—the parts that are discarded during refining. Choose from the following:

Breads. An assortment of breads can be enjoyed on the AGE-less diet, including sandwich-type breads, bagels, pita, tortillas, wraps, and rolls. Make sure to choose 100-percent whole grain breads with ingredients such as cracked or rolled grains, sprouted grains, flax seeds, and nuts, instead of airy, fluffy products made from finely ground flours. Whole-grain products like these are rich in fiber and nutrients and have a lower glycemic index, which helps keep blood sugar levels in check. Avoid breads made with refined white flour, which has had most of it nutrients and fiber removed and can cause blood sugar levels to spike. Also avoid high-fat breads such as biscuits and croissants, which have more AGEs than low-fat choices.

Cereals. Your best bets are minimally processed cereals such as cooked oatmeal, steel-cut oats, or cracked grain cereals. Muesli, made from uncooked rolled oats or other whole grains, is another good option. Some ready-to-eat cereals such as bran flakes and shredded wheat are among the lower-AGE choices. However, ready-to-eat cereals that are made with added sugar or honey and undergo extensive heat-processing, dehydration, and extrusion are much higher in AGEs.

Crackers and Snack Foods. These foods often contain added fats and sugars and are heat-processed until dry and crisp, which adds a large amount of AGEs. Many of these products are also low in nutrition and high in salt and artificial ingredients, so there are many reasons to avoid them. A good substitute for processed snacks such as crackers, chips, and pretzels is popcorn, which is a whole grain food. Choose air-popped corn or a low-fat microwave variety, not the "buttery" sorts that mimic what is available at theaters.

Pasta. For the best nutrition, choose whole grain pasta instead of refined versions. Bulk up your pasta dishes with lots of vegetables to reduce carbs and calories. Or substitute spaghetti squash or Zucchini Noodles (page 267) for high-carb pasta.

Whole Grains. Boiled or steamed whole grains such as brown rice, barley, bulgur wheat, farro, quinoa, spelt, wild rice, and others are good choices. When making grain-based salads, casseroles, and side dishes, use a high proportion of vegetables and fewer grains to reduce the carb and calorie counts of the dish.

AGE-Less Tips for Using Grain Products

❑ **Choose whole grain, lower-fat breads, and whole grain cereals and grain dishes.** This will maximize fiber and other nutrients and keep AGE levels under control.

❑ **To satisfy a taste for grilled food, try a quesadilla filled with mashed beans or grilled vegetables and reduced-fat cheese.** To minimize AGEs, coat the pan with a spritz of nonstick cooking spray instead of frying the quesadilla in butter, margarine, or oil.

Table 6.8 AGE Content of Selected Grains and Grain Products*

Food	Portion Size	100 kU or less Very Low	100–500 kU Low	501–1000 kU Medium	1001–3000 kU High	3001–5000 kU Very High	5000–12,000 kU Highest
BREADS							
Bagel	2 ounces	■					
Bagel, toasted	2 ounces	■	■				
Biscuit	2 ounces			■			
Bread, whole wheat	2 ounces	■					
Croissant	2 ounces			■			
Pita bread	2 ounces	■					
CEREALS							
Bran flakes	1 cup	■					
Corn flakes, sugar frosted	1 cup		■				
Crisp rice cereal	1 cup			■			
Granola	1/2 cup		■				
Oatmeal, cooked	1 cup	■					
CRACKERS AND SNACKS							
Popcorn, low-fat	3 cups	■					
Pretzels	1 ounce			■			
Saltines	1 ounce		■				
Toasted wheat crackers	1 ounce		■				
PASTA AND GRAINS							
Pasta, boiled	1 cup		■				
Rice, boiled	1 cup	■					

*Note that in the case of toasted bagels, two boxes—"Very Low" and "Low"—have been marked. This indicates that the food is on the "borderline" of two categories, and therefore belongs in both categories.

❑ **Substitute wedges of whole grain pita bread or thinly sliced bagel rounds for crackers.** Breads have a lower AGE count than crackers. Even better, use lettuce leaves, Belgian endive leaves, or other fresh vegetables for scooping dips and spreads.

❑ **Enjoy your bread toasted, if you like, but skip high-fat spreads.** Toasting bread increases AGEs, but the amount is still a great deal less than that of meats and fats. For instance, half of a bagel (1 ounce) contains about 30 kU AGEs. Toasting increases the amount to about 50 kU. But spreading the bagel with just one tablespoon of cream cheese adds over 1,000 kU AGEs!

❑ **Garnish salads with chickpeas, kidney beans, or a sprinkling of raw nuts or seeds instead of browned or fried croutons.** Or toss in some whole wheat penne pasta, wheat berries, farro, or other cooked whole grains.

OILS, SPREADS, DRESSINGS, NUTS, AND OTHER FAT SOURCES

Making smart fat choices—whether you're choosing an oil, a spread or dressing, or a ripe avocado—is a high priority in AGE-less eating. Fats and oils can contain very high levels of AGEs, which form during refining and processing. Avoid using refined vegetable oils and margarine as much as possible. Also avoid using butter, which contains even more AGEs than vegetable oils. As for plant foods that are high in good fats, such as nuts and seeds, use them in moderation so you can benefit from important nutrients without overloading on AGEs.

Avocado. This buttery-smooth fruit makes a sumptuous addition to salads, sandwiches, and many other foods. Since avocados are a whole natural food, they are a healthier fat choice than processed fats and oils. The fat in avocados is mostly monounsaturated, which has a favorable effect on blood cholesterol levels. Avocados also provide many important nutrients, including fiber, potassium, vitamin E, and B vitamins.

Mayonnaise. Choose light and lower-fat versions. Or use equal parts of mayo and yogurt as a dressing for chicken and potato salads.

Hummus, mashed avocado, and mustard are all good alternatives to mayonnaise on sandwiches.

Nuts and Seeds. While nuts and seeds do contain AGEs, they are among the best fat choices since they are whole foods and provide fiber, protein, and many other important nutrients. Choose raw nuts and seeds, since roasting can double AGE content, and use in moderation. Store nuts and seeds in the refrigerator or freezer to maintain freshness and slow AGE formation.

Olive Oil. Choose cold pressed "extra-virgin" olive oil, which is the least refined and most flavorful, and provides a variety of antioxidants and phytonutrients. To preserve freshness, keep olive oil away from direct light so that it does not become oxidized. Even better, store it in the refrigerator to slow oxidation and AGE formation. Pull it out a few minutes before you need it to allow it to liquefy.

Olives. Olives have been cultivated in parts of the Mediterranean for thousands of years, and are botanically classified as fruits. One ounce (about $1/4$ cup sliced) contains about the same amount of AGEs as one tablespoon of olive oil. Olives provide many different phytonutrients, some of which function as antioxidants. Use olives to perk up salads, pasta dishes, and other recipes.

Salad Dressings. Choose lower-fat dressings or a small amount of full-fat dressing. Be sure to read labels and avoid those that are high in added sugar and salt. Even better, make your own dressing with extra-virgin olive oil, vinegar or lemon juice, and herbs. For a touch of sweetness, try balsamic vinegar (which is made from grape juice), or include a splash of orange or pomegranate juice in homemade salad dressings. Above all, learn to enjoy just a light coating of dressing.

AGE-Less Tips for Using Oils, Spreads, Dressings, and Other Fat Sources

❏ **Whenever possible, choose organic cold-pressed or expeller-pressed oils.** Compared to conventionally produced oils, cold- and expeller-pressed oils are subjected to less heat and are not extracted with chemical solvents. In addition, organic foods are GMO-free.

Table 6.9 AGE Content of Selected Fats and High-Fat Foods*

Food	Portion Size	100 kU or less — Very Low	100–500 kU — Low	501–1000 kU — Medium	1001–3000 kU — High	3001–5000 kU — Very High	5000–12,000 kU — Highest
FATS AND OILS							
Butter	1 tablespoon				X	X	
Canola oil	1 tablespoon			X	X		
Margarine	1 tablespoon			X			
Mayonnaise, full-fat	1 tablespoon				X		
Mayonnaise, low-fat	1 tablespoon		X				
Olive oil	1 tablespoon		X	X			
Sesame oil, toasted	1 tablespoon					X	
HIGH-FAT FOODS							
Avocado	¼ cup		X				
Olives	¼ cup		X				
Peanut butter	2 tablespoons				X		
Peanuts, roasted	¼ cup						
Pumpkin seeds, raw	¼ cup		X				
Sunflower seeds, raw	¼ cup			X			
Sunflower seeds, roasted	¼ cup				X		

*Note that in the case of some foods, such as canola oil, two boxes—"Medium" and "High," for instance—have been marked. This indicates that the food is on the "borderline" of two categories, and therefore belongs in both categories.

❏ **Avoid roasted or toasted oils such as dark (toasted) sesame oil.** The extra heat treatment greatly increases AGEs.

❏ **Reduce AGE formation by storing your oils with care.** Exposure to heat, air, and light increases the oxidation of fats, which speeds AGE formation. Avoid storing oils for long periods in the pantry, or even worse, near the stovetop or in sunlight. To maintain freshness, keep your oils in the refrigerator.

❏ **Dress your salads smartly.** Dressings (whether reduced-fat or regular) that contain a bit of fat will increase your absorption of beta-carotene and other fat-soluble nutrients. A sprinkling of untoasted nuts, ground flaxseed, or chia; a few olives; or a few slices of avocado would be expected to provide the same benefits. Just don't go overboard, since fats do contain AGEs and are high in calories.

❏ **Avoid using high heat when cooking with oils or high-fat foods.** When fats are cooked with high heat—as when sautéing on a stovetop—they can begin to smoke and turn brown. This is a sign that more AGEs have formed. By all means, avoid browned fats, since they can have an incredibly high amount of avoidable AGEs!

SWEETENERS AND SWEETS

While sweeteners such as sugar, honey, and syrup are low in AGEs, a diet high in sugar can contribute to high blood sugar levels, obesity, and eventually, diabetes. Moreover, when sweeteners are added to foods and heated—in the making of cookies and sweetened ready-to-eat cereals, for instance—they can react with the fats and proteins in these foods to form AGEs. Sweets that tend to be lowest in AGEs include dairy desserts such as ice cream and pudding, fruit desserts such as sorbet, and baked or grilled fruits. Dark chocolate is also a good choice. Of course, all desserts should be enjoyed in moderation.

The best advice regarding added sweeteners such as sugar, corn syrup, honey, agave, maple syrup, and others is to limit them as much as possible. The guideline that's put forth by the American Heart Association (AHA) offers a reasonable upper limit for these sweeteners. The AHA recommends no more than six teaspoons of added sugar per day for most women and no more than nine teaspoons for most men. For most people, this amounts to about 5 percent of total calories eaten per day. Note that this recommendation refers only to sugar that is *added* to food, not to sugar that occurs naturally in foods such as fruits, vegetables, and milk products.

To help put these recommendations in perspective, many people consume over three times the recommended intake for added sugars. This is easy to do when you consider that sugar is added to the majority of processed foods. The biggest contributor of sugar to the American diet is sweetened beverages—one twelve-ounce soda contains about ten teaspoons of added sugars.

Table 6.10 AGE Content of Selected Sweeteners and Sweets*

Food	Portion Size	100 kU or less — Very Low	100–500 kU — Low	501–1000 kU — Medium	1001–3000 kU — High	3001–5000 kU — Very High	5000–12,000 kU — Highest
SWEETENERS							
Honey	1 table-spoon	■					
Sugar	1 table-spoon	■					
SWEETS							
Apple crumb pie	1/8 pie				■		
Biscotti with almonds	1 ounce			■			
Cheese Danish	2.5 ounces				■		
Chocolate chip cookies	1 ounce		■	■			
Chocolate, dark	1 ounce		■	■			
Frozen fruit pop	2 ounce	■					
Fruit sorbet	1/2 cup	■					
Ice cream, vanilla	1/2 cup	■					
Pudding, chocolate	1/2 cup	■					

*Note that in the case of some foods, such as chocolate chip cookies, two boxes—"Low" and "Medium," for instance—have been marked. This indicates that the food is on the "borderline" of two categories, and therefore belongs in both categories.

AGE-Less Tips for Using Sweets and Sweeteners

❏ **Minimize your use of all sweeteners.** Although they are low in AGEs, they are associated with a number of health problems, including diabetes and obesity.

❏ **Limit your intake of sweets and desserts.** This will help you rein in carbs, calories, and also AGEs. Keep in mind that AGEs tend to be highest in baked goods that are rich in sugars and fats. When sugar and other sweeteners are added to foods and heated, they can react with fats and proteins to form AGEs.

CONDIMENTS AND SEASONINGS

Condiments and seasonings are very important in the AGE-less diet since they can perk up the flavor of your foods without adding age-accelerating AGEs. Avoid condiments such as ketchup and sweet barbecue sauce, which are high in sugar.

The following seasonings and condiments can be a healthful part of a low-AGE diet:

- Bottled salsa and picante sauce
- Capers
- Condiments and hot sauces, such as Tabasco, horseradish, wasabi, chiles, and hot peppers
- Herbs and spices (fresh or dried)
- Lemon and lime juices
- Mustard
- Pickles
- Soy sauce
- Vinegar

AGE-Less Tips for Using Condiments and Seasonings

❏ **Experiment with herbs and spices to see what you like best.** These seasonings can boost the flavor of your dishes without adding AGEs. Herbs and spices are also more concentrated in antioxidants than any other food category, so they are big contributors to our antioxidant intake when used regularly.

❏ **Enjoy vinegar in a variety of foods.** So many different vinegars are available—red wine, white wine, apple cider, rice, balsamic, sherry, raspberry, malt, and more—that they can be used in far more than salad dressings. Use them in your marinades to add flavor and lower AGE formation during cooking. For added zip, splash some vinegar on a dish of cooked vegetables, chicken, or fish. Or skip the oily dressings entirely and use sweet balsamic vinegar alone to dress your salad.

❏ **Use high-sodium condiments with care.** Some condiments are high in sodium, and depending on your health needs and dietary restrictions, they may have to be used sparingly. Soy sauce, of course, is very high in sodium—even "light" versions should be used sparingly. Be aware that some prepared sauces and pickles can be high in sodium, as well, so by all means, check the label before making a purchase.

❏ **Skip high-sugar condiments like ketchup and sweet barbecue sauce.** Although they are not high in AGEs on their own, these products can boost AGE levels if they are used in excess and on a frequent basic.

Table 6.11   AGE Content of Selected Condiments

Food	Portion Size	100 kU or less — Very Low	100– 500 kU — Low	501– 1000 kU — Medium	1001– 3000 kU — High	3001– 5000 kU — Very High	5000– 12,000 kU — Highest
Ketchup	1 table-spoon						
Mustard	1 table-spoon						
Pickles	1 ounce						
Soy sauce	1 table-spoon						
Vinegar, balsamic	1 table-spoon						
Vinegar, white	1 table-spoon						

BEVERAGES

Many beverages are low-AGE choices. The trick is to avoid sugary products like sodas and sports drinks, to avoid or minimize the use of sweeteners, and to replace cream with milk.

Coffee. Coffee provides an impressive amount of antioxidants and other nutrients, including potassium, magnesium, manganese, and niacin—which is great, because for so many of us, this is a favorite beverage. Just as important, coffee is low in AGEs. When you prepare your morning cup of Joe, minimize the sugar and lighten your beverage with milk instead of cream, as cream is higher in AGEs. (See Table 6.5.)

Tea. Like coffee, tea has been found to contain antioxidants and other important nutrients. Both white and green tea are less processed than black tea and appear to be highest in beneficial substances, but all teas—green, white, and black—are healthful, and all are low in AGEs, as are herbal teas. Again, though, you'll want to minimize the sugar and lighten with milk instead of cream.

Milk. All milk, even whole, is low in AGEs and provides important nutrients, such as protein, calcium, and vitamin D. Choose nonfat and low-fat versions for drinking to reduce calories and saturated fats. You may opt to use whole milk in coffee, tea, and recipes, but be sure to skip AGE-rich cream.

Sodas. Keep in mind that it is best to avoid all sodas. Regular sodas provide far too much sugar, as well as other ingredients of questionable safety, and "diet" versions contain artificial sweeteners. However, if you must drink sodas, choose sugar-free versions and avoid dark-colored varieties. The dark color and characteristic flavor of these beverages is due to AGEs that are made by caramelizing sugars. While these sodas are not exceptionally high in preformed AGEs, they do contain very reactive pre-AGEs, which can mix with food proteins or fats in the stomach and gut, and generate additional AGEs. (For more information on sodas, see the inset on page 34.)

Juices. Fruit and vegetable juices are low in AGEs and provide a variety of vitamins and minerals. However, whole fruits and vegetables are a better choice. Fruit juices, in particular, are high in carbo-hydrates and low in fiber, and the lack of fiber causes their sugars to be rapidly absorbed. Enjoy these beverages in moderation.

Table 6.12 AGE Content of Selected Beverages

Food	Portion Size	100 kU or less Very Low	100–500 kU Low	501–1000 kU Medium	1001–3000 kU High	3001–5000 kU Very High	5000–12,000 kU Highest
Beer	8 ounces						
Coffee	8 ounces						
Cola, diet	8 ounces						
Cola, regular	8 ounces						
Milk (low-fat or whole)	8 ounces						
Orange juice	8 ounces						
Sprite, diet	8 ounces						
Sprite, regular	8 ounces						
Tea	8 ounces						
Vegetable juice	8 ounces						
Whiskey	1 ounces						
Wine, white	8 ounces						

AGE-Less Tips for Choosing Beverages

❏ **Avoid dark sodas, such as colas, which contain very reactive pre-AGEs.** While light-colored sodas may be low in these substances, keep in mind that they are still loaded with harmful ingredients.

❏ **Don't use cream in your coffee or tea.** Instead, use whole or low-fat milk.

CONCLUSION

The modern diet, rich in animal protein and industrially processed foods, brings with it an abundance of toxic, age-accelerating AGEs.

One of the most powerful tools we have to reclaim our health is a more plant-based diet built around whole, natural foods. Choosing ingredients for your AGE-less meals need not be expensive or time consuming. The foods you need are widely available in grocery stores, farmers markets, natural foods stores, and many other places.

As you already know, when controlling AGEs, the method of cooking you use is just as important as the foods themselves. Switching from dry-heat methods such as roasting, grilling, and frying to gentler moist-heat methods such as poaching, steaming, braising, and stewing, can make a huge difference in your diet's level of AGEs. Chapter 7 takes a closer look at these AGE-less cooking techniques and offers additional tips for preparing delicious, satisfying meals that can be enjoyed by the entire family.

7.

AGE-Less
Cooking Techniques

J ust a few generations ago, most of our meals were prepared at home. Foods were most often fresh, local, organic, and pasture-raised. In stark contrast, most of our food today is industrially processed, with an ever-increasing reliance on fast foods, take-out, and convenience foods. This change has added not just more sugar, salt, additives, and preservatives, but also more toxic AGEs. One of the most powerful tools we have to reclaim our health is to shop carefully and get back into the kitchen to rediscover the lost art of cooking with whole natural foods.

As we have emphasized throughout this book, to a great extent, *how you cook* determines how many AGEs end up in your food. Fortunately, it's easy to prepare delicious AGE-less meals. Many of our favorite comfort foods—including soups, stews, meatballs, skillet dinners, and sandwiches—are perfect for eating the AGE-less way. Importantly, AGE-less cooking methods are very much in tune with the needs of working people and busy families. Beginning on page 175, you will find recipes for many delicious dishes. In this chapter, you will learn how to use AGE-less cooking techniques. For the novice cook, we will explain cooking terms, temperature levels, and all the other basics you need to know. In addition, you will find practical tips for preparing some of your favorite foods with fewer AGEs.

Moist- Versus Dry-Heat Cooking

If you are an experienced cook, the terms "moist-heat" and "dry-heat" may be part of your vocabulary. To others, however, these terms may seem a bit mysterious. Let's take a look at exactly what they mean.

Dry-Heat Cooking

This term refers to any technique in which heat is transferred to the food *without* using moisture. For instance, when you roast meat in an oven, heat released from the oven coils raises the temperature inside the oven to cook the meat. When you grill a steak, heat from your barbecue grill cooks the meat. Dry-heat cooking typically involves temperatures of at least 350°F to 400°F (175°C to 204°C), but they can be even higher. Although it may seem counterintuitive since cooking oil is a liquid, deep-frying is also a dry-heat cooking method. This makes sense if you keep in mind that water and oil repel each other. For instance, if you add a few drops of water to a skillet of hot oil, you will see a fierce reaction.

The browning of food, seen when meat is roasted or bread is toasted, can be achieved only through dry-heat cooking. The brown color and the accompanying flavors and aromas are characteristic of the Maillard reaction, which also forms AGEs. (See page 11 for a further discussion of this reaction.)

Moist-Heat Cooking

This refers to any technique in which heat is transferred to food using moisture. For instance, when food is submerged in a simmering liquid, it is cooked through moist heat. Moist-heat cooking generally involves temperatures of no more that 212°F (100°C), which is the boiling point of water. Poaching, steaming, braising, and stewing are all classic moist-heat cooking methods.

Water is a powerful inhibitor of the Maillard reaction, which is why foods cooked with moist heat do not brown and form far fewer AGEs than foods cooked with dry heat. For instance, poached chicken has about 80 percent fewer AGEs than grilled chicken. Mastering moist-heat cooking methods is a key step in eating the AGE-less way.

COOKING THE AGE-LESS WAY

Cooking the AGE-less way is based on two very simple concepts— using moist heat and using the lowest cooking temperature possible. These two concepts tend to go hand-in-hand, since the temperature reached with moist-heat cooking methods such as poaching, steaming, braising, and stewing, does not exceed the boiling point (212°F, or 100°C). In contrast, the temperatures reached with dry-heat cooking methods such as roasting, grilling, broiling, and frying, can be more than twice as high. Cooking with acidic ingredients such as lemon juice, vinegar, wine, and tomatoes also reduces new AGE formation, while at the same time adding flavor. Let's take a look at some simple, time-honored techniques that can help you eat well and also avoid unwanted AGEs.

Boiling and Simmering

Boiling involves cooking food in a liquid (such as water or broth) that churns vigorously, with bubbles continuously breaking through the surface.

Boiling is well suited for pasta, since the moving water keeps the pasta from sticking together. It is also used to blanch vegetables, a technique in which fresh vegetables such as green beans or asparagus are briefly tossed into boiling water to lightly cook the food and intensify color and flavor. Shellfish such as lobster, crab, and shrimp are often boiled, sometimes with liquids such as beer or wine and flavorful spices. These delicate foods take just a few minutes to cook.

Meats and poultry are generally not cooked at a full boil, as this technique can leave them tough and tasteless. Rather, these foods benefit from lower, slower cooking through simmering, which is described below, or through braising or stewing, which are discussed later in this chapter.

Simmering is a gentler version of boiling. It is suited for dishes such as soups, stews, and pot roasts, all of which benefit from long, slow cooking. The temperature stays slightly below the boiling point, at around 185°F to 205°F (85°C to 95°C), and the surface of the liquid gently bubbles.

Simmering overlaps with other AGE-less methods such as braising and stewing, both of which traditionally involve simmering
either meat or poultry in a flavorful liquid after first browning it.
(This chapter will explain how to modify both braising and stewing
techniques to reduce the formation of AGEs.) Meats and poultry that
are simmered become savory, succulent, and fork-tender. Delicate
foods such as fish and eggs are poached just below a simmer to prevent
them from breaking apart during cooking.

Braising

This wonderfully simple "comfort food" cooking method is a main-
stay of Mediterranean cuisine. Braising is ideal for cooking tougher
cuts of meat, such as brisket, that require up to several hours of cooking to become tender and succulent. Foods such as chicken and pork
chops can also be prepared using this technique, but they are typically
cooked in less than an hour.

Standard recipes usually call for browning or searing the meat as
the first step in braising. This involves cooking the meat over high heat
for a few minutes on each side, until the surface turns deep brown and
crusty, but the interior remains uncooked. The browned meat is then
partially covered with liquid and simmered in a covered pot on the
stovetop. The meat may also be slowly cooked in a covered pot in the
oven at a low temperature, usually around 300°F to 325°F (150°C to
165°C). Braising cooks food with a combination of steam and simmering liquid.

To minimize the formation of AGEs when braising, you need to
modify the traditional browning step. Instead of deeply browning
the meat at a high temperature in a pool of fat, coat a nonstick skillet
with cooking spray and brown the meat over medium heat for only a
minute or two on each side, just to lightly brown and seal the meat.
You can also include acidic ingredients such as wine and tomatoes in
the cooking liquid, since these help reduce AGEs. Add flavor with
generous amounts of herbs, spices, and other seasonings. The recipe
section of this book provides examples of tender and flavorful meats
that are braised the AGE-less way.

En Papillote

En papillote (pah-pee-YOHT) is a simple but elegant method that involves cooking foods in parchment paper or foil packets. The packet is placed in the oven, where the food steams in its own juices, creating delicious flavor. Steaming ensures that the food does not dry out during cooking, and the high moisture level inside the packet inhibits AGE formation. This method is best suited for delicate, quick-cooking foods such as boneless skinless chicken breasts, fish fillets, and shellfish. Other ingredients such as seasonings, vegetables, lemon slices, or a splash of wine can be added to the packet contents to enhance taste.

Aluminum foil is the easiest to work with because it creates a tight seal for holding in the steam. Parchment is trickier to work with but makes a stunning presentation. This is how you can create a packet with parchment. (See Figure 7.1 on page 150.)

1. For each serving, use a 12-by-16-inch sheet of parchment paper. Fold the sheet in half to make a 12-by-8-inch rectangle and cut into a half-heart shape so that the parchment forms a heart when unfolded.

2. Open the heart and lay it on a work surface. Layer the ingredients onto one side of the heart near the fold. Fold the other half of the heart over to enclose the filling.

3. Starting at the top of the heart and using small folds, fold along the edges of the parchment to seal the packet. Each small fold should overlap and seal the previous fold.

4. When you have made the last fold at the point of the heart, twist the tip tightly to seal the packet. You can also use a metal paper clip to ensure a tight seal. Place the packets on a baking sheet, and bake as directed in the recipe.

Poaching

Poaching is frequently used in French cooking. It involves submerging food in a liquid such as water, broth, or wine. Herbs, seasonings, and aromatic vegetables like celery and onion are typically added to the liquid to infuse the food with flavor. The heat is adjusted to maintain a very low simmer in which a few bubbles reach the surface of the

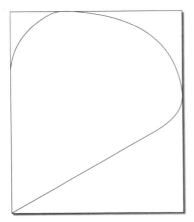

1. Fold a 12-by-16-inch sheet of parchment paper in half, and cut it into a half-heart shape so that it forms a heart when unfolded.

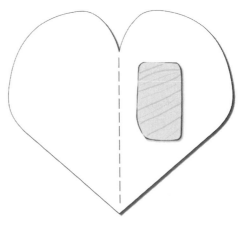

2. Lay the open heart on a work surface, and layer the ingredients on one side of the heart near the fold.

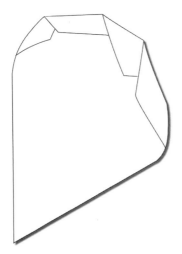

3. Fold the other half of the heart over the food. Then, starting at the top of the heart, use small overlapping folds to seal the packet.

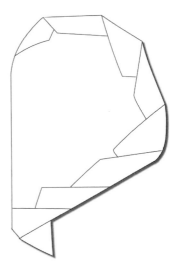

4. When you have made the last fold at the point of the heart, twist the tip tightly to seal the packet.

Figure 7.1. Enclosing Food in Parchment for En Papillote Cooking

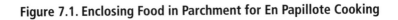

liquid every few seconds. This gentle cooking technique is particularly suited for delicate foods such as poultry, seafood, and eggs. When the food is cooked, the poaching liquid may be reduced and used as the basis for a sauce.

Poaching is perfect when you need cooked chicken or seafood for salads and sandwiches. Or you can top a piece of poached chicken or fish with a bit of fresh herb pesto or a zesty topping such as Chimichurri Sauce (page 280) or Lemon-Dill Sauce (page 281) for a simple main course. The inset on page 224 offers basic recipes for poaching poultry and seafood. The "Breakfast" section that begins on page 181 features creative ways to prepare poached eggs.

Pressure Cooking

A pressure cooker is a large deep pot with a locking lid that seals in steam. The food, along with some liquid and seasonings, is placed in the covered pot and the contents are brought to a boil on the stovetop. Once the steam builds up to the correct pressure, a release valve lets out excess steam to maintain constant pressure and a constant temperature of around 250°F (120°C) inside the pot.

Pressure-cooking is a good method for preparing moist and tender home-style meals. Foods such as whole grains, dried beans, chicken, and even pot roast can be cooked in about one-third of the usual time. Always consult your pressure cooker's directions for specific information regarding its proper use and safety procedures.

Slow Cooking

Slow cookers, or "Crock Pots," cook foods in a liquid or sauce very slowly at low temperatures, essentially braising or stewing the food. Since slow cookers allow for unattended cooking, they are great for fuss-free home-style meals. These appliances can turn just a few simple ingredients into dishes that are tender, moist, flavorful, and low in AGEs.

As with braising and stewing, many slow cooker recipes call for browning meats prior to adding them to the slow cooker. You can modify the browning step to minimize AGEs. Instead of deeply browning the meat at a high temperature in a pool of fat, coat a non-stick skillet with cooking spray and cook the meat over medium heat for a minute or two on each side, just to lightly brown and seal the food. You can also include acidic ingredients such as wine and tomatoes in the cooking liquid, since these will help reduce AGE formation. Boost flavor with herbs and aromatic vegetables such as onions, garlic, celery, and carrots.

Steaming

While most people are familiar with steaming vegetables, this AGE-less cooking method is also well suited for delicate protein foods such as chicken breasts; fish fillets; and shellfish, including clams, oysters, and mussels. Steaming is widely used to prepare Asian cuisine such as steamed dumplings or fish steamed over a bed of aromatic vegetables. Steam is a good choice when you want foods to retain their shape, color, and texture. Unlike boiling, where nutrients can leach into the cooking water, steaming allows most of the nutrients to remain in the food.

Steaming is easily done on the stovetop with an inexpensive collapsible steam basket that fits into a standard 6-quart cooking pot. Some cookware sets and woks come with steamer inserts. Another option is a bamboo steamer, which has two or three tiers that can be stacked, allowing you to cook several foods at the same time.

As with poaching, a variety of liquids—including water, broth, wine, and beer—can be used to cook the food. Seasonings such as green tea leaves, ginger, and lemongrass can be added to the liquid, or seasonings can be sprinkled over the food itself. As the steam rises, the food is infused with flavors. When steaming, keep the level of liquid below the holes or slats in the steamer so that liquid does not bubble up through the holes. Check the liquid level occasionally and add more if needed to keep the pot from drying out.

Stewing

Like braising, stewing is an ideal cooking method for tenderizing tough cuts of meat. The main difference is that braising is most often used to cook large pieces of meat, such as those used to make pot roast, while stewing is generally used for cooking small pieces of meat, such as the cubes used in beef stew. Also, in a stew, the ingredients are totally submerged in liquid, while in braising, they are only partially submerged.

As with braising, stewing recipes typically call for browning the meat as a first step. The meat is then immersed in liquid in a covered pot and gently simmered either on the stovetop or in the oven. Stewing can take one or more hours, depending on the recipe.

Again, you can reduce AGEs when stewing by minimizing the browning step. Coat a nonstick skillet with cooking spray and brown the meat over medium heat for a couple of minutes, just to lightly brown and seal the meat. You can also include wine, tomatoes, or a splash of vinegar or lemon juice in the cooking liquid to help deter AGE formation during stewing. Note that if too much of an acidic ingredient is used, grains and vegetables in the stew may toughen and not cook properly. The recipes included in Part Two will guide you in using acidic liquids with delicious and healthful results.

TIPS FOR REDUCING AGEs
WHEN GRILLING, BROILING, AND ROASTING

The moist-heat methods described above are the best way to deter AGE formation during cooking and should be used to prepare the majority of your meals. Dry-heat cooking methods like grilling and broiling should be minimized, particularly when preparing meat and poultry. However, when you do choose to grill or broil, here are some steps you can take to reduce AGEs.

❑ When making meats, chicken, and turkey, choose lean meats and skinless poultry. Keep in mind, though, that although leaner foods produce less AGEs, all cells in meats contain not only proteins, but also certain reactive fats and sugars that can trigger AGE formation. So even lean meats can form many AGEs when cooked with dry heat.

❑ Marinate meats and poultry with low-sugar, low-oil marinades made with acidic ingredients such as lemon juice, lime juice, and vinegar. For tips on making and using marinades, see the inset on page 286. Recipes for making AGE-less marinades can be found in Part Two of this book.

❑ Use small pieces of meat, poultry, or seafood, as they cook faster than large pieces. Skewers or grill baskets can be used to cook shrimp, scallops, and chunks of steak or chicken. When cooking skewers of meat and vegetables, space the chunks of meat and vegetables about $1/2$ inch apart on the skewer. This helps the food cook more quickly. Remember that the less time the food spends on the grill, the fewer AGEs will generally form.

❑ When grilling burgers, shape them with the sides slightly thicker than the center to promote faster, more even cooking. Avoid pressing down on the burgers during cooking, as this removes moisture. Flip burgers every couple of minutes to prevent charring and promote more even cooking.

❑ Avoid overcooking meats. Rare or medium-rare cooked steaks are lower in AGEs than well-done steaks. Just be sure to cook the meats to the recommended safe minimum cooking temperatures in order to protect against foodborne illnesses such as salmonella and *E. coli*. (See Table 7.1.)

❑ Cook meat en papillote (page 149) in foil packets on the grill. Or cook meat in a foil packet (to conserve moisture) until almost done, and then remove the food from the foil and place it on the grill for just a few minutes to finish cooking. Another lower-AGE method is to partially pre-cook the meat by simmering it in liquid so it does not need to be on the grill as long.

❑ Use ceramic and other nonstick cooking surfaces—as opposed to stainless steel, cast iron, and other metals—to help to reduce AGE formation.

❑ As often as possible, choose seafood for dry-heat cooking methods such as grilling, broiling, and baking. Seafood cooks quickly and forms fewer AGEs than meats and poultry.

❑ Choose vegetables and fruits for grilling, broiling, and roasting, since they form far fewer AGEs than meats and poultry.

❏ Have a grilled sandwich or quesadilla made with vegetables and reduced-fat cheese. Again, the amount of AGEs found in the grilled bread or tortilla is much less than the amount that would be found in grilled meat.

❏ Minimize AGEs at every meal by serving plenty of healthy side dishes made with vegetables, fruits, and whole grains, which are naturally low in AGEs.

Table 7.1 Safe Minimum Cooking Temperatures

Food	Temperature (degrees F)
Fish and shellfish	145°F
Ground beef, pork, veal, or lamb	160°F
Poultry (whole or parts) or ground turkey or chicken	165°F
Steaks, roasts, or chops (beef, veal, lamb, or pork)	145°F plus 3-minute rest time*

*During the rest time, the temperature remains constant or continues to rise, which destroys harmful microorganisms.

REHEATING FOODS

As you know, when you cook raw foods, the level of heat generated and the amount of time that the food is exposed to the heat helps determine its AGE content. The same principles apply to reheating leftovers. For reasons of food safety, it is recommended that leftovers be reheated to 165°F. Soups, sauces, and gravies should be brought to a boil.

Leftover soup or stew can simply be reheated on a stovetop. Since these foods contain a lot of water, there will be minimal formation of new AGEs during reheating. Foods such as leftover pot roast can be reheated in a covered pot on the stove along with some of the pot roast juices or sauce. Microwaving is also a good option for reheating because it tends to heat foods without drying them out. For foods without liquid, add some broth, sauce, or gravy, and reheat just long enough to bring the food to the desired temperature.

GIVE YOUR RECIPES AN AGE-LESS MAKEOVER

By mastering the techniques presented in this chapter, you will take a huge step toward preparing a variety of easy and delicious AGE-less meals. But your choice of ingredients will also affect your AGE load because certain foods and ingredients—especially those that are fatty and overly processed—deliver more AGEs than their leaner, less-processed counterparts. Chapter 6 offers more details on the best foods for stocking your AGE-less pantry. Table 7.2 puts it all together and offers tips for transforming your favorite recipes into new AGE-less dishes.

Table 7.2 Strategies for Lowering AGEs in Different Foods

Type of Recipe	To Lower AGEs . . .
Burgers	• Use lean ground meat (at least 93% lean).
	• Add some finely chopped mushrooms, onions, or other vegetables to the burger mixture. This will increase moisture, boost nutritional value, and make meat portions go further.
	• Shape the center of burgers slightly thinner than the edges. This will promote faster, more even cooking.
	• Avoid pressing down on the burgers during cooking, as this will remove moisture.
	• Cook on nonstick surfaces such as a nonstick skillet or a tabletop grill (such as a George Foreman Grill) with a nonstick coating. Direct contact with a metal cooking or grilling surface enhances AGE formation.
Casseroles	• If the recipe includes browned ground beef or turkey, use a nonstick skillet and cook the meat just until done. Minimize browning.
	• If the recipe calls for cooked chicken, use poached chicken instead of grilled or roasted.
	• Use unprocessed, reduced-fat cheese, and add any cheese toppings during the last minute of cooking so they are heated just long enough to melt. Do not brown.

Grilled Meats and Poultry	• Marinate your food in an acidic marinade before grilling.
	• Wrap meats or poultry in a foil pouch for the first part of cooking, or pre-cook by poaching or steaming until the food is almost done. Then finish cooking on a grill surface.
	• Cook steaks rare or medium-rare to lower AGE formation.
Meatballs	• Use lean ground meat (at least 93% lean).
	• Use fresh untoasted breadcrumbs or rolled oats instead of dried toasted crumbs.
	• Omit the browning step and simply simmer the meatballs in the sauce until cooked through.
Meatloaf	• Use lean ground meat (at least 93% lean).
	• Use fresh untoasted breadcrumbs or rolled oats instead of dried toasted crumbs.
	• Add lots of finely chopped vegetables such as mushrooms, peppers, spinach, carrots, and onion to the meatloaf mixture to boost nutritional value, add moisture and flavor, and make meat portions go further.
Omelets and Frittatas	• Cook omelets and frittatas in a nonstick skillet, using cooking spray or a small amount of olive oil instead of butter.
	• Use unprocessed reduced-fat cheese.
	• When making cheese-topped frittatas, sprinkle the cheese on last and cook just long enough to melt. Do not brown.
Pizza	• Feature vegetable toppings instead of high-fat meats like sausage and ground beef.
	• Use lower-fat mozzarella and add it only during the last minute of baking—just long enough to melt. Do not brown.
Salads	• For main dish salads, add poached chicken, steamed seafood, or legumes instead of grilled or roasted chicken and meat.
	• Use unprocessed reduced-fat cheeses.
	• Use lower-fat mayonnaise and salad dressings.
	• Substitute canned chickpeas or kidney beans for croutons. Or toss in some leftover cooked penne or rotini pasta, or some cooked grain such as farro, wheat berries, or quinoa.
	• Instead of having crackers as an accompaniment to a salad, enjoy wedges of whole grain pita bread.

Type of Recipe	To Lower AGEs . . .
Sandwiches	• Use lower-AGE fillings like poached chicken, canned tuna or salmon, grilled or fresh vegetables, or eggs instead of roasted or grilled meats.
	• Limit the amount of meat in sandwiches to a couple of ounces. Add bulk with lots of lettuce, tomato, onion, and other vegetables.
	• Use low-fat spreads and dressings, or spread sandwiches with hummus, mashed avocado, or mustard instead of mayonnaise.
	• Use reduced-fat, unprocessed cheeses.
	• When making grilled sandwiches, lightly coat the outside of the bread with cooking spray instead of spreading it with butter or margarine.
Soups and Stews	• Include acidic ingredients like tomatoes or wine in the cooking liquid. Note that if too much of an acidic ingredient is added, grains and vegetables may toughen and not cook properly, so use in moderation.
	• Minimize or omit the browning step.

CONCLUSION

You can drastically reduce the amount of AGEs in foods simply by changing the way you cook. By choosing moist-heat cooking methods such as poaching, braising, stewing, and steaming, you can decrease AGE formation while creating great meals. In fact, these time-honored techniques are featured in tasty cuisines all over the world.

You now know how to select leaner, less-processed foods; how to make smart substitutions in recipes; how to use acidic ingredients, like lemon and tomatoes, to reduce AGE formation; and, of course, how to use different AGE-less cooking techniques. But can you continue AGE-less eating away from home? Absolutely. Chapter 8 will help you stay AGE-less when dining out in a variety of different restaurants.

8.

AGE-Less Eating Away from Home

The proportion of foods eaten away from home has steadily risen over the past several decades. The average American family now spends close to half of its food budget on meals and snacks eaten away from home. Restaurants and stores that sell fast food, takeout, and convenience foods have become so popular that many people have literally replaced home cooking with meals prepared by restaurants, supermarkets, and other establishments. It's no secret that these foods are often much higher in calories and lower in nutritional quality than home-cooked meals. However, most people are unaware that a steady diet of these foods also makes AGE-overload a near certainty.

The good news is that many restaurants also offer delicious choices that are both nutritious and low in AGEs. Some of the world's finest cuisines feature AGE-less cooking techniques such as poaching, steaming, braising, and stewing, and an increasing number of restaurants feature beautifully presented meals built around fresh, locally grown produce. Many are also expanding their menus with creative and delicious meatless meals.

Eating out is one of the pleasures of life, and it can remain so while you are following the AGE-less plan. This chapter offers tips to guide you to the best choices when eating out, enabling you to make the most of the menu's offerings in a wide variety of settings while keeping your AGE load at a modest level.

GENERAL TIPS

When you eat in a restaurant, it's not always possible to know exactly what you are getting. However, a few general tips can go a long way toward helping you remain on a low-AGE diet whenever you dine away from home.

Inspect the Menu Ahead of Time

Many restaurants post their menus online and/or have printed copies of their menus that you can keep on file for planning restaurant meals or ordering takeout. This provides an opportunity to study the menu ahead of time and determine the best choices. It also prepares you to ask questions about ingredients and cooking methods and to make special requests, such as asking the restaurant to omit a melted cheese topping, a creamy sauce, or a high-fat dressing.

Be Wise About Size

A major trend in restaurant cuisine is oversized food portions. Because of this, many of us frequently ingest too many AGEs simply because we eat too much food. In addition to overloading the body with pre-formed AGEs, restaurant meals often provide an excess of highly processed carbohydrates that can raise blood sugar levels. The following tips will help you deal with restaurant-size portions.

❏ Ask if you can order a smaller (often more reasonable) portion. Some restaurants offer half-portions or "senior" portions for a reduced price. This will double your bargain, as you'll also be getting less calories and fewer AGEs.

❏ Split the main course with someone, or take half of it home for another meal.

❏ Dine out more often for lunch than dinner. Portions (and prices) tend to be substantially smaller at lunch than they are at dinner, so you can cut down on AGEs as well as save money.

❏ Create a meal out of appetizers and side dishes, such as a shrimp cocktail, a cup of vegetable soup, and a salad.

❏ Choose generous portions of vegetables and salads and smaller portions of meat and cheese.

Choose Poached, Steamed, Stewed, or Braised Main Courses

As you know by now, meats—especially grilled, broiled, seared, roasted, fried, and processed meats—are the main contributors to an overload of AGEs. A major key to success is choosing food that has been prepared with a method that uses moist heat. Dishes like soups and stews, which feature simmered meat, chicken, or seafood with lots of vegetables, are perfect for the AGE-less way. Foods cooked en papillote (steamed in a parchment or foil packet) can also be a good choice.

Downsize Dessert

Everyone knows that high-calorie cakes, pastries, and other rich desserts should be saved for an occasional treat. It's no secret that these foods contain unhealthy amounts of sugar, white flour, and fat, among other things. But not everyone knows that these foods are also full of AGEs. So when you do have a rich dessert, share it with others and enjoy just a few bites. Or opt for a lighter treat such as a small dish of fruit (fresh, poached, roasted, or grilled), sorbet, granita, frozen yogurt, or pudding.

Ask for Olive Oil Instead of Butter

Dishes with buttery and creamy sauces can be very high in AGEs. Instead, choose dishes made with ingredients like tomatoes, wine, and a splash of olive oil. Also choose olive oil-based dressings for salads. Another critically important move is to request that dressings and sauces be served on the side so you can control how much is added. Then use as little as necessary for taste.

Balance a High-AGE Restaurant Meal With Lower AGE Choices Throughout the Day

If you plan to have grilled or roasted meat at one meal, keep your daily AGE intake in check by choosing lower-AGE foods at other meals. For example, when you are scheduled for a high-AGE meal at lunch, enjoy oatmeal, fruit, and milk for breakfast, and have bean or lentil soup and a salad for dinner.

Be Mindful of Mindless Eating and Drinking

Sometimes, we eat out of boredom or routine. This often becomes a "mindless" ritual when we stop at a coffee shop for that morning double-whipped latte or grab a mid-afternoon "treat" at work. These are just a few ways that mindless eating can sneak into daily life.

The major problem with mindless eating is that creamy, sweet supersized coffee drinks, sugary sodas, pastries, and other grab-and-go fare can add greatly to your AGE load, not to mention your intake of calories. Strangely, many people think that snack foods must be something processed to be satisfying. Examples include protein or cereal bars, chips, crackers, pretzels, and cookies. Unfortunately, these highly processed foods bear no resemblance to the natural foods from which they were derived. Moreover, most of these foods are heat-treated, which makes them disproportionately rich in AGEs compared with "real food." So snack smartly with choices like fresh fruit, yogurt, or a low-fat latte with a sprinkling of cocoa. Or choose a cup of soup, fresh vegetables with bean dip, or leftovers from a low-AGE meal. In other words, when you are hungry, think "real" food, not "processed" food.

MULTICULTURAL MENU OPTIONS

Just about every type of restaurant has tasty lower-AGE options. Ethnic restaurants offer many delicious possibilities, since some of the world's finest cuisines use AGE-less cooking methods such as steaming, poaching, braising, and stewing. Trying new foods can expand your choices and open up a whole new world of flavors! Here are some ideas to get you started.

■ CHINESE FOOD

Chinese dishes, with their ample portions of vegetables and modest helpings of meat, are a good example of right-sized AGE-less meals. Many dishes featured on traditional Chinese menus are also steamed, which is perfect for AGE-less eating. Think dim sum—tiny portions of foods such as dumplings and buns that are steamed and served fresh.

Unfortunately, American-style Chinese food is often prepared by cooking foods in oil over high heat and adding heavy sauces that feature unhealthy amounts of sugar and sodium. To avoid AGEs, steer clear of fried egg rolls and wontons; battered and deep-fried meats; sugary sauces, like sweet and sour; roast duck and pork; fried rice; and toasted sesame oil, which is very high in AGEs. Instead, select foods cooked with AGE-less methods and enhance their flavors with hot mustard, soy sauce (in moderation), or ginger sauce.

Keep in mind that some Chinese restaurants will be happy to steam (rather than stir-fry) many of their dishes. In this case, you could opt for many combinations of seafood or chicken and vegetables. While steaming is your best option, even stir-frying is better than American-style deep-fried foods. If you do get a stir-fried dish, choose seafood, tofu, or chicken, which will have about half as many AGEs as stir-fried beef.

The following dishes fit well within an AGE-less diet:

- Dim sum

- Broth-based soups such as egg drop, hot and sour, and wonton

- Steamed dumplings

- Steamed fish, tofu, and vegetable dishes

- Hot pot meals made with seafood, tofu, or chicken and vegetables (cooked at the table fondue-style in a pot of simmering broth)

- Egg Foo Yung made with seafood, tofu, or vegetables

- Steamed or boiled brown rice

- Steamed or boiled noodles

■ FRENCH FOOD

There is a perception that French people remain slim despite a diet of creamy sauces and buttery croissants. The fact is that French food is not as rich and calorie-laden as many people think. To begin, portions tend to be more reasonably sized in France than in the United States. And although some dishes are definitely high in fat, those foods make up only a small part of French cuisine. Moreover, many classic dishes use AGE-less cooking methods such as poaching, en papillote cooking, steaming, and braising in wine or tomato sauce. Roasted or grilled vegetables may also be featured, which are much lower in AGEs than roasted or grilled meats. Also keep in mind that fresh, beautifully presented salads are extremely popular in French cuisine, as is fresh raw seafood. Finally, the French seldom barbecue their meat, and frying is frowned upon.

How can you keep your meals light and AGE-less when dining in a French restaurant? Here are some items to look for:

- Mussels simmered in tomato, wine, or mustard sauce

- Crab or shrimp cocktail

- Smoked salmon

- Consommé and broth-based soups

- Bean and lentil soups and stews

- Grilled or roasted vegetables

- Steamed or poached seafood and poultry (order sauces on the side)

- Seafood or chicken cooked en papillote (steamed in parchment paper packets) with vegetables, wine, and olive oil

- Seafood or chicken provençal (cooked in tomato or tomato-wine sauce)

- Seafood or vegetable stews such as bouillabaisse and ratatouille

- Salads with light vinaigrette dressing (even better, ask for cruets of oil and vinegar)

■ GREEK FOOD

Several key principles of the Greek diet, the originator of the Mediterranean diet, are important to grasp. The Greeks make good use of olive oil rather than butter, often opt for vegetable-based main courses, and prefer fresh fish to fatty red meats. They also include flavorful herbs, yogurt, and lemon in their dishes. Enjoy these foods often on your AGE-less plan, and save the high-AGE foods such as buttery filo-crusted pies and roasted meats for an occasional indulgence. Keep in mind that feta is high in AGEs, so have just a sprinkling. Fortunately, a little bit of this flavorful cheese goes a long way.

A number of Greek favorites are served in pita bread, which is also a highly popular accompaniment for salads and main dishes. Fortunately, pitas are low in AGEs. Even grilled pitas are a lower-AGE food—as long as they're not basted with oil or cooked in a pool of oil on the grill. Be sure to ask for whole wheat pitas if available.

Some lower-AGE items that you may find on Greek menus include:

- Dips and spreads made with vegetables, beans, and yogurt, such as tzatziki (yogurt, cucumber, garlic, and herbs) and melintzano-salata (eggplant, garlic, olive oil, and lemon)

- Soups such as avgolemono (egg, lemon, and rice in chicken broth), fasolada (white bean and vegetable), lentil, and seafood

- Baked fish dishes such as plaki (fish baked with tomatoes, onions, and garlic), and fish baked in grape leaves

- Dolmades (grape leaves stuffed with seasoned rice, ingredients such as pine nuts and currants, and sometimes minced meat, and then cooked in water and lemon)

- Lamb dishes that are braised, stewed, or cooked en papillote

- White beans baked with tomatoes and herbs

- Pita sandwiches filled with grilled or roasted vegetables such as eggplant, portabella mushrooms, and zucchini

- Greek salad topped with steamed seafood and a light sprinkling of feta

■ INDIAN FOOD

Like Mediterranean and Middle Eastern food, Indian cuisine is rich in vegetables, legumes, and plenty of herbs and spices. The liberal use of herbs and spices is a critical point, since much of the flavor that we crave is due to AGEs, and this craving could be satisfied by a smart use of these antioxidant-rich seasonings! Authentic Indian cuisine also showcases many delicious vegetarian options, which are compatible with AGE-less eating. Other items you may want to include in your meal are chutney, a spicy condiment; pickles; and onion salad.

Paneer, a mild-tasting fresh cheese, is used in many traditional Indian dishes. It is made by curdling hot milk with an acid such as lemon juice or vinegar. It is then drained and pressed into a block. Paneer is a good choice when cubed and simmered in curries or stews, or crumbled and added to dishes. Avoid Paneer that has been sautéed, fried, grilled, baked, or browned, as this will increase AGEs. In fact, any Indian food that is fried may contain a large amount of AGEs.

As with all cuisines, roasted and grilled poultry and red meat should be limited, and braised and stewed dishes should be favored instead. Best bets at your favorite Indian restaurant include:

- Dal (bean, pea, or lentil) stews, soups, or patties

- Broth- or bean-based soups with vegetables, seafood, or chicken

- Chapati and roti (whole wheat flatbreads)

- Raita (cold yogurt-based side dish with cucumbers or other vegetables)

- Vegetable and seafood dishes such as curry or vindaloo (a spicy dish that may include tomato, vinegar, and wine)

- Biriyani (rice dishes) made with vegetables or seafood (ask if brown rice is available)

■ ITALIAN

Within the European family of diets, Mediterranean foods have proven to be the healthiest over many years and in hundreds of studies. Included in this group is Italian cuisine. Pasta is a great low-AGE staple—as long as it's eaten in moderation. (Choose whole-wheat pasta when possible.) Pair it with red sauce, a glass of red wine, and plenty of colorful veggies to punch up meals with health-promoting phytonutrients. Traditional Italian cuisine also features lots of seafood, which is lower in AGEs than poultry and meat.

Of course, Italian restaurants also offer foods high in AGEs, such as pork sausage and poultry and meat cutlets that have been breaded and fried. You'll want to avoid these menu choices as much as possible. (To learn about the effects of breading and frying, see page 91.) Gobs of melted mozzarella cheese—like those found on most pizzas—and piles of Parmesan will also put you over your AGE limit, so be sure to go easy on the cheese. Here are some lower-AGE items that you might find on the menu of your local Italian eatery.

- Vegetable and bean soups like pasta fagioli and minestrone

- Steamed clams or mussels in tomato or wine sauce

- Whole grain pasta with tomato sauce, such as pasta arrabbiata, marinara, or puttanesca

- Pasta with red clam sauce

- Seafood Fra Diavolo (in a spicy red sauce)

- Seafood stews such as cioppino

- Garden salad with vinaigrette dressing

- Grilled or roasted vegetables

- Cappuccino made with low-fat milk

■ JAPANESE FOOD

Traditional Japanese cuisine is among the healthiest cuisines in the world. Steamed or simmered seafood and soy foods—such as tofu and edamame—are often featured, along with plenty of vegetables, whole grain noodles or brown rice, and antioxidant-rich green tea. However, be aware that Japanese food, like many other cuisines, can deliver very high amounts of salt. It pays to peruse the nutritional information when available. Examples of lower-AGE dishes include:

- Miso and other broth-based soups with vegetables, seafood, chicken, or noodles

- Sashimi (raw slivered fish)

- Edamame (boiled green soybeans)

- Salads made with seaweed, cucumber, vegetables, or steamed seafood

- Sushi made with seafood (not fried) or vegetables

- Steamed or boiled vegetable or seafood dumplings

- Boiled soba (buckwheat) noodles or udon (wheat) noodles simmered in broth with vegetables, tofu, or seafood

- Steamed brown rice

■ MEXICAN FOOD

From deep-fried tortilla chips to steak strips browned in oil, modern Mexican restaurant dining can be a challenge on the AGE-less diet. Fortunately, many restaurants serving traditional Mexican cuisine now offer a good selection of vegetarian and lighter options. Most also have an excellent à la carte menu, which allows you to create a meal to suit your needs.

Be aware that most Mexican dishes, from salads to burritos and enchiladas, come loaded with cheese. Be sure to tell your server that instead of cheese, you'd like your dish topped with crisp shredded lettuce, diced tomatoes, salsa, or guacamole. Also opt for red sauce or verde (green) sauce instead of cheese or sour cream sauces.

A number of Mexican dishes come wrapped in or accompanied by tortillas, so this is another area in which you'll want to ask for the healthiest product available. Instead of white flour tortillas, choose corn tortillas, many of which are made from whole grain corn and contain about half the calories and carbs of white flour tortillas. Another option is whole grain flour tortillas, when available. Of course, tortillas should be eaten soft, not fried.

Best bets on Mexican menus include:

- Marinated seafood salad such as ceviche and shrimp cocktail

- Broth-based or vegetable soups such as chicken tortilla soup and chilled gazpacho

- Posole (hominy stew) with vegetables or chicken

- Bean soups made with, for instance, black beans or pinto beans

- Bean burritos or enchiladas with red or green sauce

- Spinach, vegetable, or seafood enchiladas with red or green sauce

- Shrimp or fish tacos in soft corn tortillas

- Grilled vegetable fajitas (ask for a minimum of oil to be used)

- Grilled or roasted vegetables (ask for a minimum of oil to be used)

- Salads made with black or pinto beans, grilled vegetables, guacamole, salsa, and a light sprinkling of cheese

- Brown rice, if available

■ MIDDLE EASTERN FOOD

Encompassing a number of different countries and a wide range of cuisines, Middle Eastern fare offers many tasty AGE-less selections. Bulgur wheat, chickpeas, eggplant, yogurt, olive oil, parsley, and aromatic herbs and spices are among the many healthful ingredients featured. Some AGE-less items that you may find on menus include:

- Vegetable and bean dips and spreads such as hummus (blended chickpeas with tahini, lemon, olive oil, and seasonings) and baba ganoush (roasted eggplant with lemon, olive oil, tahini, garlic, and herbs)

- Soups and stews made with lentils, chickpeas, fava beans, vegetables, seafood, chicken, and lamb

- Wraps and pitas filled with with hummus, baba ganoush, or falafel (Note that falafel patties are traditionally deep-fried, but some restaurants offer baked falafel.)

- Tabbouleh salad (bulgur wheat with tomatoes, cucumber, lemon, olive oil, parsley, and mint) and other salads made with vegetables, whole grains, and legumes

- Stuffed cabbage rolls with rice and ground chicken or lamb (Note that they are cooked using moist heat.)

- Couscous with stewed vegetables, beans, seafood, chicken, or lamb

FAST FOOD RESTAURANTS

Fast food restaurants specialize in foods that can be prepared and served quickly, often at a drive-through window. These establishments present a big challenge to the AGE-less diner. Menu offerings such as burgers, fried fish sandwiches, deep-fried chicken nuggets, and French fries are definitely not on the AGE-less diet. Since these foods are nutritionally bad on so many levels, they should quite simply be avoided.

Grilled chicken, often considered to be the "healthy" go-to item at most fast food restaurants, may be lower in fat and calories than other fast foods, but one serving can deliver an entire day's worth of AGEs. So grilled chicken should also be limited. Keep in mind, though, that if you do get grilled chicken, you can balance out the rest of your day with low-AGE options such as oatmeal or yogurt and fruit at breakfast, and a bean dish or soup at dinner.

Fast food restaurants that offer vegetarian options, such as bean burritos or veggie burgers, are the best bet. Fast food subs and sandwiches can also be a good choice. Some of these establishments also offer salads and soups. Breakfast can be one of the better choices, since many offer oatmeal, yogurt, and egg sandwiches. Best bets include:

- Vegetarian burgers
- Bean burritos (with shredded lettuce, salsa, and/or guacamole instead of cheese and sour cream)
- Vegetarian sandwiches or subs on whole grain bread, piled high with vegetables, not overloaded with cheese, and spread with mustard or a drizzle of light salad dressing instead of full-fat mayonnaise
- Tuna subs or sandwiches (only if made with light mayonnaise)
- Salads with light dressing
- Broth-based soups such as vegetable, bean, or chicken noodle
- Oatmeal with fruit and nuts
- Yogurt and fruit parfaits
- Egg white sandwiches on English muffins, bagels, or buns (preferably whole grain)

- Scrambled egg burritos

- Low-fat lattes or iced coffees (without sugary syrups or whipped cream toppings)

SENSATIONAL SALADS

Loaded with antioxidants and other important nutrients, crisp fresh salads are key to any anti-aging plan. Many restaurants specialize in salads, and some allow you to create your own by choosing from a wide variety of ingredients. But do take care when ordering, or you might end up with a lot more calories, fat, and AGEs than you think you are getting. Whether you are ordering a main dish salad from the menu or selecting ingredients at a salad bar, there are plenty of ways to create a dish that is both healthful and delicious.

■ FROM THE MENU

When ordering salads from the menu, choose main dish salads that are topped with steamed, poached, or lightly grilled shrimp, scallops, or fish. Ask that they be cooked until done, but not overdone. If you do not find what you are looking for in the salad section of the menu, peruse the listings of side dishes and entrees for ingredients that could be added to your greens, and ask if you can have a salad made to order. Examples of healthy add-ins include grilled or roasted vegetables, edamame, assorted beans (lima, cannellini, black, garbanzo, etc.), hard-boiled eggs, and tuna packed in spring water. Finally, ask for oil and vinegar rather than one of the restaurant's prepared dressings, which are likely to contain lots of fat and sugar.

■ AT THE SALAD BAR

Always start with a pile of fresh greens such as spinach, mesclun, kale, or romaine lettuce, along with plenty of colorful fresh vegetables. Add chickpeas, kidney beans, edamame, tofu, hard-boiled eggs, or steamed seafood for low-AGE protein. You can top your creation with a sprinkling of cheese, but go easy, since AGEs can add up. Garnish with some chopped olives and a sprinkling of nuts or seeds.

Then opt for a light dressing or a drizzle of vinaigrette, or ask for cruets of oil and vinegar.

Try to completely avoid mayonnaise-based salads such as tuna salad or coleslaw, since they will most likely be prepared with large amounts of oily dressing. Limit your portion of oily marinated vegetables, draining off as much of the marinade as possible before putting the veggies on your plate. Finish off with some fresh fruit for dessert.

CONCLUSION

The AGE-less lifestyle does not sentence you to a lifetime in the kitchen, cooking every meal that you eat. On the contrary, countless delicious foods are available for your dining pleasure in a wide variety of restaurants. A two-pronged approach will help you make the most of your meals whether eaten in a restaurant or at home. First, favor wholesome, unprocessed ingredients such as vegetables, fruits, legumes, and whole grains, as these foods are naturally low in AGEs. Then, pay attention to how the foods are cooked so that you can minimize cooking-related AGEs. By doing this, you can fill up on low-AGE dishes while getting plenty of health-promoting fiber and nutrients. The result will be fresh food that will enhance your well-being as it pleases your palate.

Conclusion

eginning in the womb, our mother's diet begins to shape our food preferences. As children, our food choices are further influenced by what our parents feed us, and we begin to decide which foods we like or dislike. These decisions are further affected by our culture, our peers, our budget, and by ever-present exposure to advertising, among other factors. Our diets ultimately become a part of who we are, and we use phrases like "I'd like that well done," "Extra cheese, please," or "Supersize that" to make sure our food is served to us the way we prefer it. Over time, we simply become creatures of habit when it comes to what we eat.

Most people are acutely aware that the "modern" diet or "Standard American Diet"—the diet that most of us have chosen—is a root cause of the epidemics of obesity and poor health. Despite an abundance of weight-loss programs, health websites, and self-help books that cause us to make occasional detours into healthier eating, most of us ultimately return to our old eating habits. There is no doubt that changing what we consume can be very difficult. However, if you have gotten this far into the book, we hope that you can see that *Dr. Vlassara's AGE-Less Diet* is a game-changer on so many levels.

As scientists, we believe that what we have uncovered about AGEs and their profound negative effects on health and aging is one of the most exciting discoveries of the twenty-first century. We know unequivocally that the chemical compounds known as AGEs are a key driver of inflammation in the body. This chronic, systemic inflammation fuels cardiovascular disease, diabetes, kidney disease, dementia, and many other health problems. We also know that, over time, AGEs make tissues stiff and brittle—one of the underlying reasons our organs begin to fail and our skin begins to wrinkle. And all we have to do to avoid the devastating effects of AGEs is choose the right foods and pay attention to the way we cook them.

Why did it take so long to find out about AGEs? Perhaps investigators were immersed in issues such as "low-carb" versus "low-fat." Perhaps they were focused on single foods such as red meat or sugar, or preoccupied with deficiencies or excesses of single nutrients such as unsaturated or saturated fats. Perhaps it was unthinkable to believe that the way we cook nearly all of our food could be a contributor to the epidemics of disease we are seeing today. Whatever the reasons, despite a huge preoccupation with what may constitute "the best diet," many food experts did not recognize the very profound and harmful effects of excessive amounts of AGEs formed by the heat processing of foods.

In Part One, we provided the information you need to reduce your own AGE intake through simple adjustments to your diet. We understand that some people will take our diet to extremes. This is something we do not advocate. We also understand that for some people, modifying established cooking and eating habits may seem a daunting task. But with the tools offered in this book, you have the ability to make changes gradually and, as you do so, to reduce the destructive effects of AGEs. In Part Two, we provide dozens of recipes to help you make the transition. You'll find that the AGE-less diet can be easy to prepare, delicious, and also economical. And perhaps best of all, AGE-less principles can be applied to any type of eating plan.

We believe that AGEs will come to be recognized as a leading cause of many degenerative diseases—as our research has shown. Perhaps one day, all you will need to do to lower your AGE levels will be to take a pill. But in the meantime, you have it within your power to take control of what you and your loved ones consume. We hope the information in this book gives you all the inspiration and guidance you need to get started.

PART TWO

AGE-Less
Recipes

About the Recipes

When people first learn about AGEs, they may fear that AGE-less food will be bland or boring or that they will have to go on an extreme raw diet to avoid them. This is far from the truth. Once you understand the secrets of AGE-less cooking and meal planning, you will find that your meals can be as delicious and as easy to prepare as they have always been. As explained earlier in the book, the AGE-less diet resembles Mediterranean cuisine, featuring savory soups and stews, braised dishes, succulent poached and *en papillote* meals, and other comfort-style foods.

Keep in mind that AGEs *do not need to be completely eliminated*; they just need to be reduced to a level the body can safely handle. This can be accomplished by following the three principles of the AGE-less diet outlined in Chapter 4: Learn which foods are lowest in AGEs; choose cooking methods that prevent the formation of AGEs; and include ingredients that deter the formation of AGEs. The recipes in this book are based on these principles. There is no need to meticulously count AGEs, as this has already been done for you.

The following recipes feature an abundance of low-AGE plant foods such as vegetables, fruits, and whole grains. As for foods that add the most AGEs to the diet—meats, cheeses, and fats—these are not eliminated but are used judiciously and in right-size portions. Importantly, these foods are prepared using the AGE-less cooking methods described in Chapter 7. These techniques have been featured in cuisines throughout the world to create simple and delicious dishes for many generations. But the proof is in the pudding. So here we offer over 100 recipes to get you started on your AGE-less path. As you choose from among these recipes for each day's meals, it is important to remember that at least three-quarters of your AGE-less diet should be comprised of plant foods. For that reason, you should be sure to include plenty of sides and salads in your diet. As you know, in addition to being low in AGEs, vegetables, fruits, and grains are a rich source of fiber, antioxidants, vitamins, and minerals—nutrients that will benefit your body in many ways.

One thing to consider is that while our taste for food is socially and culturally ingrained, new tastes can be learned even after many years of eating a particular way. Remember how it once seemed so difficult to "go organic," to opt for whole grain bread instead of white bread, or to reduce saturated fat or sugar? Once you become accustomed to a lighter, fresher, cleaner, and healthier way of eating, you may wonder how you could have eaten any other way.

THE NUTRITION FACTS

The Nutrihand PRO recipe analysis program, along with the USDA National Nutrient Database and product information from manufacturers, was used to calculate the nutrition information for the recipes in this book. For each recipe, information on calories, carbohydrates, dietary fiber, protein, fat, saturated fat, cholesterol, sodium, and calcium is provided. Nutrients are always listed per one single serving— one bowl of soup, one helping of salad, one portion of a main dish, etc. This gives you the information you need to choose recipes that meet any special needs or limitations you may have regarding fat, cholesterol, sodium, and other important nutrients.

Sometimes, the ingredients lists give you different options. For instance, you might be able to choose between 93-percent lean ground beef or ground turkey, or between nonfat or low-fat milk. This will help you create dishes that suit your tastes, your nutrition goals, and the ingredients you typically keep in your pantry and fridge. Just keep in mind that the nutritional analysis is always based on the first ingredient listed.

VARIATIONS AND EXPERIMENTATION

Most people get bored eating the same dishes day in and day out. Fortunately, the pages that follow offer dozens of recipes, so you already have a wide range of choices; and, as explained above, the ingredients lists often suggest different options. In addition, at the end of a number of recipes, you'll find "Variation" suggestions that highlight ingredient substitutions, give you a twist on an old favorite, or help you tune up a recipe so that it better suits your preferences. For instance, you can "change up" Cinnamon-Apple Oatmeal by replacing the apples with peaches or pears (page 193), you can make Waldorf Chicken Salad more flavorful through the simple addition of curry powder (page 227), or you can turn Cinnamon Roasted Pears into a special-occasion dish by topping each pear with a small scoop of ice cream and a sprinkling of chopped walnuts (page 291). Want to create a sophisticated spin on Chicken Dijon? Instead of cooking individual servings in foil packets, enclose the ingredients in elegant parchment packets (page 202). The possibilities are endless.

While this book provides plenty of options, at the heart of the recipes are healthy ingredients, easy cooking techniques, and instructions that can be successfully followed by virtually any cook. As you prepare these dishes, you will find yourself becoming more comfortable with AGE-less techniques, and you will see how you can take many of your own favorite recipes and transform them into healthier meals by modifying cooking methods and making simple ingredient adjustments. We wish you many satisfying AGE-less meals to come.

Breakfast

Starting your day the AGE-less way is a snap, since many favorite breakfast foods are naturally low in AGEs. Fresh and frozen fruits, hearty whole grain breads, whole grain cereals (especially porridge-type cereals such as oatmeal and uncooked cereals such as muesli), milk, and yogurt are all good options. Eggs, whether scrambled, steam-basted, poached, or boiled, are also good choices. If you want your eggs without the cholesterol, fat-free egg substitutes and liquid egg whites are convenient alternatives.

AGE-less breakfasts such as yogurt and fruit, oatmeal, or a scrambled egg sandwich are so simple to prepare that no recipe is needed. When you have a few minutes more, try the recipes presented in this chapter. All are easy, AGE-less, and perfect for a tasty breakfast, a satisfying brunch, or even a light dinner.

EGGS IN SPICY TOMATO SAUCE

YIELD: 4 SERVINGS

14$^1/_2$-ounce can no-salt-added tomatoes, undrained, or 3 cups chopped fresh tomatoes

$^1/_2$ cup chopped yellow onion

1 tablespoon extra-virgin olive oil

1 teaspoon crushed garlic

$^1/_4$ teaspoon salt

$^1/_8$ teaspoon ground black pepper

$^1/_8$ teaspoon crushed red pepper flakes

4 large eggs

2 tablespoons chopped fresh basil

1. Place the first 7 ingredients (tomatoes through crushed red pepper) in a blender, and blend until smooth.

2. Pour the blended mixture into a large nonstick skillet, and bring to a boil. Adjust the heat to maintain a simmer, and cook uncovered, stirring frequently, for about 15 minutes, or until the mixture is reduced to about 1$^1/_4$ cups and has cooked down to the consistency of marinara sauce. (To reduce splatters, use a splatter screen or place a lid on the skillet, leaving it partially ajar to allow the steam to escape.)

3. Break one egg into a custard cup. Hold the cup close to the surface of the simmering sauce, and slip the egg into the sauce. Repeat with the remaining eggs. Cover and cook for 3 to 5 minutes, or until the whites are set and the yolks have thickened.

4. To serve, spoon one-fourth of the sauce onto each of four serving plates. Top each serving with an egg and, if desired, sprinkle with some additional black pepper. Top each serving with a sprinkling of basil, and serve immediately.

VARIATIONS

❑ Serve over polenta if desired.

❑ Substitute 2 teaspoons of chopped seeded jalapeño pepper for the crushed red pepper flakes and top with fresh cilantro instead of basil.

NUTRITION FACTS (PER SERVING)

Calories: 140   Carbohydrates: 7 g   Fiber: 2 g   Protein: 8.4 g

Fat: 9 g   Sat. Fat: 2.3 g   Cholesterol: 208 mg   Sodium: 232 mg   Calcium: 51 mg

POACHED EGGS WITH ASPARAGUS AND RED ONION

YIELD: 4 SERVINGS

1 pound fresh asparagus, with tough ends snapped off

4 slices red onion, cut into half-rings

1 pinch salt

1 pinch ground black pepper

Water for cooking

4 large eggs, poached (see page 188)

DRESSING

2 tablespoons extra-virgin olive oil

1 tablespoon orange juice

1 tablespoon white wine vinegar

1 teaspoon Dijon mustard

$1/4$ teaspoon salt

$1/4$ teaspoon ground black pepper

1. Combine all of the dressing ingredients in a small bowl and whisk to mix. Set aside.

2. Coat a large nonstick skillet with cooking spray and add the asparagus, onion, salt, pepper, and 1 tablespoon of water. Cover and cook over medium-high heat for 3 minutes. Reduce the heat to medium and cook for about 3 minutes more, shaking the pan occasionally, just until the asparagus are tender. Add a little water during cooking, if needed, but only enough to prevent scorching.

3. Remove the skillet from the heat. Drizzle the vegetable mixture with 2 tablespoons of the dressing and toss to coat.

4. Divide the vegetable mixture among 4 serving plates. Top each serving with a poached egg and drizzle with $1^{1}/_{2}$ teaspoons of the remaining dressing. Sprinkle with additional black pepper, if desired, and serve immediately.

NUTRITION FACTS (PER SERVING)

Calories: 160   Carbohydrates: 7 g   Fiber: 2.2 g   Protein: 8.5 g

Fat: 11.6 g   Sat. Fat: 2.5 g   Cholesterol: 185 mg   Sodium: 361 mg   Calcium: 49 mg

ARUGULA WITH PORTABELLA AND POACHED EGGS

YIELD: 4 SERVINGS

8 ounces sliced baby portabella mushrooms (about 3 cups)

1 medium yellow onion, sliced and cut into half-rings

$1/4$ teaspoon salt

$1/4$ teaspoon ground black pepper

Water for cooking

6 cups fresh baby arugula (about 6 ounces)

$1/4$ cup quartered grape tomatoes

4 large eggs, poached (see page 188)

DRESSING

2 tablespoons extra-virgin olive oil

1 tablespoon lemon juice

1 tablespoon white wine vinegar

1 teaspoon Dijon mustard

$1/4$ teaspoon salt

$1/4$ teaspoon ground black pepper

1. Coat a large nonstick skillet with cooking spray. Add the mushrooms, onion, salt, pepper, and 1 tablespoon of water. Cover and cook over medium heat for about 5 minutes, or until the vegetables are tender. If necessary, remove the lid and cook for another minute or 2, until any excess liquid has evaporated and the vegetables are lightly browned. Remove the skillet from the heat and set aside.

2. Combine all of the dressing ingredients in a small bowl and whisk to mix.

3. Combine the arugula and tomatoes in a large bowl. Drizzle with 3 tablespoons of the dressing, and toss to mix. Add the mushrooms and onions and toss gently. Divide the mixture among 4 serving plates.

4. Top each serving with one poached egg, and drizzle with 1 teaspoon of the remaining dressing. Sprinkle each serving with some additional black pepper, if desired, and serve immediately.

NUTRITION FACTS (PER SERVING)

Calories: 164   Carbohydrates: 7 g   Fiber: 2 g   Protein: 9 g

Fat: 12 g   Sat. Fat: 2.6 g   Cholesterol: 185 mg   Sodium: 461 mg   Calcium: 87 mg

BROCCOLI OMELET WITH FRESH TOMATO SALSA

Yield: 1 serving

$3/_4$ to 1 cup thinly sliced (lengthwise) fresh broccoli florets and peeled stems

3 tablespoons scallions, thinly sliced on the bias

Water for cooking

$3/_4$ teaspoon extra-virgin olive oil

$1/_2$ cup fat-free egg substitute or liquid egg whites, or 1 large egg plus 2 egg whites, beaten

1 tablespoon crumbled reduced-fat feta or goat cheese

SALSA

$1/_4$ cup chopped seeded fresh tomato

1 tablespoon finely chopped scallions

1 tablespoon chopped black olives

$1/_8$ teaspoon crushed red pepper flakes

1. Combine the salsa ingredients in a small bowl and toss to mix. Set aside.

2. Coat an 8-inch nonstick skillet with cooking spray. Add the broccoli, scallions, and one tablespoon of water. Cover and cook over medium heat for about 4 minutes, or just until the broccoli is tender. Transfer the vegetables to a bowl and cover to keep warm.

3. Coat the skillet with the olive oil and preheat over medium heat. Add the eggs and reduce the heat to medium-low. Cook without stirring for a couple of minutes, or until the eggs are set around the edges. Use a spatula to lift the edges of the omelet, allowing the uncooked egg to flow below the cooked portion. Cook for another minute or until the eggs are almost set.

4. Arrange the broccoli mixture over half of the omelet and sprinkle with the cheese. Fold the omelet over to enclose the filling. Cook for another minute or until set. Slide the omelet onto a serving plate and top with the salsa. Serve immediately.

Nutrition Facts (Per Serving)

Calories: 167   Carbohydrates: 12 g   Fiber: 3.4 g   Protein: 17 g

Fat: 6.4 g   Sat. Fat: 0.5 g   Cholesterol: 0 mg   Sodium: 444 mg   Calcium: 96 mg

---

CAULIFLOWER AND SUN-DRIED TOMATO FRITTATA

YIELD: 2 SERVINGS

1$^1/_2$ cups sliced fresh cauliflower florets (sliced about $^1/_4$-inch thick)

$^1/_4$ cup water

$^1/_8$ teaspoon ground black pepper

2 tablespoons chopped sun-dried tomatoes (not packed in oil)

1$^1/_2$ teaspoons extra-virgin olive oil

$^1/_2$ teaspoon crushed garlic

1 cup fat-free egg substitute, or 2 large eggs plus 4 egg whites, beaten

2 tablespoons crumbled reduced-fat feta cheese

2 tablespoons finely chopped fresh parsley

1. Coat a 9-inch nonstick skillet with cooking spray. Add the cauliflower, water, and pepper. Place over medium heat, cover, and cook for about 5 minutes or until the cauliflower is tender. If there is any liquid remaining in the skillet, cook uncovered briefly to let it evaporate.

2. Stir the tomatoes, olive oil, and garlic into the cauliflower, and cook for 10 seconds.

3. Pour the eggs over the cauliflower mixture, and cook without stirring for a couple of minutes, or until the edges start to set. Continue to cook for a few minutes more, lifting the edges with a spatula and allowing uncooked egg to flow beneath the cooked portion until the frittata is almost set.

4. Slide the frittata onto a large plate (wet side up). Using oven mitts or pot-holders, place the skillet upside down over the frittata, and invert the frittata back into the skillet. Cook for another minute or until the bottom of the frittata is set.

5. Cut the frittata in half, top each serving with half of the feta cheese and parsley, and serve immediately.

NUTRITION FACTS (PER SERVING)

Calories: 140   Carbohydrates: 9 g   Fiber: 2 g   Protein: 16 g

Fat: 5 g   Sat. Fat: 1 g   Cholesterol: 2 mg   Sodium: 430 mg   Calcium: 69 mg

---

EGG SKILLET WITH SPINACH, POTATOES, AND MUSHROOMS

YIELD: 4 SERVINGS

$^3/_4$ cup thinly sliced leeks (white and light green parts), or 1 medium yellow onion, cut into thin wedges

1 tablespoon plus 1 teaspoon extra-virgin olive oil

Water for cooking

3 cups sliced fresh mushrooms

2 cups cooked new potatoes, halved and sliced about $^3/_8$-inch thick*

1$^1/_2$ teaspoons crushed garlic

$^1/_2$ teaspoon salt, divided

$^1/_2$ teaspoon ground black pepper, divided

5 cups (moderately packed) sliced fresh spinach

4 large eggs

$^3/_4$ teaspoon ground paprika

---

*To cook the potatoes, steam or boil them for about 10 minutes, or until easily pierced with a sharp knife. Cook the day before or let them sit until cool enough to handle before slicing.

1. Place the leek or onion, olive oil, and 2 tablespoons of water in a large non-stick skillet. Cover and cook over medium heat, stirring occasionally, for about 4 minutes, or until the leek or onion starts to soften.

2. Add the mushrooms, potatoes, garlic, and $^1/_4$ teaspoon each of the salt and pepper to the skillet. Cover and cook, stirring occasionally, for about 4 minutes, or until the mushrooms are tender.

3. Add the spinach to the skillet mixture, and cook uncovered for 1 minute, or until the spinach wilts. Use a spoon to make 4 wells in the vegetable mixture.

4. Crack 1 egg into each well and sprinkle the eggs with the remaining salt and pepper. Sprinkle the paprika over the top of the skillet mixture. Reduce the heat to medium-low, cover, and cook for 3 to 4 minutes, or until the eggs are set. Serve immediately.

NUTRITION FACTS (PER SERVING)
Calories: 206   Carbohydrates: 19 g   Fiber: 3.6 g   Protein: 11.1 g
Fat: 9.7g   Sat. Fat: 2.2 g   Cholesterol: 212 mg   Sodium: 526 mg   Calcium: 80 mg

Eggs With an AGE-Less Style

From elegant omelets and frittatas to simple poached and scrambled dishes, eggs make a quick meal any time of the day or night. And among protein-rich foods, eggs are one of the lowest in AGEs. This chapter includes several recipes for omelets and frittatas, which can be used as inspiration for your own creations. Below, you'll find a simple guide to other AGE-less cooking methods for eggs.

Scrambled Eggs

Whisk the desired number of eggs until well blended. (Whisk briefly for denser curds or vigorously for lighter, fluffier curds.) Coat a skillet with cooking spray, and place over medium heat until a drop of water sizzles when added. Reduce the heat to medium-low, add the eggs, and cook until they begin to set around the edges. As the eggs begin to set, gently pull a spatula across the bottom and sides of the pan, forming large curds. Cook for about a minute, or just until set.

Steam-Basted Eggs

Coat a nonstick skillet with cooking spray, and preheat over medium heat until a drop of water sizzles when added. Use a large skillet for 4 eggs or a medium skillet for 2 eggs. Break the eggs and slip them into the pan. Immediately reduce the heat to medium-low, and add 1 teaspoon of water per egg. Place a lid on the pan to hold in the steam. Cook for a couple of minutes or until the whites are set and the yolks thicken.

Poached Eggs

Fill a pot or deep skillet with 3 inches of water. Bring the liquid to a boil; then reduce the heat to keep the water gently simmering. Break one egg into a custard cup, hold it close to the water's surface, and slip the egg into the water. Repeat with the remaining eggs. Cook until the whites are set and the yolks thicken, 3 to 5 minutes. Use a slotted spoon to lift the eggs out of the water. If desired, trim away any straggling pieces of egg white before serving.

Hard-Boiled Eggs

Place eggs in a single layer in a pot. Add enough water to cover the eggs by at least 1 inch. Cover the pot, bring to a boil, and turn off the heat. Allow the eggs to stand, covered, for 12 to 15 minutes. A good way to tell when an egg is hard-boiled is to place it on a flat surface and give it a spin. A fully-cooked egg will spin rapidly while an uncooked egg will spin slowly and unevenly. Drain and place in cool water for several minutes to stop the cooking. Refrigerate for up to one week before serving.

Note that while many people prefer their egg yolks "runny," food safety guidelines recommend cooking eggs until both the yolk and the white are firm, whether poached, boiled, or steam-basted. Scrambled eggs should also be cooked until firm.

SOUTHWESTERN-STYLE EGGS

YIELD: 4 SERVINGS

$1/4$ cup finely chopped yellow onion

2 teaspoons extra-virgin olive oil

Water for cooking

1 cup canned black beans, undrained and coarsely mashed

$1/2$ teaspoon ground cumin

$1/2$ teaspoon chili powder

$1/4$ cup plus 2 tablespoons chunky-style salsa, divided

4 corn tortillas (5-inch rounds)

4 large eggs, steam-basted or poached (see page 188)

$1/4$ cup shredded reduced-fat Mexican blend or Monterey Jack cheese

$1/4$ cup thinly sliced scallions

1. Place the onion, olive oil, and 1 tablespoon of water in a 1-quart saucepan. Cover and cook over medium heat for about 4 minutes to soften.

2. Stir the beans, cumin, chili powder, and 2 tablespoons of the salsa into the onion mixture. Cook uncovered, stirring frequently, for several minutes, or until the mixture has the thick consistency of refried beans. Cover and set aside to keep warm.

3. Heat the tortillas according to package directions. For each serving, place one tortilla on each of 4 plates. Spread a quarter of the beans over each tortilla and top with an egg and 1 tablespoon each of the salsa, cheese, and scallions. Serve immediately.

NUTRITION FACTS (PER SERVING)

Calories: 217   Carbohydrates: 21 g   Fiber: 6.5 g   Protein: 13 g

Fat: 9.2 g   Sat. Fat: 2.8 g   Cholesterol: 190 mg   Sodium: 392 mg   Calcium: 176 mg

SPINACH, EGG AND CHEESE QUESADILLA

YIELD: 1 SERVING

2 tablespoons thinly sliced scallions or leeks

Water for cooking

$1/_2$ cup (packed) chopped fresh spinach

$1/_8$ teaspoon ground black pepper

$1/_4$ cup fat-free egg substitute, 2 egg whites, or 1 large egg, beaten

1 whole grain flour tortilla (9-inch round)

$1/_4$ cup shredded reduced-fat Monterey Jack or Mexican blend cheese

Olive oil cooking spray

2 tablespoons chunky-style salsa (optional)

1. Coat a 10-inch nonstick skillet with cooking spray, and add the scallions or leeks and 1 teaspoon of water. Cover and cook over medium heat for about 3 minutes to soften. Add the spinach and black pepper, and cook uncovered for another minute or until the spinach is wilted.

2. Distribute the vegetables evenly over the bottom of the skillet, and pour the egg over the vegetables. Reduce the heat to medium-low, cover, and cook without stirring for about $1^1/_2$ minutes or until the egg is set. Fold the egg in half like an omelet.

3. Lay the tortilla on a flat surface, and place the egg over the bottom half of the tortilla. Sprinkle the cheese over the egg and fold the tortilla over to enclose the filling.

4. Wipe out and respray the skillet and place over medium heat. Lay the filled tortilla in the skillet and spray the top lightly with the cooking spray. Cook for about $1^1/_2$ minutes on each side, or until the tortilla is lightly browned and the cheese is melted. Cut into wedges and serve hot, accompanied by the salsa if desired.

NUTRITION FACTS (PER SERVING)

Calories: 267   Carbohydrates: 27 g   Fiber: 3.7 g   Protein: 19 g

Fat: 9.4 g   Sat. Fat: 3.6 g   Cholesterol: 15 mg   Sodium: 437 mg   Calcium: 385 mg

---

BUCKWHEAT PORRIDGE WITH APPLES AND WALNUTS

YIELD: 6 SERVINGS

$^1/_2$ cup uncooked brown rice

$2^1/_2$ cups nonfat or low-fat milk

$1^1/_2$ cups water

$^1/_2$ cup uncooked roasted buckwheat groats (kasha)

$^1/_4$ plus 2 tablespoons dark raisins or chopped dates

$1^1/_2$ cups Steamed Apples (see page 295)

$^1/_2$ cup plus 1 tablespoon chopped walnuts (unroasted)

1 to $1^1/_2$ teaspoons ground cinnamon (optional)

2 tablespoons maple syrup (optional)

1. Place the rice in a blender and process for about 15 seconds, or just until it has the texture of coarse grits. (Depending on the power of your blender, this may take more or less time.) Set aside.

2. Place the milk and water in a $2^1/_2$-quart nonstick pot, and bring to a boil. Stir in the ground rice and the buckwheat, and reduce the heat to maintain a simmer. Cover and cook, stirring occasionally, for about 15 minutes, or until the mixture is thick and the grains are tender.

3. Stir the raisins or dates into the porridge, and cook for another minute. Remove the pot from the heat, and allow it to sit covered for 5 minutes.

4. For each serving, place $^3/_4$ cup of the buckwheat mixture in a serving bowl, and top with $^1/_4$ cup of apples and $1^1/_2$ tablespoons of walnuts. Sprinkle with some of the cinnamon and/or drizzle with 1 teaspoon of maple syrup, if desired. Serve immediately.

NUTRITION FACTS (PER SERVING)
Calories: 248   Carbohydrates: 42 g   Fiber: 3.5 g   Protein: 8.1 g
Fat: 6.9 g   Sat. Fat: 0.8 g   Cholesterol: 2 mg   Sodium: 71 mg   Calcium: 146 mg

MIXED BERRY MUESLI

YIELD: 4 SERVINGS

1¼ cups uncooked old-fashioned oatmeal (5-minute cooking time)

⅓ cup sliced almonds or chopped walnuts or pecans (unroasted)

⅓ cup wheat bran, raw (untoasted) wheat germ, or finely shredded unsweetened coconut

¼ cup dried cranberries or blueberries

2 cups plain nonfat or low-fat yogurt or milk

2 cups fresh mixed berries

1. Place the first 4 ingredients (oats through berries) in a bowl, and stir to evenly mix.

2. For each serving, place ½ cup of the oat mixture in a serving bowl, and stir in ½ cup of yogurt or milk.

3. Allow the mixture to sit for 10 to 15 minutes, or refrigerate for several hours or overnight for a thicker texture. Stir in a little more yogurt or milk if needed, and top with ½ cup of berries. Serve immediately.

VARIATIONS

❏ Substitute Steamed Apples (see page 295) for the mixed fresh berries.

❏ Substitute chopped pitted dates for the dried cranberries or blueberries, and sliced bananas for the mixed berries.

NUTRITION FACTS (PER SERVING)

Calories: 267   Carbohydrates: 46 g   Fiber: 8 g   Protein: 12 g
Fat: 6.1 g   Sat. Fat: 0.6 g   Cholesterol: 3 mg   Sodium: 94 mg   Calcium: 233 mg

---

STRAWBERRY-BANANA BREAKFAST BAGEL

YIELD: 1 SERVING

½ of a whole grain bagel

¼ cup low-fat, no-added-salt cottage cheese, part-skim ricotta cheese, or farmer's cheese

1 tablespoon chopped walnuts (unroasted)

5 slices banana

1 medium strawberry, cut into 5 slices

1 teaspoon honey

1. Lightly toast the bagel if desired. Spread the cheese over the bagel.

2. Top with the walnuts first, and then the banana and strawberry slices. Drizzle the honey over the top and serve.

NUTRITION FACTS (PER SERVING)
Calories: 239   Carbohydrates: 37 g   Fiber: 4 g   Protein: 14 g
Fat: 5.3 g   Sat. Fat: 0.9 g   Cholesterol: 5 mg   Sodium: 238 mg   Calcium: 60 mg

---

CINNAMON-APPLE OATMEAL

YIELD: 4 SERVINGS

2 cups chopped peeled apple

2 cups water, divided

2 cups nonfat or low-fat milk

2 cups uncooked old-fashioned oatmeal
(5-minute cooking time)

$1/2$ to 1 teaspoon ground cinnamon

$1/4$ cup plus 2 tablespoons chopped walnuts or pecans (unroasted)

$1/4$ cup raisins or chopped dates (optional)

4 teaspoons maple syrup

1. Place the apples and $1/4$ cup of the water in a 3-quart pot. Cover and cook over medium heat for about 2 minutes, or just until the apples begin to soften.

2. Add the remaining $1^3/4$ cups of water to the pot along with the milk and oats, and bring to a boil. Adjust the heat to maintain a simmer. Cover and cook, stirring occasionally, for about 5 minutes or until the liquid is absorbed. Turn off the heat and allow the pot to sit for 2 minutes.

3. For each serving, place a quarter of the oatmeal mixture (about $1^1/3$ cups) in a serving bowl. Sprinkle with $1/8$ to $1/4$ teaspoon of cinnamon, $1^1/2$ tablespoons of nuts, and, if using, 1 tablespoon of raisins or dates. Top with a drizzle of maple syrup and serve immediately.

VARIATION

❑ Substitute peaches or pears for the apples.

NUTRITION FACTS (PER SERVING)
Calories: 296   Carbohydrates: 46 g   Fiber: 6 g   Protein: 11 g
Fat: 9 g   Sat. Fat: 1.1 g   Cholesterol: 2 mg   Sodium: 52 mg   Calcium: 174 mg

---

QUINOA WITH BANANAS AND BLUEBERRIES

Yield: 5 servings

1 cup uncooked quinoa

1 1/2 cups nonfat or low-fat milk (dairy, almond, or coconut)

1 1/2 cups water

1 1/4 cups sliced banana (about 1 1/4 large)

1 cup fresh blueberries

1/2 cup chopped pecans or sliced almonds (unroasted)

2 1/2 tablespoons shredded unsweetened coconut

5 teaspoons honey (optional)

1. Place the quinoa in a wire strainer and rinse well with cool running water.

2. Place the rinsed quinoa in a 2 1/2-quart nonstick pot, and add the milk and water. Bring to a boil; then reduce the heat to maintain a simmer. Cover and cook, stirring occasionally, for about 25 minutes, or until the quinoa is soft and the liquid is absorbed. Remove the pot from the heat and allow the pot to sit covered for 5 minutes.

3. For each serving, place about 3/4 cup of the quinoa in a serving bowl. Top each serving with a fifth of the bananas, blueberries, nuts, and coconut. Top with a drizzle of honey, if desired, and serve immediately.

Nutrition Facts (Per Serving)

Calories: 315   Carbohydrates: 41 g   Fiber: 5.8 g   Protein: 9 g

Fat: 14.2 g   Sat. Fat: 2.6 g   Cholesterol: 2 mg   Sodium: 34 mg   Calcium: 120 mg

---

FROSTY FRUIT SMOOTHIE

Yield: 1 serving

1 1/2 cups frozen strawberries, blueberries, mixed berries, or pitted dark sweet cherries

1/2 cup nonfat or low-fat milk or pomegranate juice

1/2 cup plain nonfat or low-fat Greek-style yogurt

1/2 cup crushed ice

2 tablespoons chopped walnuts or almonds (unroasted)

1 to 1 1/2 tablespoons raw (untoasted) wheat germ, oat bran, flax meal, or chia seeds (optional)

Low-calorie sweetener to taste (optional)

1. Place all of the ingredients in a blender, and blend until smooth.

2. Pour into a 16-ounce glass and serve immediately.

VARIATIONS

❏ Substitute frozen mandarin orange sections or frozen pineapple chunks for the berries. If using juice instead of milk, use orange juice instead of pomegranate juice.

❏ Substitute frozen banana slices for $\frac{1}{2}$ cup of the berries.

NUTRITION FACTS (PER SERVING)

Calories: 305   Carbohydrates: 33 g   Fiber: 6.7 g   Protein: 22 g
Fat: 11.7 g   Sat. Fat: 0.9 g   Cholesterol: 2 mg   Sodium: 108 mg   Calcium: 372 mg

---

MOCHA-BANANA SMOOTHIE

YIELD: 1 SERVING

$\frac{3}{4}$ cup nonfat or low-fat milk

$\frac{1}{2}$ cup frozen banana slices

$\frac{1}{2}$ cup black coffee, frozen into ice cubes

2 tablespoons sliced almonds (unroasted)

Low-calorie sweetener to taste

$1\frac{1}{2}$ tablespoons shredded unsweetened coconut (optional)

1 tablespoon unsweetened cocoa powder

$\frac{1}{8}$ teaspoon ground cinnamon (optional)

1. Place all of the ingredients in a blender, and blend until smooth.

2. Pour into a 16-ounce glass and serve immediately.

NUTRITION FACTS (PER SERVING)

Calories: 208   Carbohydrates: 32 g   Fiber: 5.1 g   Protein: 11 g
Fat: 6.9 g   Sat. Fat: 1.1 g   Cholesterol: 4 mg   Sodium: 82 mg   Calcium: 268 mg

---

Main Courses

The main course, or entrée, typically adds more AGEs to the daily diet than any other food. This is because the main course often features a large portion of meat or poultry cooked with dry-heat methods such as grilling, broiling, frying, or roasting. But even meatless entrées can be loaded with AGEs if made with gobs of high-fat cheese, butter, and oil.

Fortunately, AGE-less main dishes can be tasty, filling, and simple to prepare. In fact, the two magic meal words in the average working household—fast and easy—are also central to the AGE-less way. Poaching, steaming, stewing, and other moist-heat cooking methods, which require very little attention, are the keys to making AGE-less meals. Convenient oven-braised and slow cooker meals can also fit the bill. Moreover, many family favorites such as meatloaf, meatballs, and skillet dinners can be enjoyed on the AGE-less diet.

The AGE-less main dishes offered in the following pages feature right-size portions of lean protein along with nutrient-rich vegetables and wholesome whole grains. Ingredients such as lemon juice, wine, and tomatoes, along with aromatic herbs and spices, enhance the flavor of foods instead of age-accelerating AGEs.

As you peruse this chapter, keep in mind that you will find many more delicious main courses in other sections of this book. A selection of savory soups and stews begins on page 237, a collection of hearty main dish salads starts on page 221, and recipes for satisfying sandwiches can be found on page 249.

BRAISED CHICKEN AND VEGETABLES

YIELD: 4 SERVINGS

1 pound boneless skinless chicken breast, cut into 4 equal pieces

$^1/_2$ teaspoon ground black pepper

Scant $^1/_2$ teaspoon salt

$^1/_4$ teaspoon ground paprika

1 cup no-salt-added chicken broth

1 cup dry white wine

1$^1/_2$ tablespoons chopped fresh thyme, or 1$^1/_2$ teaspoons dried

1 teaspoon crushed garlic

8 ounces unpeeled new potatoes or fingerling potatoes, cut into halves or quarters

12 baby carrots

1 medium yellow onion, cut into $^3/_8$-inch-thick wedges

$^3/_4$ cup frozen green peas

1 tablespoon extra-virgin olive oil

2 tablespoons finely chopped fresh parsley

1. If necessary, cut the chicken breasts in half horizontally or butterfly them so they are no more than $^3/_4$-inch thick. Sprinkle both sides of the chicken with some of the pepper, salt, and paprika, and set aside.

2. Combine the broth, wine, thyme, and garlic, and set aside.

3. Coat a large, deep nonstick skillet with cooking spray, and preheat over medium heat. Add the chicken and cook for about 1 minute on each side, or just long enough to lightly brown and seal the meat. Add the potatoes, carrots, and onion to the skillet.

4. Pour the broth mixture over the chicken and vegetables, and bring to a boil. Adjust the heat to maintain a simmer, cover, and cook for 10 minutes. Turn the chicken over and cook for 10 additional minutes, or until the chicken is cooked through and the vegetables are tender. (An instant-read thermometer inserted in the thickest part of the chicken should registerat least 165°F.) Add the peas, cover, and simmer for about 3 minutes to heat through.

5. Use a slotted spoon to transfer the chicken and vegetables to a large warmed bowl. Cover and set aside to keep warm. Bring the liquid in the skillet to a boil over medium heat. Stir in the olive oil and cook uncovered for about 5 minutes, or until reduced to about $^1/_2$ cup.

6. To serve, place a quarter of the chicken and vegetables in each of 4 shallow bowls. Drizzle with 2 tablespoons of the sauce and top with a sprinkling of parsley. Serve hot.

NUTRITION FACTS (PER SERVING)

Calories: 293   Carbohydrates: 20 g   Fiber: 4 g   Protein: 28 g

Fat: 6.6 g   Sat. Fat: 1.2 g   Cholesterol: 73 mg   Sodium: 448 mg   Calcium: 47 mg

---

CHICKEN WITH LEMON-CAPER SAUCE

YIELD: 4 SERVINGS

1 pound boneless skinless chicken breast, cut into 4 equal pieces

1 cup no-salt-added chicken broth

3 tablespoons lemon juice

2 teaspoons crushed garlic

$1/_2$ teaspoon ground black pepper

Scant $1/_2$ teaspoon salt

2 tablespoons capers, drained

1 tablespoon extra-virgin olive oil

1. If necessary, cut the chicken breasts in half horizontally or butterfly them so they are no more than $3/_4$-inch thick.

2. Place the broth, lemon juice, garlic, pepper, and salt in a large nonstick skillet. Add the chicken, cover, and bring to a simmer over medium heat. Adjust the heat to maintain a simmer, cover, and cook for 10 minutes. Then turn the chicken and cook for 10 minutes more. (An instant-read thermometer inserted in the thickest part should register at least 165°F.) Transfer the chicken to a warmed plate, and cover to keep warm.

3. Bring the liquid in the skillet to a boil over medium heat, and cook uncovered for about 8 minutes, or until it is reduced to about $1/_3$ cup. Stir in the capers and olive oil during the last minute of cooking.

4. To serve, slice the chicken thinly at an angle and drizzle with the sauce. Serve hot.

VARIATION

❏ Omit the capers, and add 2 teaspoons each of chopped fresh rosemary and chopped fresh thyme to the liquid. If using dried herbs, add $2/_3$ teaspoon each.

NUTRITION FACTS (PER SERVING)

Calories: 167   Carbohydrates: 2 g   Fiber: 1.1 g   Protein: 25 g

Fat: 6.4 g   Sat. Fat: 1.1 g   Cholesterol: 72 mg   Sodium: 494 mg   Calcium: 15 mg

---

BISTRO CHICKEN WITH OLIVES AND TOMATOES

YIELD: 4 SERVINGS

1 pound boneless skinless chicken breast, cut into 4 equal pieces

$^1/_2$ teaspoon ground black pepper

1 cup chopped yellow onion

$^1/_2$ cup chopped celery

1 teaspoon crushed garlic

2 tablespoons water

$^1/_4$ cup dry white wine

1 tablespoon capers, drained

1 tablespoon finely chopped fresh basil, or 1 teaspoon dried

1 tablespoon finely chopped fresh parsley, or 1 teaspoon dried

1 can (14$^1/_2$ ounces) diced tomatoes, undrained

$^1/_4$ cup chopped black or green olives

1 tablespoon extra-virgin olive oil

1. If necessary, cut the chicken breasts in half horizontally or butterfly them so they are no more than $^3/_4$-inch thick. Sprinkle both sides of the chicken breasts with pepper.

2. Coat a large nonstick skillet with cooking spray and preheat over medium heat. Add the chicken and cook for about 1 minute on each side, or just long enough to lightly brown and seal the meat. Remove the chicken from the pan and set aside.

3. Add the onion, celery, garlic, and 2 tablespoons of water to the skillet. Cover and cook for 5 minutes, or until tender. Add the wine, cover, and cook for 2 minutes.

4. Add all of the remaining ingredients except for the olive oil to the skillet, and bring to a boil. Return the chicken to the skillet, and adjust the heat to maintain a simmer. Cover and cook for 20 minutes, turning the chicken after 10 minutes. (An instant-read thermometer inserted in the thickest part should register at least 165°F.) Then uncover and cook for about 5 minutes to thicken the sauce. Stir in the olive oil during the last minute of cooking.

5. Serve hot, if desired, spooning the chicken and sauce over whole grain angel hair pasta, spaghetti squash, or Zucchini Noodles (see page 267).

NUTRITION FACTS (PER SERVING)

Calories: 230   Carbohydrates: 12 g   Fiber: 2.6 g   Protein: 26 g

Fat: 7.9 g   Sat. Fat: 1.2 g   Cholesterol: 73 mg   Sodium: 482 mg   Calcium: 62 mg

---

STEAMED CHICKEN WITH HOT MUSTARD SAUCE

YIELD: 4 SERVINGS

1 pound boneless skinless chicken breast, cut into 4 equal pieces

$1/_2$ teaspoon ground black pepper

$1/_4$ teaspoon salt

2 green tea bags

3 cups fresh sugar snap peas or snow peas

1 cup diagonally sliced carrots

1 tablespoon plus 1 teaspoon sesame seeds (unroasted)

SAUCE

2 tablespoons rice vinegar

2 tablespoons reduced-sodium soy sauce

2 tablespoons Chinese hot mustard

1 tablespoon plus 1 teaspoon frozen (thawed) orange juice concentrate

2 teaspoons canola oil or untoasted sesame oil

1. Combine all of the sauce ingredients in a bowl and whisk to mix. Set aside.

2. If necessary, cut the chicken breasts in half horizontally or butterfly them so they are no more than $3/_4$-inch thick. Sprinkle the chicken with the pepper and salt, and set aside.

3. Cut open the tea bags and sprinkle the tea into a 6-quart pot. Add a steamer basket and fill with enough water to reach within $1/_2$ inch of the bottom of the basket.

4. Arrange the chicken in the steamer basket, cover, and bring to a boil. Allow the chicken to steam for 10 minutes.

5. Arrange the peas and carrots over the chicken, cover, and steam for 5 additional minutes, or until the chicken is cooked through and the vegetables are tender. (An instant-read thermometer inserted in the thickest part of the chicken should register at least 165°F.)

6. For each serving, place one piece of chicken and a quarter of the vegetables in a shallow bowl. Drizzle one-fourth of the sauce over each serving and sprinkle with one-fourth of the sesame seeds. Serve hot.

VARIATION

❑ To make Ginger-Garlic Sauce, omit the mustard in the sauce and add 1 tablespoon plus 1 teaspoon finely grated fresh ginger and 1 teaspoon crushed garlic.

NUTRITION FACTS (PER SERVING)

Calories: 243   Carbohydrates: 14 g   Fiber: 3.7 g   Protein: 28 g

Fat: 7.2 g   Sat. Fat: 1.1 g   Cholesterol: 73 mg   Sodium: 557 mg   Calcium: 69 mg

---

STEAMED CHICKEN WITH CILANTRO SAUCE

YIELD: 4 SERVINGS

2 green tea bags

4 medium-large collard green, kale, or Chinese cabbage leaves

1 pound boneless skinless chicken breast, cut into 4 equal pieces and pounded to an even $1/_2$-inch thickness

2 tablespoons matchstick-size pieces fresh ginger

SAUCE

2 tablespoons reduced-sodium soy sauce

2 teaspoons rice vinegar

1 teaspoon Sriracha sauce or Asian-style chili sauce with garlic

1 tablespoon canola oil

2 teaspoons crushed garlic

$1/_2$ cup finely chopped fresh cilantro

1. Cut open the tea bags and place the tea leaves in a 6-quart pot. Add a steamer basket and pour in enough water to reach within $1/_2$ inch of the bottom of the basket.

2. Line the basket with the collard, kale, or cabbage leaves. Arrange the chicken over the leaves, and scatter the ginger evenly over the chicken.

3. Cover the pot and bring to a boil. Steam for about 15 minutes, or until the chicken is done. (An instant-read thermometer inserted in the chicken should register at least 165°F.)

4. Remove $1/_4$ cup of the liquid from the pot (excluding the tea leaves), and set aside to use in the sauce. Return the chicken to the pot and cover to keep warm.

5. To make the sauce, add the soy sauce, vinegar, and Sriracha to the reserved cooking liquid. Stir, and set aside. Place the oil and garlic in a small nonstick skillet, and cook over medium heat for about 30 seconds, or until the garlic begins to turn color and smells fragrant. Add the soy sauce mixture to the skillet, and bring a boil. Cook uncovered for about 3 minutes, or until reduced in volume to one-third cup. Add the cilantro and cook for an additional 30 seconds, or until the cilantro is wilted.

6. To serve, place one collard, kale, or cabbage leaf on each serving plate, and top with a piece of chicken. Drizzle each piece of chicken with one-fourth of the sauce, and serve hot.

NUTRITION FACTS (PER SERVING)

Calories: 181   Carbohydrates: 4 g   Fiber: 1 g   Protein: 25 g

Fat: 6.6 g   Sat. Fat: 0.6 g   Cholesterol: 73 mg   Sodium: 513 mg   Calcium: 41 mg

---

CHICKEN DIJON

YIELD: 4 SERVINGS

1 pound boneless skinless chicken breast, cut into 4 equal pieces

2 cups sliced fresh mushrooms

1 medium yellow onion, thinly sliced and separated into rings

$^1/_4$ cup dry white wine

$^1/_2$ teaspoon ground black pepper

$^1/_4$ teaspoon salt

3 tablespoons Dijon mustard

1 tablespoon finely chopped fresh rosemary, or 1 teaspoon dried

1. Preheat the oven to 350°F.

2. If necessary, cut the chicken breasts in half horizontally or butterfly them so they are no more than $^3/_4$-inch thick. Set aside.

3. Cut 4 sheets of aluminum foil, each about 16 inches long. Arrange the sheets of foil on a work surface, and center one-fourth of the mushrooms and onions on the lower half of each sheet. Drizzle 1 tablespoon of the wine over the vegetables, and sprinkle with one-fourth of the pepper and salt. Top the vegetable mixture with a piece of chicken. Spread one-fourth of the mustard over each piece of chicken, and sprinkle with the rosemary.

4. Fold the top part of the foil over the lower part. Double-fold the edges together to tightly seal the packets. Arrange the packets on a large baking sheet.

5. Bake for 30 minutes, or until the chicken is done and the vegetables are tender. (Open one packet with care, as steam will escape, and test for doneness. An instant-read thermometer inserted in the thickest part of the chicken should register at least 165°F. Reseal the packet if further cooking is necessary.)

6. Allow the packets to sit for 5 minutes before opening with care. Serve hot over brown rice or whole wheat couscous, if desired.

VARIATIONS

❏ Add $^1/_2$ cup of thinly sliced unpeeled potatoes to each packet. Place the potatoes on the foil first, and layer the mushrooms, onions, and other ingredients over the potatoes.

❏ For an impressive presentation at the table, enclose the chicken and vegetables in parchment rather than aluminum foil. (See page 149 for directions.)

SOBA NOODLE BOWL

YIELD: 4 SERVINGS

3 cups no-salt-added chicken broth

$1/4$ cup reduced-sodium soy sauce

2 teaspoons grated fresh ginger

$1 1/2$ teaspoons crushed garlic

$1/4$ teaspoon ground white pepper

12 ounces thinly sliced boneless skinless chicken breast

$1 1/4$ cups sliced fresh mushrooms

4 ounces dried soba (Japanese buckwheat) noodles

$1 1/4$ cups julienne-cut carrots

$1 1/4$ cups bias-sliced snow peas or thinly sliced broccoli florets

1 tablespoon untoasted sesame oil

$1/2$ cup very thinly bias-sliced scallions

1. Place the broth, soy sauce, ginger, garlic, and white pepper in a 4-quart pot, and bring to boil over medium heat.

2. Add the chicken to the pot, and allow the liquid to return to a boil. Adjust the heat to maintain a simmer, cover, and cook for 2 minutes.

3. Add the mushrooms to the pot, cover, and simmer for one minute. Add the soba noodles, cover, and simmer for 3 minutes, or until the noodles are almost tender.

4. Add the carrots and snow peas or broccoli to the pot, cover, and cook for 1 to 2 minutes, or until the vegetables are crisp-tender. Stir in the sesame oil.

5. Divide the mixture among 4 shallow bowls, and top each serving with about 2 tablespoons of the scallions. Serve immediately.

PICADILLO

YIELD: 5 SERVINGS

1 pound ground beef, chicken,
or turkey (at least 93% lean)

1 medium yellow onion, chopped

1 medium green bell pepper
or 2 mild banana peppers,
seeded and chopped

1 teaspoon crushed garlic

1 teaspoon ground cumin

$1/2$ teaspoon dried oregano

1 can (15 ounces) no-salt-added
tomato sauce

$1/3$ cup sliced pimento-stuffed
green olives

$1/4$ cup raisins

$1/4$ teaspoon salt

$1/4$ teaspoon cayenne pepper

1. Coat a large nonstick skillet with cooking spray, and add the ground beef, onion, bell or banana peppers, garlic, cumin, and oregano. Cover and cook over medium heat, stirring occasionally to crumble the meat, for about 8 minutes, or until the meat is no longer pink and the vegetables are tender.

2. Stir in the remaining ingredients and bring to a boil. Adjust the heat to maintain a simmer, cover, and cook for 5 minutes. Remove the lid, and simmer uncovered for 5 to 8 additional minutes, or until most of the liquid has evaporated and the sauce is thick.

3. Serve hot with warm corn tortillas and shredded lettuce, use to fill crisp leaves of romaine lettuce, or serve over polenta or quinoa.

NUTRITION FACTS (PER $3/4$-CUP SERVING, MEAT MIXTURE ONLY)
Calories: 211   Carbohydrates: 15 g   Fiber: 2.1 g   Protein: 19 g
Fat: 7.2 g   Sat. Fat: 2.7 g   Cholesterol: 57 mg   Sodium: 333 mg   Calcium: 18 mg

AGE-*LESS* TIP—USING GROUND MEAT

Animal protein—especially red meat—is the biggest contributor of AGEs to many diets. The good news is that using moist-heat cooking methods significantly limits the creation of further AGEs. When making a skillet dish, instead of browning the ground meat in a pool of fat over high heat, coat the pan with cooking spray, cover the pan, and place the meat over medium heat just until it is cooked through.

SPANISH-STYLE SPAGHETTI SAUCE

YIELD: 4 SERVINGS

8 ounces ground beef, chicken, or turkey (at least 93% lean)

1 cup chopped yellow onion

$^1/_2$ cup finely chopped celery

1$^1/_2$ teaspoons crushed garlic

$^1/_2$ teaspoon ground black pepper

$^1/_4$ to $^1/_2$ teaspoon crushed red pepper flakes

1 can (14$^1/_2$ ounces) diced no-salt-added tomatoes, undrained

$^1/_4$ cup chopped fresh parsley

1 tablespoon chopped fresh oregano, or 1 teaspoon dried

$^1/_2$ cup sliced pimento-stuffed green olives

1 tablespoon plus 1 teaspoon capers, drained

1. Coat a large nonstick skillet with cooking spray, and add the ground meat, onion, celery, garlic, black pepper, and crushed red pepper. Cover and cook over medium heat, stirring occasionally to crumble the meat, for about 6 minutes, or until the meat is no longer pink and the vegetables soften.

2. Place the tomatoes, parsley, and oregano in a blender, and blend until smooth. Pour the mixture into the skillet, and stir in the olives and capers.

3. Bring the mixture to a boil. Adjust the heat to maintain a simmer, cover, and cook, stirring occasionally, for 5 minutes. Remove the lid and simmer uncovered, stirring occasionally, for 10 additional minutes, or until the mixture has thickened and reduced to about 3 cups in volume.

4. Serve hot over Zucchini Noodles (see page 267), spaghetti squash, polenta, or whole grain pasta.

NUTRITION FACTS (PER $^3/_4$-CUP SERVING, SAUCE ONLY)

Calories: 140   Carbohydrates: 10 g   Fiber: 2.5 g   Protein: 14 g

Fat: 5.4 g   Sat. Fat: 1.9 g   Cholesterol: 36 mg   Sodium: 314 mg   Calcium: 40 mg

CHIPOTLE MEATBALLS

YIELD: 5 SERVINGS

MEATBALLS

1 pound ground turkey, chicken, or beef (at least 93% lean)

2 cups chopped fresh mushrooms (about $1/_4$-inch pieces)

$1/_2$ cup quick-cooking oatmeal (1-minute cooking time)

2 egg whites or 1 large egg, beaten

1 teaspoon crushed garlic

$1/_2$ teaspoon salt

$1/_2$ teaspoon ground black pepper

CHIPOTLE SAUCE

1 can (4 ounces) chipotle chile peppers in adobo sauce

2 cans (14$1/_2$ ounces each) no-salt-added diced tomatoes, undrained

$3/_4$ cup chopped yellow onion

$1/_2$ cup chicken or beef broth

$1/_4$ cup fresh cilantro leaves

1 teaspoon crushed garlic

1 tablespoon extra-virgin olive oil

1. To make the sauce, drain the sauce from the canned chile peppers into a blender. Wearing protective gloves, cut open the chiles and remove and discard all or part of the seeds and the inner membranes (this tones down the heat). Add the chiles to the blender, and purée until smooth. Pour into a bowl and set aside.

2. Place the tomatoes, onion, broth, cilantro, garlic, and olive oil in the blender. Add 2 tablespoons of the chile purée, and blend until smooth. (Reserve the remaining purée for another use.)

3. Pour the sauce into a large deep skillet, and bring to a boil over medium heat. Adjust the heat to maintain a simmer, cover, and cook for 5 minutes.

4. While the sauce simmers, place all of the meatball ingredients in a large bowl, and mix until evenly combined. Shape $1/_4$-cup portions of the mixture into a total of 15 meatballs.

5. Add the meatballs to the sauce, adjust the heat to maintain a simmer, and cover. Cook for 15 minutes, turning the meatballs every 5 minutes. Remove the lid and simmer uncovered, turning every 5 minutes, for an additional 15 minutes, or until the meatballs are cooked through and the sauce is the consistency of marinara sauce. (An instant-read thermometer inserted in the center of a meatball should register at least 160°F.) To reduce splatters, use a splatter screen or place a lid on the skillet, leaving it partially ajar to let steam escape.

6. If desired, serve over Zucchini Noodles (see page 267), or serve with warm corn tortillas, shredded lettuce, and avocado slices.

NUTRITION FACTS (PER SERVING)
Calories: 242   Carbohydrates: 17 g   Fiber: 4 g   Protein: 23 g
Fat: 9.8 g   Sat. Fat: 3.3 g   Cholesterol: 64 mg   Sodium: 425 mg   Calcium: 24 mg

---

MEATBALLS WITH MARINARA SAUCE

YIELD: 5 SERVINGS

MEATBALLS

1 pound ground turkey, chicken, or beef (at least 93% lean)

2 cups chopped fresh mushrooms (about $1/4$-inch pieces)

$1/2$ cup quick-cooking oatmeal (1-minute cooking time)

2 egg whites or 1 large egg, beaten

$1^1/2$ teaspoons crushed garlic

$1^1/2$ teaspoons whole fennel seeds

1 teaspoon dried Italian seasoning

$1/2$ teaspoon salt

$1/2$ teaspoon ground black pepper

SAUCE

$2^1/2$ cups ready-made marinara sauce

$1/2$ cup beef or vegetable broth

1. To make the meatballs, place all of the meatball ingredients in a large bowl, and mix until evenly combined. Shape $1/4$-cup portions of the mixture into a total of 15 meatballs, and set aside.

2. To make the sauce, pour the ready-made sauce and broth into a large deep skillet, and bring to a boil over medium heat. Add the meatballs to the sauce, and adjust the heat to maintain a simmer. Cover and simmer, turning the meatballs every 6 to 8 minutes, for 30 minutes, or until the meatballs are cooked through and the sauce is thick. (An instant-read thermometer inserted in the center of a meatball should register at least 160°F.)

3. If desired, serve hot over Zucchini Noodles (see page 267), spaghetti squash, or whole grain pasta, or use to make meatball sandwiches.

NUTRITION FACTS (PER SERVING)
Calories: 225   Carbohydrates: 20 g   Fiber: 4.3 g   Protein: 23 g
Fat: 7.7 g   Sat. Fat: 2.9 g   Cholesterol: 64 mg   Sodium: 627 mg   Calcium: 49 mg

---

MUSHROOM AND HERB MEATLOAF

Yield: 6 servings

1¼ pounds ground beef or turkey (at least 93% lean)

2 cups chopped fresh mushrooms (about ¼-inch pieces)

½ cup finely chopped yellow onion

¼ cup finely chopped green bell pepper

½ cup quick-cooking oatmeal (1-minute cooking time)

2 egg whites or 1 large egg

1 tablespoon plus 1 teaspoon Dijon or spicy mustard

1 tablespoon plus 1 teaspoon dried parsley

1 teaspoon dried thyme

1½ teaspoons crushed garlic

½ teaspoon ground black pepper

1 can (8 ounces) no-salt-added tomato sauce, divided

½ teaspoon plus ⅛ teaspoon salt, divided

1. Preheat the oven to 350°F. Place the first 11 ingredients (the ground meat through black pepper) in a large bowl. Add 1 tablespoon of the tomato sauce and ½ teaspoon of the salt, and mix until evenly combined.

2. Coat a 9-x-5-inch meatloaf pan with cooking spray, and press the mixture evenly into the pan. Combine the remaining tomato sauce with the remaining ⅛ teaspoon of salt, and pour the mixture over the meatloaf.

3. Bake uncovered for 1 hour, or until an instant-read thermometer inserted in the center of the loaf reads at least 160°F for ground beef, or at least 165°F for ground turkey. Allow to sit for 10 minutes before slicing and serving.

Nutrition Facts (Per Serving)

Calories: 219   Carbohydrates: 14 g   Fiber: 2.4 g   Protein: 24 g

Fat: 7.4 g   Sat. Fat: 2.9 g   Cholesterol: 60 mg   Sodium: 411 mg   Calcium: 28 mg

---

SPICY BEEF AND POTATO SKILLET

YIELD: 4 SERVINGS

1 pound ground beef (at least 93% lean)

1 cup chopped yellow onion

1 tablespoon ground paprika

1/4 teaspoon cayenne pepper

1/4 teaspoon ground black pepper

3 cups unpeeled new potatoes, sliced 1/4-inch thick

3 cups sliced fresh mushrooms

1 cup beef broth

1 tablespoon chopped fresh thyme, or 1 teaspoon dried

1 tablespoon chopped fresh rosemary, or 1 teaspoon dried

2 teaspoons crushed garlic

1/4 teaspoon salt

1. Coat a large nonstick skillet with cooking spray, and add the beef, onion, paprika, cayenne pepper, and black pepper. Cover and cook over medium heat, stirring occasionally to crumble the beef, for about 6 minutes, or until the meat is no longer pink and the onion softens.

2. Add all of the remaining ingredients to the skillet, and bring to a boil. Adjust the heat to maintain a simmer, cover, and cook, stirring occasionally, for about 15 minutes, or until the potatoes are tender. If necessary, cook uncovered for a few minutes, or until most of the liquid has evaporated. Serve hot.

NUTRITION FACTS (PER 1¹/₂-CUP SERVING)

Calories: 291   Carbohydrates: 26 g   Fiber: 4.1 g Protein 28 g

Fat: 8.5 g   Sat. Fat: 3.5 g   Cholesterol: 71 mg   Sodium: 454 mg   Calcium: 50 mg

AGE-*LESS* TIP—
USING MUSHROOMS AS A MEAT EXTENDER

You can replace part of the meat in many recipes with chopped mushrooms, which have a meaty taste and texture but are very low in AGEs. Up to half of the ground meat in recipes such as tacos can be replaced. A fourth to a third of the ground meat in meatloaf, burger, and meatball recipes can be replaced. When making a skillet dish, simply add sliced mushrooms to the pan along with other flavorful ingredients.

TUSCAN PORK WITH WHITE BEANS

YIELD: 6 SERVINGS

$1^1/_2$ cups dried white beans, such as navy or cannellini, soaked for 8 hours or overnight and drained

1 teaspoon dried sage

1 teaspoon dried rosemary

$^3/_4$ teaspoon whole fennel seeds

2 to 3 teaspoons crushed garlic

$^3/_4$ teaspoon salt

$^1/_2$ teaspoon ground black pepper

2 cups no-salt-added chicken or vegetable broth

$1^3/_4$-pound pork loin roast, trimmed of visible fat

1. Place the beans in a 3-quart slow cooker.

2. Combine the sage, rosemary, fennel seeds, garlic, salt, and pepper in a small bowl, and stir to mix. Add half of the herb mixture to the beans, reserving the rest. Pour the broth over the bean mixture, and stir to mix.

3. Spread the remaining herb mixture over the roast, and place the roast over the beans. Cover the pot and cook at high power for 4 hours or at low power for 8 hours, or until the beans are soft and the roast is so tender that it can be easily pulled apart with a fork. (An instant-read thermometer inserted in the center of the roast should register at least 145°F.)

4. To serve, remove the pork roast from the slow cooker, place it on a plate, and pull the pork apart into chunks. Serve hot with the beans.

NUTRITION FACTS (PER SERVING, 3 OUNCES PORK WITH $^3/_4$ CUP BEANS)

Calories: 360   Carbohydrates: 35 g   Fiber: 8 g   Protein: 36 g

Fat: 8.5 g   Sat. Fat: 3.1 g   Cholesterol: 67 mg   Sodium: 332 mg   Calcium: 113 mg

CAJUN SHRIMP BOIL

YIELD: 4 SERVINGS

24 ounces beer, light or regular

Water for cooking

12 ounces unpeeled red new potatoes (about 6 medium), cut into $1^1/_2$-inch pieces

3 tablespoons Cajun or Creole seasoning

3 medium ears fresh-shucked corn, each cut into 3 pieces

$2^1/_2$ cups fresh broccoli or cauliflower florets (2-inch pieces)

$1^1/_4$ pounds large unpeeled raw shrimp

1. Pour the beer into a 6-quart pot. Then add water until the pot is filled halfway.

2. Add the potatoes and the seasoning to the pot, and bring to a boil over medium-high heat. Cover, leaving the lid slightly ajar, and boil for 4 minutes. Add the corn, and boil for 4 minutes more, or until the potatoes are nearly done. Add the broccoli or cauliflower, and boil for 1 additional minute.

3. Add the shrimp to the pot, and boil for 2 to 3 minutes, or just until the shrimp turn opaque and are cooked through. Drain well and serve hot.

Nutrition Facts (Per Serving)

Calories: 213   Carbohydrates: 30 g   Fiber: 4.9 g   Protein: 24 g

Fat: 1.9 g   Sat. Fat: 0.4 g   Cholesterol: 168 mg   Sodium: 515 mg   Calcium: 68 mg

---

PORK CARNITAS

Yield: 8 servings

2 teaspoons crushed garlic	1 teaspoon salt
2 teaspoons dried oregano	$2\frac{1}{4}$-pound pork loin or pork sirloin roast, trimmed of visible fat
1 teaspoon ground cumin	
$1\frac{1}{2}$ teaspoons ground black pepper	1 cup beer, light or regular

1. Preheat the oven to 325°F.

2. Combine the garlic, oregano, cumin, pepper, and salt in a small dish, and stir to mix. Rub the mixture over all sides of the roast.

3. Coat a 9-by-13-inch pan with cooking spray, and place the roast in the pan. Pour the beer around the meat.

4. Cover the pan with aluminum foil and bake for $2\frac{1}{2}$ hours, or until the roast can be easily pulled apart with a fork. (An instant-read thermometer inserted in the center of the roast should register at least 145°F.) Remove from the oven and allow the roast to sit, covered loosely with the foil, for 10 minutes.

5. Pull the meat into chunks and toss in some of the cooking liquid to moisten. Serve with warm corn tortillas, salsa, and avocado slices, or spoon over brown rice and top with chopped cilantro or tomato salsa.

Nutrition Facts (Per 3-ounce Serving, Meat Only)

Calories: 171   Carbohydrates: 1 g   Fiber: 0.3 g   Protein: 26 g

Fat: 4.6 g   Sat. Fat: 1.7 g   Cholesterol: 74 mg   Sodium: 369 mg   Calcium: 11 mg

---

GREEK-STYLE SKILLET DINNER

YIELD: 4 SERVINGS

12 ounces ground beef or lamb (at least 93% lean)

1 cup chopped yellow onion

$3/_4$ cup chopped carrot ($1/_4$-inch dice)

2 teaspoons crushed garlic

1 teaspoon dried oregano

$1/_4$ teaspoon ground cinnamon

$2^1/_4$ cups reduced-sodium beef broth, divided

1 cup vegetable juice, such as V-8

$1/_4$ teaspoon ground black pepper

1 cup uncooked quick-cooking barley or whole wheat orzo

$1/_4$ cup finely chopped fresh parsley

2 tablespoons finely chopped fresh mint

$1^1/_2$ teaspoons lemon juice

1. Coat a large nonstick skillet with cooking spray, and add the ground meat and onion. Cover and cook over medium heat, stirring occasionally to crumble the meat, for about 6 minutes, or until the meat is no longer pink.

2. Add the carrots, garlic, oregano, cinnamon, and 1 cup of the broth to the skillet. Cover and cook over medium heat for 5 minutes, or until the carrots start to soften.

3. Add the remaining $1^1/_4$ cups of broth and the vegetable juice, pepper, and barley or orzo to the skillet. Cover and cook over medium heat for about 15 minutes, or until the barley or orzo is tender. Add a little more broth if the mixture seems too dry.

4. Stir the parsley, mint, and lemon juice into the skillet mixture. Turn off the heat and allow the pan to sit covered for 5 minutes before serving.

NUTRITION FACTS (PER $1^1/_2$-CUP SERVING)

Calories: 297   Carbohydrates: 37 g   Fiber: 6 g   Protein: 23 g

Fat: 7 g   Sat. Fat: 2.7 g   Cholesterol: 53 mg   Sodium: 552 mg   Calcium: 52 mg

---

STEAMED FISH WITH GINGER SAUCE

YIELD: 2 SERVINGS

1 green tea bag

5 thin slices fresh ginger

2 large leaves napa or Chinese cabbage

2 fish fillets (4 to 5 ounces each), such as halibut, cod, pollock, or salmon

$^1/_3$ cup thinly sliced leek (white and light green parts)

$^1/_2$ cup julienne-cut carrots

2 teaspoons reduced-sodium soy sauce

SAUCE

1 tablespoon reduced-sodium soy sauce

1 teaspoon finely grated fresh ginger

$^1/_2$ teaspoon canola or untoasted sesame oil

1. Combine the sauce ingredients in a small bowl, and set aside.

2. Cut the tea bag open and sprinkle the tea into a 6-quart pot. Add the ginger slices. Then add a steamer basket and fill with enough water to reach within $^1/_2$ inch of the bottom of the basket.

3. Line the steamer basket with the cabbage leaves, and arrange the fish fillets over the leaves. Sprinkle half of the leeks and carrots over each fish fillet, and drizzle each one with 1 teaspoon of soy sauce.

4. Cover the pot and bring to a boil. Allow the fish to steam for about 10 minutes, or until it flakes easily with a fork.

5. Use a spatula to transfer the cabbage and fish to serving plates. Stir the sauce, and drizzle half over each fish fillet. Serve immediately.

NUTRITION FACTS (PER SERVING)

Calories: 129   Carbohydrates: 6 g   Fiber: 0.7 g   Protein: 23 g

Fat: 2.2 g   Sat. Fat: 0.6 g   Cholesterol: 54 mg   Sodium: 417 mg   Calcium: 40 mg

---

FISH PACKETS WITH PESTO AND PLUM TOMATOES

YIELD: 4 SERVINGS

4 white fish fillets (5 ounces each), such as cod, halibut, or grouper

¹/₄ cup Basil Pesto (page 282) or ready-made pesto

12 slices plum tomato (about 2 medium tomatoes)

¹/₂ teaspoon ground black pepper

1. Preheat the oven to 400°F.

2. Cut 4 sheets of aluminum foil, each about 15 inches long. Arrange the sheets of foil on a work surface, and center a fish fillet on the lower half of each sheet. Spread each fillet with a tablespoon of pesto, and top with 3 plum tomato slices and some black pepper.

3. Fold the top part of the foil over the lower part. Double-fold the edges together to tightly seal the packets. Arrange the packets on 2 rimmed baking sheets, spacing them evenly apart.

4. Bake for about 15 minutes, or until the packets are puffed and the fish flakes easily with a fork. (Open one packet with care, as very hot steam will escape, and test for doneness. The fish should be easy to flake with a fork. Reseal the packet if further cooking is necessary.)

5. Open the packets with care. Serve the fish and juices over whole wheat orzo or couscous, if desired.

VARIATIONS

❏ Substitute Lemon-Dill Sauce (see page 281) for the pesto.

❏ For an impressive presentation at the table, enclose the fish and tomatoes in parchment rather than aluminum foil. (See page 149 for directions.)

NUTRITION FACTS (PER SERVING)

Calories: 177   Carbohydrates: 2 g   Fiber: 0.6 g   Protein: 22 g

Fat: 8.6 g   Sat. Fat: 1.9 g   Cholesterol: 53 mg   Sodium: 188 mg   Calcium: 82 mg

---

WHITE FISH WITH TOMATOES, PEAS, AND PARSLEY SAUCE

YIELD: 2 SERVINGS

3 or 4 lemon slices

$1/2$ teaspoon coarsely ground black pepper

2 white fish fillets (4 ounces each), such as halibut or cod

1 medium fresh tomato, chopped

1 cup frozen green peas, thawed

$1/2$ cup chopped sweet white or red onion

1 teaspoon capers, drained

$1^1/2$ cups fresh arugula

SAUCE

1 tablespoon very finely chopped fresh parsley

1 tablespoon extra-virgin olive oil

$1/2$ teaspoon crushed garlic

2 tablespoons lemon juice

$1/8$ teaspoon salt

1. Pour 1 inch of water into a 6-quart pot, and add the lemon slices and pepper to the water. Place a steamer basket in the pot, and arrange the fish fillets in a single layer in the basket.

2. Cover the pot and bring it to a boil. Allow the fish to steam for 6 to 8 minutes, or until it turns opaque and flakes easily with a fork.

3. While the fish is cooking, combine the sauce ingredients in a small bowl and stir to mix. Set aside.

4. Place the fish in a bowl, and use a fork to break it into chunks. Add the tomato, peas, onion, and capers, and toss gently to mix.

5. Arrange half of the arugula leaves on each of two serving plates, and top each serving with half of the fish mixture. Drizzle the sauce over the top, and serve immediately.

NUTRITION FACTS (PER SERVING)

Calories: 275   Carbohydrates: 18 g   Fiber: 5.1 g   Protein: 29 g

Fat: 9.9 g   Sat. Fat: 1.4 g   Cholesterol: 36 mg   Sodium: 339 mg   Calcium: 101 mg

---

PRESTO PAELLA

YIELD: 5 SERVINGS

8 ounces turkey or chicken Italian sausage (hot or mild), with casings removed

$3/4$ cup chopped yellow onion

2 cups reduced-sodium chicken broth

$3/4$ cup diced fresh plum tomato

$1/2$ cup dry white wine

$1^1/2$ cups uncooked whole wheat orzo (about 9 ounces)

1 teaspoon crushed garlic

Scant $1/2$ teaspoon loosely packed saffron threads

$1/4$ teaspoon dried oregano

$3/4$ cup frozen green peas

12 ounces peeled and deveined medium raw shrimp

1. Coat a large deep skillet with cooking spray, and add the sausage and onion. Cover and cook over medium heat for about 5 minutes, stirring occasionally to crumble the sausage, until the meat is no longer pink and the onion softens.

2. Stir the broth, tomato, wine, orzo, garlic, saffron, and oregano into the sausage mixture, and bring to a boil. Adjust the heat to maintain a simmer, cover, and cook for about 10 minutes, or until most of the liquid has been absorbed and the orzo is almost tender.

3. Stir the peas into the skillet mixture, and return to a simmer. Cover and cook for 2 minutes. Stir in the shrimp and cook uncovered, stirring occasionally, for about 4 minutes, or until the shrimp turn opaque and are cooked through. Add a little more broth if needed.

4. Turn off the heat, cover the skillet, and allow the paella to sit for 5 minutes before serving.

NUTRITION FACTS (PER $1^1/2$-CUP SERVING)

Calories: 355   Carbohydrates: 43 g   Fiber: 8 g   Protein: 30 g

Fat: 5.3 g   Sat. Fat: 1.2 g   Cholesterol: 149 mg   Sodium: 649 mg   Calcium: 114 mg

---

WHITE BEAN CASSOULET

YIELD: 5 SERVINGS

2 tablespoons extra-virgin olive oil

3 cups sliced fresh mushrooms

2 medium yellow onions, thinly sliced and cut into quarter rings (about 1 1/2 cups)

2 carrots, halved lengthwise and thinly sliced (1 cup)

3/4 cup thinly sliced celery

2 teaspoons crushed garlic

2 teaspoons dried sage

1 teaspoon whole fennel seeds

1 teaspoon dried thyme

1/2 teaspoon salt

1/2 teaspoon ground black pepper

2 cups chopped fresh plum tomatoes (about 10 ounces)

3/4 cup vegetable juice, such as V-8

2 cans (15 ounces each) cannellini beans, drained

TOPPING

1 slice whole grain bread, torn into pieces

2 teaspoons crushed garlic

2 teaspoons extra-virgin olive oil

1. Preheat the oven to 350°F.

2. Place the olive oil in a large nonstick skillet, and add the next 10 ingredients (mushrooms through pepper). Cover and cook over medium heat for about 10 minutes, stirring occasionally, until the vegetables are tender.

3. Add the chopped tomato and vegetable juice to the skillet, cover, and cook for about 10 minutes, or until the tomatoes have cooked down into a sauce. Stir in the beans and cook uncovered for 3 to 5 minutes to thicken the sauce. Set aside.

4. To make the topping, place the bread, garlic, and olive oil in a food processor, and process into crumbs. Set aside.

5. Coat five 12-ounce ramekins with cooking spray, and divide the bean mixture among the ramekins. Top the bean mixture in each ramekin with some of the crumbs.

6. Bake uncovered for about 12 minutes, or until the crumbs are lightly toasted. Allow to sit for 5 minutes before serving. (Alternatively, bake in a 2-quart casserole dish for about 15 minutes.)

NUTRITION FACTS (PER 1 1/4-CUP SERVING)

Calories: 268   Carbohydrates: 38 g   Fiber: 10.4 g   Protein: 11.3 g

Fat: 9.1 g   Sat. Fat: 1.1 g   Cholesterol: 0 mg   Sodium: 406 mg   Calcium: 104 mg

RICE BOWL WITH EGGS AND EDAMAME

YIELD: 4 SERVINGS

1 cup uncooked brown rice

2¹/₂ cups no-salt-added vegetable broth, chicken broth, or coconut milk*

2 large eggs, beaten

2 cups sliced fresh mushrooms

1¹/₂ teaspoons finely grated fresh ginger

1 teaspoon crushed garlic

2 cups (moderately packed) thinly sliced fresh spinach

1¹/₂ cups cooked shelled edamame

2 to 3 tablespoons reduced-sodium soy sauce

¹/₃ cup thinly sliced scallions

¹/₃ cup julienne-cut carrots

---

*Use lower-fat coconut milk, with 4 to 5 grams of fat per cup. This is usually sold in cartons in the dairy case of grocery stores.

1. Cook the rice with the broth or coconut milk according to package directions, and set aside. Alternatively, make the rice the day before and refrigerate until needed.

2. Coat a large nonstick skillet with cooking spray, and preheat over medium heat. Pour the eggs into the skillet and swirl to evenly coat the bottom of the pan. Cook without stirring for a couple of minutes, or until firm. Slide the eggs onto a large cutting board, slice into thin strips, and set aside.

3. Respray the skillet and add the mushrooms. Cook uncovered over medium heat for about 4 minutes, or until the mushrooms are lightly browned. Add the ginger and garlic, and cook for 15 seconds more. Stir in the spinach and edamame, and cook for a couple of additional minutes, or just long enough to wilt the spinach and heat the edamame.

4. Add the reserved rice and eggs to the skillet mixture. Cook for a couple of minutes, stirring occasionally, to heat through.

5. Divide the mixture among 4 shallow bowls. Drizzle each serving with some of the soy sauce, and top with some of the scallions and carrots. Serve hot.

NUTRITION FACTS (PER 1¹/₂-CUP SERVING)

Calories: 341   Carbohydrates: 48 g   Fiber: 7 g   Protein: 20 g

Fat: 8 g   Sat. Fat: 1.2 g   Cholesterol: 104 mg   Sodium: 400 mg   Calcium: 97 mg

LENTILS WITH PORTABELLAS AND BROWN RICE

YIELD: 4 SERVINGS

1 cup dried brown lentils

2 1/4 cups no-salt-added chicken or vegetable broth

3/4 cup chopped yellow onion

Water for cooking

3 cups sliced baby portabella (cremini) mushrooms (8 ounces)

2 teaspoons crushed garlic

2 cups chopped fresh tomatoes (about 10 ounces)

1 teaspoon dried thyme

3/4 teaspoon salt

1/2 teaspoon ground black pepper

1 tablespoon extra-virgin olive oil

2 cups hot cooked brown rice (about 2/3 cup uncooked)

1/3 cup thinly sliced scallions

1. Place the lentils and broth in a 2-quart pot, and bring to a boil. Adjust the heat to maintain a simmer, cover, and cook for about 20 minutes, or until the lentils are tender but not mushy. Remove from the heat and set aside. (Do not drain.)

2. While the lentils are cooking, coat a large nonstick skillet with cooking spray, and add the onion and 2 tablespoons of water. Cover and cook over medium heat for about 4 minutes, or until the onion starts to soften.

3. Add the mushrooms to the skillet, cover, and cook for 3 minutes, or until the mushrooms soften. Remove the lid from the skillet, and cook for 3 additional minutes, or until the mushrooms are lightly browned. Add the garlic and cook for about 15 seconds, or just until fragrant.

4. Add the tomatoes, thyme, salt, and pepper to the skillet. Cover and cook for 3 minutes or until the tomatoes soften. Add the reserved undrained lentils and adjust the heat to maintain a simmer. Cook uncovered for about 8 minutes, or until most of the liquid evaporates. Stir in the olive oil.

5. For each serving, spread 1/2 cup of the rice in a shallow bowl and top with about 1 cup of the lentil mixture. Sprinkle with a quarter of the scallions, and serve hot.

VARIATION

❏ Serve the lentil mixture over Zucchini Noodles (page 267). spaghetti squash, or polenta instead of brown rice.

NUTRITION FACTS (PER SERVING)

Calories: 357   Carbohydrates: 60 g   Fiber: 19 g   Protein: 19 g

Fat: 5.3 g   Sat. Fat: 0.8 g   Cholesterol: 0 mg   Sodium: 362 mg   Calcium: 61 mg

MEXICAN BLACK BEAN AND RICE BOWL

YIELD: 4 SERVINGS

1½ teaspoons crushed garlic

2 cans (15 ounces each) reduced-sodium black beans, undrained

1 teaspoon chili powder

1 teaspoon ground cumin

2 cups hot cooked brown rice (about ⅔ cup uncooked)

1 cup diced avocado

1⅓ cups Cilantro Salsa (see page 282)

1½ cups shredded romaine lettuce

½ cup shredded reduced-fat Monterey Jack cheese or crumbled queso fresco

1. Coat a large nonstick skillet with cooking spray and add the garlic. Cook over medium heat for about 20 seconds, or until the garlic smells fragrant. Add the beans, chili powder, and cumin. Cook uncovered, stirring frequently, for 6 to 8 minutes, or until most of the liquid evaporates. Remove the skillet from the heat and cover to keep warm.

2. For each serving, place ½ cup of the rice in a shallow bowl and top with one-fourth of the beans. Place ¼ cup of the diced avocado on one side of the beans, and one-fourth of the salsa on the other side. Sprinkle a quarter of the lettuce and cheese over the top, and serve immediately.

NUTRITION FACTS (PER SERVING)

Calories: 441 Carbohydrates: 62 g Fiber: 16 g Protein: 21 g

Fat: 12.5 g Sat. Fat: 2.5 g Cholesterol: 10 mg Sodium: 468 mg Calcium: 230 mg

---

AGE-*LESS* TIP—
CHOOSING THE BEST FOODS FOR YOUR PANTRY

Although it is generally best to choose foods that have been processed as little as possible, not all processed foods are high in AGEs. Don't hesitate to use plant-based products such as canned beans, brown rice, frozen vegetables, rolled oats, and whole grain pasta, which are convenient, high in nutrients, and very appropriate for your AGE-less diet.

Main Event Salads

I t's hard to beat the ease and versatility of a main dish salad. Many colorful and delicious salads can be created in a matter of minutes using a variety of handy ingredients. Salads are perfect for the AGE-less diet, since plant foods are naturally very low in AGEs. Additionally, plant foods are chock-full of age-defying nutrients and antioxidants that boost the benefits of your AGE-less lifestyle.

This chapter offers an array of sensational main dish salads that are perfect for an AGE-less lunch or dinner. AGEs are kept within reasonable limits by starting out with generous amounts of vegetables and then adding other wholesome ingredients such as fresh fruits, whole grains, and whole grain pasta. Light dressings, herbs, and spices infuse delectable flavors. Notably, these recipes also feature reduced-fat cheeses as well as lean meats, poultry, and seafood prepared the AGE-less way, with moist-heat cooking methods. Just as important, several salads cast legumes such as chickpeas, cannellini beans, edamame (young soybeans), or lentils in starring roles. These low-AGE ingredients provide generous amounts of high-quality protein, making them satisfying and delicious alternatives to higher-AGE meats, poultry, and fish.

FRESH HERB CHICKEN SALAD

YIELD: 4 SERVINGS

2 cups shredded or chopped Basic Poached Chicken (page 224)

1$\frac{1}{2}$ cups frozen green peas, thawed

$\frac{1}{2}$ cup finely chopped celery

$\frac{1}{2}$ cup thinly sliced scallions

$\frac{1}{2}$ cup finely chopped fresh parsley

1 to 2 teaspoons finely chopped fresh lemon thyme or other thyme

DRESSING

2 tablespoons extra-virgin olive oil

1$\frac{1}{2}$ tablespoons white wine vinegar

1$\frac{1}{2}$ tablespoons lemon juice

1 tablespoon orange juice

2 teaspoons Dijon mustard

$\frac{1}{4}$ teaspoon salt

$\frac{1}{4}$ teaspoon ground black pepper

1. Place the chicken, peas, celery, scallions, parsley, and thyme in a large bowl, and toss to mix.

2. Place the dressing ingredients in a small bowl, and whisk to combine. Pour the dressing over the chicken mixture, and toss to coat evenly.

3. Set the salad aside for 15 minutes, or cover the bowl and chill until ready to serve. If desired, serve the salad in leaves of butterhead lettuce.

NUTRITION FACTS (PER SERVING)

Calories: 228   Carbohydrates: 12 g   Fiber: 3.5 g   Protein: 24 g
Fat: 9.5 g   Sat. Fat: 1.6 g   Cholesterol: 55 mg   Sodium: 338 mg   Calcium: 5 mg

AGE-*LESS* TIP—PREPARING CHICKEN FOR YOUR SALADS AND SANDWICHES

When cooking chicken for healthy AGE-less salads and sandwiches, poach a boneless skinless chicken breast in a liquid that includes lemon juice. The liquid and acidic juice will reduce the creation of further AGEs while making the meat moist and flavorful.

GREEK CHICKEN CHOPPED SALAD

YIELD: 2 SERVINGS

6 cups chopped or shredded romaine lettuce

1 cup chopped tomato

1 cup chopped cucumber

1 cup chopped or shredded Basic Poached Chicken (page 224)

$1/_2$ cup chopped red onion

$1/_4$ cup chopped Kalamata or black olives

3 tablespoons chopped Greek salad peppers (pepperoncini) or banana peppers

3 tablespoons crumbled reduced-fat feta cheese

2 teaspoons capers, drained

DRESSING

2 tablespoons extra-virgin olive oil

2 tablespoons red wine vinegar

$1/_4$ teaspoon coarsely ground black pepper

$1/_4$ teaspoon salt

1. Place the lettuce, tomato, cucumber, chicken, onion, olives, peppers, feta cheese, and capers in a large bowl, and toss to mix.

2. Place the dressing ingredients in a small bowl, and whisk to combine. Pour the dressing over the salad mixture, and toss to coat evenly. Serve immediately.

VARIATIONS

❏ Substitute Shrimp Poached in White Wine (page 226) for the chicken.

❏ Substitute grilled chicken marinated in Lemon-Caper Marinade (page 285) or Lemon-Pepper Marinade (page 287).

NUTRITION FACTS (PER SERVING)

Calories: 342   Carbohydrates: 15 g   Fiber: 4.9 g   Protein: 26 g

Fat: 20 g   Sat. Fat: 2.6 g   Cholesterol: 54 mg   Sodium: 683 mg   Calcium: 75 mg

Perfectly Poached Chicken and Seafood

Delectable poached foods are featured in the world's finest cuisines. One of the easiest cooking methods, poaching is also ideal for keeping AGE formation to a minimum. Below you'll find the basic steps for preparing poached chicken and seafood that can be used in tempting main course salads.

BASIC POACHED CHICKEN

Follow this recipe whenever you need cooked chicken for salads, sandwiches, or other recipes. Poached chicken can also be thinly sliced and served as a simple entrée with a zesty topping such as Chimichurri Sauce (page 280) or Cilantro Salsa (page 282).

YIELD: 4 SERVINGS (EACH ABOUT $1/2$ CUP CHOPPED)

1 pound boneless skinless chicken breast halves, cut into 4 equal pieces

$1/4$ cup lemon juice

$3/4$ teaspoon salt

$3/4$ teaspoon coarsely ground black pepper

1. Place the chicken in a nonreactive pot or a deep skillet (such as non-stick, ceramic, enamel, or stainless steel) that is large enough to hold the chicken in a single layer. Add enough water to completely cover the chicken (about 2 cups), and add the lemon juice, salt, and pepper.

2. Bring the water to a simmer over medium heat. Adjust the heat to maintain a low simmer so that a few bubbles rise to the surface of the liquid every few seconds. Cover and cook for about 20 minutes or until done. (An instant-read thermometer inserted in the thickest part should register at least 165°F.) During cooking, periodically skim off and discard any froth that rises to the surface.

3. Transfer the chicken to a plate, draining off the poaching liquid, and allow the chicken to sit for at least 5 minutes. Then dice or shred as needed for your recipe.

VARIATIONS

❏ To make Classic French Poached Chicken, add 1 medium carrot (quartered), 1 medium rib celery with leaves (quartered), 3 sprigs flat-leaf parsley (or 1 teaspoon dried), 3 sprigs fresh thyme (or 1 teaspoon dried), and 2 bay leaves to the poaching liquid, and cook as directed.

❑ To make Green Tea and Ginger Poached Chicken, add 6 thin slices (each about $\frac{1}{8}$-inch thick) fresh ginger plus the contents of 1 green tea bag to the poaching liquid. Substitute $\frac{1}{4}$ teaspoon ground white pepper for the black pepper, and cook as directed.

❑ To make Southwestern Poached Chicken, substitute lime juice for the lemon juice, and add 2 teaspoons of ground cumin and 1 sprig of fresh oregano (or $\frac{1}{4}$ teaspoon dried) to the poaching liquid. Cook as directed.

NUTRITION FACTS (PER SERVING)
Calories: 129 Carbohydrate: 0 g   Fiber: 0 g   Protein: 24 g

Fat: 2.9 g   Sat. Fat: 0.6 g   Cholesterol: 73 mg   Sodium: 349 mg   Calcium: 6 mg

---

FISH POACHED IN WHITE WINE

Use this basic recipe when you need cooked seafood for salads or other recipes. Or serve the fish as a simple entrée with a zesty topping such as Lemon-Dill Sauce (page 281), Lemon-Parsley Sauce (page 280), or Tomato and Caper Salsa (page 283).

YIELD: 4 SERVINGS

1$\frac{1}{2}$ cups dry white wine	$\frac{1}{4}$ teaspoon salt
1 cup water	4 slices of lemon (each $\frac{1}{4}$-inch thick)
2 to 3 bay leaves	4 firm-fleshed fish fillets or steaks (4 to 5 ounces each), such as salmon or grouper
$\frac{1}{2}$ teaspoon coarsely ground black pepper	

1. Place the wine, water, bay leaves, pepper, salt, and lemon slices in a large nonstick skillet. Cover and bring to a boil. Reduce the heat to maintain a low simmer, and cook covered for 5 minutes.

2. Add the fish to the skillet. Cover and cook for 6 to 8 minutes, or until the fish turns opaque throughout and flakes easily with a fork.

3. Using a spatula, transfer the fish to a plate, draining off any poaching liquid. Serve warm or chilled.

NUTRITION FACTS (PER SERVING)
Calories: 161   Carbohydrates: 0 g   Fiber: 0 g   Protein: 22.5 g

Fat: 7.2 g   Sat. Fat: 1.1 g   Cholesterol: 62 mg   Sodium: 207 mg   Calcium: 16 mg

VARIATION

❏ To make Shrimp Poached in White Wine, substitute 1 pound peeled and deveined raw shrimp for the fish fillets. Poach for about 4 minutes or until the shrimp turn opaque and are cooked through. Drain and serve warm or chilled.

NUTRITION FACTS (PER SERVING)

Calories: 96   Carbohydrates: 0 g   Fiber: 0 g   Protein: 23 g

Fat: 0.6 g   Sat. Fat: 0.1 g   Cholesterol: 182 mg   Sodium: 122 mg   Calcium: 73 mg

BERRY DELICIOUS CHICKEN SALAD

YIELD: 4 SERVINGS

12 cups mixed baby salad greens

2 cups shredded or thinly sliced Basic Poached Chicken (page 224)

1 cup sliced fresh strawberries

$1/_2$ cup fresh blueberries

$1/_4$ cup plus 2 tablespoons chopped walnuts (unroasted)

$1/_4$ cup plus 2 tablespoons crumbled reduced-fat feta or blue cheese

DRESSING

$1/_4$ cup extra-virgin olive oil

2 tablespoons balsamic vinegar

2 tablespoons orange juice

2 teaspoons Dijon mustard

$1/_2$ teaspoon salt

$1/_2$ teaspoon ground black pepper

1. Place all of the dressing ingredients in a small bowl, and whisk to combine. Set aside.

2. Place the salad greens, chicken, and berries in a large bowl. Drizzle with the dressing, and toss to coat evenly.

3. Divide the salad greens mixture among 4 serving plates. Top each serving with one-fourth of the walnuts and cheese, and serve immediately.

VARIATIONS

❏ Substitute 1 cup thinly sliced apple plus $1/_2$ cup halved seedless grapes for the berries, and white wine vinegar for the balsamic vinegar in the dressing.

❑ Substitute grilled chicken marinated in Lemon-Pepper Marinade (page 287) or Zesty Herb Marinade (page 285) for the poached chicken.

NUTRITION FACTS (PER SERVING)
Calories: 357   Carbohydrates: 12 g   Fiber: 3 g   Protein: 26 g
Fat: 23 g   Sat. Fat: 3 g   Cholesterol: 54 mg   Sodium: 584 mg   Calcium: 48 mg

WALDORF CHICKEN SALAD

YIELD: 4 SERVINGS

2 cups shredded or chopped Basic or Green Tea and Ginger Poached Chicken (pages 224 and 225)

1 cup diced unpeeled red-skinned apple

$^1/_2$ cup thinly sliced celery

$^1/_3$ cup dark raisins

$^1/_3$ cup chopped walnuts (unroasted)

$^1/_4$ cup nonfat or low-fat plain Greek-style yogurt

$^1/_4$ cup low-fat mayonnaise

12 leaves butterhead lettuce

1. Place the chicken, apple, celery, raisins, and walnuts in a medium-size bowl, and toss to mix.

2. Place the yogurt and mayonnaise in a small bowl, and stir to combine. Add the yogurt mixture to the chicken mixture, and toss to coat evenly.

3. For each serving, arrange 3 lettuce leaves on a serving plate and top with $1^1/_8$ cups of the chicken salad. Alternatively, fill the leaves with the chicken salad to make lettuce wraps, or serve the salad in whole grain pita pockets.

VARIATIONS

❑ Omit the raisins and substitute seedless red grapes for the apples.

❑ Add a teaspoon of curry powder to the mayonnaise mixture.

NUTRITION FACTS (PER SERVING)
Calories: 244   Carbohydrates: 19 g   Fiber: 2.5 g   Protein: 23 g
Fat: 9.1 g   Sat. Fat: 1.4 g   Cholesterol: 56 mg   Sodium: 200 mg   Calcium: 39 mg

SHRIMP COBB SALAD

YIELD: 4 SERVINGS

12 cups torn or shredded romaine lettuce or torn Boston lettuce

$1/_2$ cup plus 2 tablespoons bottled light olive oil vinaigrette salad dressing

1 recipe Shrimp Poached in White Wine (page 226), or 2 cups boiled or steamed shrimp, chilled

$1^1/_3$ cups frozen (thawed) or fresh-cooked whole kernel corn

$1^1/_3$ cups diced tomatoes (about 2 medium)

$1^1/_3$ cups diced avocado (about 2 medium)

$2/_3$ cup chopped red onion

$1/_4$ cup plus 2 tablespoons crumbled reduced-fat blue cheese

2 hard-boiled eggs

1. Place the lettuce in a large bowl and toss with $1/_2$ cup of the dressing.

2. Divide the lettuce among 4 serving plates. Top each salad with one-fourth of the shrimp, corn, tomatoes, avocado, onion, blue cheese, and egg.

3. Drizzle $1^1/_2$ teaspoons of the remaining dressing over each salad, and serve immediately.

NUTRITION FACTS (PER SERVING)

Calories: 408   Carbohydrates: 27 g   Fiber: 8 g   Protein: 33 g

Fat: 21 g   Sat. Fat: 4.7 g   Cholesterol: 281 mg   Sodium: 627 mg   Calcium: 201 mg

AGE-Less-Style Grilled Salad Toppers

Poaching or steaming is the very best option for cooking meats, poultry, and seafood. But sometimes you want a piece of grilled chicken or fish to top a main dish salad. Here is where marinades can come to the rescue. Not only do they add delicious flavor, but they can also reduce AGEs in grilled foods by up to 50 percent. AGE-less marinade recipes begin on page 285.

A tabletop grill (such as a George Foreman Grill) is a good option for grilling. Its nonstick surface forms fewer AGES than a metal surface, and it cooks food in about half the time compared with a broiler or barbecue grill. Boneless skinless chicken breasts will cook in about 4 to 5 minutes (the thickest part should reach at least 165°F). Fish filets will take 3 to 4 minutes, depending on the thickness. You'll know the fish is done when it turns opaque and can be easily flaked with a fork.

SPEEDY TACO SALAD

YIELD: 4 SERVINGS

12 ounces ground turkey, chicken, or beef (at least 93% lean)

$1/_2$ cup chopped yellow onion

1 cup cooked or canned black or pinto beans, drained

1 to $1^1/_4$ cups chunky-style salsa

10 cups shredded romaine lettuce

$1^1/_3$ cups chopped tomato

$1^1/_3$ cups frozen (thawed) or fresh-cooked whole kernel corn

1 cup sliced scallions

1 medium-large avocado, coarsely mashed

$1/_2$ cup shredded reduced-fat Monterey Jack cheese

1. Coat a large nonstick skillet with cooking spray. Add the ground meat and onion, and use a spatula to break up the meat. Cover and cook over medium heat, stirring occasionally to crumble, for about 6 minutes, or until the meat is no longer pink.

2. Add the beans and salsa to the skillet and bring the mixture to a boil. Adjust the heat to maintain a simmer, cover, and cook for 5 minutes. Remove the lid and cook for an additional 2 minutes, or until any excess liquid has evaporated. Set aside.

3. Place the lettuce, tomato, corn, and scallions in a large bowl, and toss to mix. For each salad, transfer one-fourth of the lettuce mixture to a shallow serving bowl. Top with one-fourth of the taco mixture (about $7/_8$ cup), and garnish with one-fourth of the avocado and cheese. Serve immediately.

NUTRITION FACTS (PER SERVING)

Calories: 362   Carbohydrates: 34 g   Fiber: 12.1 g   Protein: 29 g
Fat: 15.6 g   Sat. Fat: 5.2 g   Cholesterol: 70 mg   Sodium: 624 mg   Calcium: 199 mg

---

AGE-*LESS* TIP—
CHOOSING AND USING CHEESE

Since cheese is relatively high in AGEs, care must be taken in choosing and using this flavorful product. Whenever possible, select "light" or "reduced-fat" cheese, as it is lower in AGEs than its full-fat counterpart. Then heat the cheese just until it melts—or not at all—to limit the creation of further AGEs.

QUINOA SHRIMP SALAD

YIELD: 5 SERVINGS

1 cup uncooked quinoa

1 recipe Shrimp Poached in White Wine (page 226), or 2 cups boiled or steamed medium-size shrimp, chilled

3 cups (moderately packed) thinly sliced fresh spinach

1 cup diced grape tomatoes

$^3/_4$ cup thinly sliced scallions

2 tablespoons finely chopped fresh dill

$^1/_3$ cup crumbled reduced-fat feta cheese

DRESSING

3 tablespoons lemon juice

3 tablespoons extra-virgin olive oil

$1^1/_2$ teaspoons crushed garlic

$^1/_2$ teaspoon salt

$^1/_2$ teaspoon ground black pepper

1. Prepare the quinoa according to package directions. Chill before proceeding with the recipe.

2. Place the quinoa, shrimp, spinach, tomatoes, scallions, and dill in a large bowl, and toss to mix.

3. Place all of the dressing ingredients in a small bowl, and whisk to combine. Pour the dressing over the salad, and toss to coat evenly. Serve immediately, or cover and refrigerate until ready to serve. Toss in the feta cheese just before serving.

VARIATION

❑ Substitute whole wheat couscous or orzo for the quinoa.

❑ Substitute 2 cups canned or cooked (drained) cannellini beans for the shrimp.

❑ Substitute 2 cups cooked (drained) French green lentils (lentils du Puy) for the shrimp.

NUTRITION FACTS (PER SERVING)

Calories: 288   Carbohydrates: 26 g   Fiber: 3.6 g   Protein: 19 g

Fat: 12.4 g   Sat. Fat: 1.5 g   Cholesterol: 100 mg   Sodium: 461 mg   Calcium: 92 mg

TUSCAN TUNA SALAD

YIELD: 4 SERVINGS

4 ounces uncooked whole grain penne pasta (about 1$^1/_2$ cups), or $^2/_3$ cup uncooked farro

10 cups torn romaine lettuce or escarole

1$^1/_4$ cups grape tomatoes, quartered lengthwise

1$^1/_4$ cups coarsely chopped marinated artichoke hearts, drained

$^3/_4$ cup thin slivers red onion

$^1/_3$ cup chopped Kalamata or black olives

2 cans (5 ounces each) tuna in water, drained

DRESSING

3 tablespoons extra-virgin olive oil

2 tablespoons white wine vinegar

1 tablespoon lemon juice

1 teaspoon Dijon mustard

$^1/_2$ teaspoon coarsely ground black pepper

$^1/_4$ teaspoon salt

1. Cook the pasta or farro according to package directions. Drain and chill before proceeding with the recipe.

2. Place the lettuce, tomatoes, artichoke hearts, onion, olives, and cooked pasta or farro in a large bowl, and toss to mix.

3. Place the dressing ingredients in a small bowl, and whisk to combine. Pour the dressing over the salad, and toss to coat evenly.

4. Separate the tuna into chunks. Add to the salad, and toss gently to mix. Divide the salad among 4 serving plates and serve immediately.

NUTRITION FACTS (PER SERVING)

Calories: 341   Carbohydrates: 31 g   Fiber: 6.8 g   Protein: 21 g
Fat: 16 g   Sat. Fat: 1.5 g   Cholesterol: 20 mg   Sodium: 603 mg   Calcium: 54 mg

---

SALMON SALAD NIÇOISE

YIELD: 4 SERVINGS

2$^1/_2$ cups $^3/_4$-inch chunks unpeeled new potatoes (about 12 ounces)

2 cups (1$^1/_2$-inch pieces) fresh green beans

10 cups torn Boston, romaine, or escarole lettuce

1 cup halved cherry or grape tomatoes

4 slices red onion, cut into quarter-rings

2 cans (5 ounces each) low-sodium water-packed boneless, skinless salmon, drained, or 2 cups poached salmon (see Fish Poached in White Wine, page 225)

2 hard-boiled eggs, quartered lengthwise

$^1/_3$ cup coarsely chopped Niçoise or Kalamata olives

2 tablespoons capers, drained

DRESSING

$^1/_4$ cup extra-virgin olive oil

2 tablespoons lemon juice

1 tablespoon Dijon mustard

$^1/_2$ teaspoon salt

$^1/_2$ teaspoon ground black pepper

1. Place the dressing ingredients in a small bowl, and whisk to combine. Set aside.

2. Place a steamer basket in a 4-quart pot, and fill with enough water to reach within $^1/_2$ inch of the bottom of the basket. Place the potatoes in the basket, cover, and bring to a boil. Steam the potatoes for about 10 minutes, or until tender when pierced with a fork. Transfer to a bowl, toss with 2 teaspoons of the dressing, and set aside.

3. Place the green beans in the steamer basket, and cook for about 4 minutes, or until crisp-tender. Transfer to a bowl, toss with 2 teaspoons of the dressing, and set aside.

4. Place the lettuce, tomatoes, and onion in a large bowl. Drizzle with $^1/_4$ cup of the dressing, and toss to coat evenly.

5. For each serving, place one-fourth of the lettuce mixture on a plate. Separate the salmon into chunks, and mound one-fourth of the salmon in the center of the lettuce. Drizzle the salmon with a quarter of the remaining dressing (about 1 teaspoon). Then mound one-fourth of the potatoes and green beans on opposite sides of the salmon, and place 2 egg quarters on the other sides. Sprinkle one-fourth of the olives and capers over each salad, and serve immediately.

NUTRITION FACTS (PER SERVING)

Calories: 346   Carbohydrates: 25 g   Fiber: 5 g   Protein: 18 g

Fat: 20.5 g   Sat. Fat: 3.3 g   Cholesterol: 113 mg   Sodium: 693 mg   Calcium: 94 mg

GREAT GARBANZO SALAD

YIELD: 4 SERVINGS

$1/_2$ cup uncooked whole wheat orzo

1 can (15 ounces) reduced-sodium chickpeas (garbanzo beans), drained, or $1^1/_2$ cups cooked chickpeas

1 cup diced peeled and seeded cucumber

1 cup chopped plum tomatoes or diced grape tomatoes

$3/_4$ cup chopped red onion

$1/_3$ cup chopped Kalamata olives

$1/_4$ cup finely chopped fresh basil

1 cup diced fresh mozzarella cheese (4 ounces)

8 cups torn or shredded romaine lettuce

DRESSING

3 tablespoons extra-virgin olive oil

3 tablespoons lemon juice

1 teaspoon crushed garlic

$1/_2$ teaspoon salt

$1/_2$ teaspoon ground black pepper

1. Cook the orzo according to package directions. Drain, rinse with cool water, and drain again.

2. Place the orzo in a large bowl. Add the chickpeas, cucumber, tomato, onion, olives, and basil, and toss to mix.

3. Place the dressing ingredients in a small bowl, and whisk to combine. Pour the dressing over the orzo mixture, and toss to coat evenly. Allow to sit for 5 minutes.

4. Toss the mozzarella cheese and lettuce into the salad. Divide the mixture among 4 shallow bowls or serving plates, and serve immediately.

NUTRITION FACTS (PER SERVING)

Calories: 348   Carbohydrates: 32 g   Fiber: 8.3 g   Protein: 13 g

Fat: 19 g   Sat. Fat: 4.6 g   Cholesterol: 20 mg   Sodium: 581 mg   Calcium: 212 mg

WARM WHITE BEAN SALAD

YIELD: 2 SERVINGS

1 cup sliced leeks (white and light green parts) or sliced yellow onion, cut into quarter rings

1 medium-large red bell pepper, cut into quarter rings

$1/4$ teaspoon ground black pepper

Water for cooking

$1^1/4$ teaspoons crushed garlic

1 cup canned or cooked cannellini beans, drained

6 cups spinach or arugula

$1/4$ cup chopped Kalamata olives

3 tablespoons crumbled reduced-fat feta or goat cheese

DRESSING

2 tablespoons extra-virgin olive oil

1 tablespoon white wine vinegar

1 tablespoon orange juice

1 teaspoon Dijon mustard

$1/4$ teaspoon salt

$1/4$ teaspoon ground black pepper

1. Place all of the dressing ingredients in a small bowl, and whisk to combine. Set aside.

2. Coat a large nonstick skillet with cooking spray, and add the leek or onion, bell pepper, black pepper, and 2 tablespoons of water. Cover and cook over medium heat, stirring occasionally, for about 6 minutes, or until the vegetables are tender and just beginning to brown. Watch closely during the last few minutes of cooking, and reduce the heat if necessary to prevent scorching.

3. Add the garlic to the skillet mixture, and cook for about 15 seconds or until the garlic smells fragrant. Stir in the beans, cover, and cook for another minute to heat through. Set aside.

4. Place the salad greens in a large bowl, and toss with 3 tablespoons of the dressing. Divide the mixture between 2 serving plates. Top the greens on each plate with half of the warm bean mixture, and drizzle with half of the remaining dressing. Sprinkle each salad with half of the olives and cheese, and serve immediately.

NUTRITION FACTS (PER SERVING)

Calories: 352   Carbohydrates: 36 g   Fiber: 9 g   Protein: 11 g

Fat: 19 g   Sat. Fat: 3.5 g   Cholesterol: 5 mg   Sodium: 766 mg   Calcium: 136 mg

---

EDAMAME SPINACH SALAD

Yield: 2 servings

1 cup fresh or frozen shelled edamame

6 cups (moderately packed) fresh baby spinach leaves

²/₃ cup chopped fresh broccoli florets or julienne-cut carrots

¹/₂ cup diagonally sliced scallions

2 tablespoons dried sweetened cranberries

2 tablespoons pumpkin seeds (unroasted)

2 tablespoons sunflower seeds (unroasted)

¹/₄ cup plus 2 tablespoons shredded reduced-fat white Cheddar or Gouda cheese, or 3 tablespoons crumbled reduced-fat goat cheese

DRESSING

1 tablespoon plus 1 teaspoon extra-virgin olive oil

1 tablespoon plus 1 teaspoon lemon juice

1 tablespoon plus 1 teaspoon orange juice

¹/₄ teaspoon salt

¹/₄ teaspoon ground black pepper

1. Cook the edamame according to package directions. Drain and set aside for about 10 minutes to cool.

2. Place the spinach, edamame, broccoli or carrots, and scallions in a large bowl, and toss to mix.

3. Place all of the dressing ingredients in a small bowl, and whisk to combine. Pour the dressing over the salad, and toss to coat evenly.

4. Divide the salad between 2 serving plates. Top each salad with half of the dried cranberries, pumpkin and sunflower seeds, and cheese. Serve immediately.

Nutrition Facts (Per Serving)

Calories 394   Carbohydrates: 25 g   Fiber: 9 g   Protein: 26 g

Fat: 23.8 g   Sat. Fat: 4.7 g   Cholesterol: 15 mg   Sodium: 565 mg   Calcium: 335 mg

---

COLORFUL LENTIL SALAD

YIELD: 4 SERVINGS

1 cup dried French green lentils (lentils du Puy) or brown lentils, or $2^{1}/_{2}$ cups precooked lentils, drained

$2^{1}/_{4}$ cups no-salt-added vegetable or chicken broth

1 cup chopped fresh parsley, or 2 cups (moderately packed) thinly sliced fresh spinach

1 cup sliced scallions

1 cup julienne-cut carrots

$^{1}/_{4}$ cup chopped walnuts (unroasted)

3 tablespoons crumbled reduced-fat feta cheese

DRESSING

2 tablespoons extra-virgin olive oil

2 tablespoons lemon juice

1 teaspoon crushed garlic

1 teaspoon Dijon mustard

$^{1}/_{2}$ teaspoon salt

$^{1}/_{2}$ teaspoon ground black pepper

1. If using dried lentils, place the lentils and broth in a 2-quart pot, and bring to a boil. Reduce the heat to maintain a simmer, cover, and cook for about 30 minutes for French green lentils or 20 minutes for brown lentils, or until the lentils are tender but not mushy. Drain off the excess liquid and allow to cool before proceeding with the recipe.

2. Place the cooked lentils, parsley or spinach, scallions, and carrots in a large bowl, and toss to mix.

3. Place the dressing ingredients in a small bowl, and whisk to combine. Pour the dressing over the salad, and toss to coat evenly.

4. Divide the salad among 4 serving plates. Top each serving with one-fourth of the walnuts and feta cheese, and serve immediately.

NUTRITION FACTS (PER SERVING)

Calories: 325   Carbohydrates: 37 g   Fiber: 17 g   Protein: 17 g

Fat: 13.4 g   Sat. Fat: 1.5 g   Cholesterol: 2 mg   Sodium: 476 mg   Calcium: 85 mg

---

﴾oups and Stews

It's hard to beat a steaming bowl of soup or stew for a versatile, economical, and comforting meal. Now you can add AGE-less to this list of virtues. In fact, soups and stews are naturals for AGE-less dining. Simmering meats, poultry, or seafood in a savory broth is an ideal cooking method for minimizing AGE formation. Just as important, these tempting dishes often have the perfect balance of ingredients for AGE-less meal planning—moderate portions of lean protein combined with generous amounts of nutrient-packed vegetables, legumes, whole grains, and flavorful herbs and spices. And, of course, many soups develop great taste without including any meat, poultry, or fish at all. This keeps AGEs super-low.

The following pages provide a variety of soups and stews. All are easy to prepare, and some even make use of the slow cooker, which can create a full-flavored meal while you enjoy time outside the kitchen. So whether you are looking for a cup of soup to pair with a sandwich or salad, or a hearty stew for a one-dish meal, here you will find a wealth of ideas that are perfect for your AGE-less plan.

HOME-STYLE CHICKEN SOUP

YIELD: 8 SERVINGS

1¹/₂ cups diced carrots

¹/₂ cup chopped onion

¹/₂ cup chopped celery

4¹/₂ cups no-salt-added chicken broth

2 teaspoons crushed garlic

1 teaspoon salt

¹/₄ teaspoon ground white pepper

12 ounces boneless skinless chicken breast, cut into 2 pieces

3 ounces whole grain rotini pasta (about 1¹/₂ cups), orzo (about ¹/₂ cup), or broken spaghetti or fettuccini (about 1¹/₂ cups)

³/₄ cup frozen green peas

3 tablespoons finely chopped fresh parsley, or 1 tablespoon dried parsley

1. Place the first 7 ingredients (carrots through white pepper) in a 4-quart pot, and bring the mixture to a boil.

2. Add the chicken to the pot, and adjust the heat to maintain a simmer. Cover and cook for 25 minutes. (An instant-read thermometer inserted in the thickest part of the chicken should read at least 165°F.) Transfer the chicken to a cutting board, and set aside.

3. Use a slotted spoon to transfer 1 cup of the vegetables to a blender. Add about 1¹/₂ cups of the broth, and carefully blend at low speed until smooth. Return the mixture to the pot.

4. Bring the soup to a boil and add the pasta. Adjust the heat to maintain a simmer, cover, and cook for 5 minutes.

5. While the pasta is cooking, use two forks to pull the chicken into small pieces. Add the shredded chicken to the pot along with the peas. Cover and simmer until the pasta is done and the peas are heated through.

6. Sir the parsley into the soup, and remove the pot from the heat. Allow to sit covered for 2 minutes before serving.

NUTRITION FACTS (PER 1-CUP SERVING)

Calories: 136   Carbohydrates: 16 g   Fiber: 3.2 g   Protein: 14.5 g

Fat: 1.8 g   Sat. Fat: 0.3 g   Cholesterol: 31 mg   Sodium: 427 mg   Calcium: 30 mg

---

CHICKEN TORTILLA SOUP

YIELD: 6 SERVINGS

1 medium yellow onion, cut into thin wedges (about 1 cup)

$^1/_2$ cup diced carrots

$2^1/_2$ cups no-salt-added chicken broth, divided

1 can (14$^1/_2$ ounces) Mexican-style tomatoes with green chilies, undrained and puréed in a blender

$^3/_4$ teaspoon ground cumin

$^3/_4$ teaspoon dried oregano

Scant $^1/_2$ teaspoon salt

$^1/_4$ teaspoon ground black pepper

10 ounces boneless skinless chicken breast, cut into 2 pieces

1 cup fresh or frozen whole kernel corn

1 medium zucchini, quartered lengthwise and sliced (about 1 cup)

TORTILLA STRIPS

4 corn tortillas (5-inch rounds), cut into 1 x $^1/_2$-inch strips

Olive oil cooking spray

$^1/_8$ teaspoon salt

1. To make the tortilla strips, preheat the oven to 350°F. Coat a baking sheet with cooking spray, and arrange the strips in a single layer on the sheet. Spray the strips lightly with the cooking spray and sprinkle with the salt. Bake for about 8 minutes, or just until crisp. Remove from the oven and set aside.

2. Place the onion, carrots, and $^1/_2$ cup of the broth in a 4-quart pot. Cover and cook over medium heat for 5 minutes, or until the vegetables soften.

3. Add the remaining 2 cups of broth and the tomatoes, cumin, oregano, salt, and pepper to the pot, and bring to a boil.

4. Add the chicken to the boiling soup, and adjust the heat to maintain a simmer. Cover and cook for 25 minutes. (An instant-read thermometer inserted in the thickest part of the chicken should read at least 165°F.) Transfer the chicken to a cutting board, and set aside.

5. Add the corn and zucchini to the pot, cover, and simmer for about 7 minutes, or until tender. While the vegetables are cooking, use two forks to pull the chicken into small pieces. Add the shredded chicken to the pot.

6. Serve the soup hot, topping each serving with some of the prepared tortilla strips.

NUTRITION FACTS (PER 1-CUP SERVING WITH TORTILLA STRIPS)

Calories: 141   Carbohydrates: 18 g   Fiber: 3.1 g   Protein: 13 g

Fat: 2 g   Sat. Fat: 0.4 g   Cholesterol: 30 mg   Sodium: 392 mg   Calcium: 41 mg

---

FIESTA CHILI

YIELD: 8 SERVINGS

1 pound ground beef or turkey (at least 93% lean)

1 cup chopped yellow onion

1 can (14$^1/_2$ ounces) diced tomatoes with green chilies, undrained

2 cans (8 ounces each) no-salt-added tomato sauce

2 tablespoons chili powder

1 teaspoon ground cumin

$^3/_4$ teaspoon dried oregano

Scant $^1/_2$ teaspoon salt

2 cans (15 ounces each) dark red kidney beans, drained (reserve $^1/_2$ cup of the liquid)

1$^1/_4$ cups fresh or frozen whole kernel corn

1. Coat a 4-quart pot with cooking spray, and add the ground meat and onion. Cover and cook over medium heat, stirring occasionally to crumble, for about 8 minutes, or until the meat is no longer pink.

2. Add the tomatoes, tomato sauce, chili powder, cumin, oregano, and salt to the pot, and bring the mixture to a boil. Adjust the heat to maintain a simmer, cover, and cook for 20 minutes, stirring occasionally.

3. Stir the beans, corn, and $^1/_4$ cup of the reserved bean liquid into the soup. Cover and simmer for 10 minutes, adding more of the reserved liquid if needed. Taste the chili and add a little more salt, if needed. Serve hot.

NUTRITION FACTS (PER 1-CUP SERVING)

Calories: 217   Carbohydrates: 27 g   Fiber: 6 g   Protein: 18 g

Fat: 4.6 g   Sat. Fat: 1.8 g   Cholesterol: 36 mg   Sodium: 390 mg   Calcium: 85 mg

---

AGE-*LESS* TIP—
ADDING FLAVOR TO YOUR AGE-LESS FOOD

To keep AGE-less dishes from being bland and boring, boost their flavor by using plenty of herbs and spices, all of which are low in AGEs. The chili powder, cumin, and oregano that spark our Fiesta Chili not only make the dish flavorful but, like all herbs and spices, also supply lots of healthful antioxidants.

PASTA FAGIOLI

YIELD: 8 SERVINGS

1 pound ground beef or turkey (at least 93% lean)

$^3/_4$ cup chopped yellow onion

$^1/_4$ cup plus 2 tablespoons bias-sliced celery

$^1/_4$ cup plus 2 tablespoons julienne-cut carrots

2 teaspoons crushed garlic

1 can (14$^1/_2$ ounces) diced Italian-style tomatoes, undrained and puréed in a blender

2 cups no-salt-added beef broth

1 cup low-sodium vegetable juice, such as V-8

1$^1/_2$ teaspoons dried basil

$^3/_4$ teaspoon dried oregano

$^3/_4$ teaspoon coarsely ground black pepper

$^1/_4$ teaspoon salt

1 can (15 ounces) red kidney beans, drained

3 ounces whole grain penne pasta (about 1$^1/_4$ cups)

1. Coat a 3-quart pot with cooking spray, and add the ground meat, onion, celery, carrots, and garlic. Cover and cook over medium heat, stirring occasionally to crumble, for about 8 minutes, or until the meat is no longer pink and the vegetables have softened.

2. Add the tomatoes, broth, vegetable juice, basil, oregano, pepper, and salt to the pot, and bring to a boil. Adjust the heat to maintain a simmer, cover, and cook for 5 minutes.

3. Add the beans and pasta to the pot, and return the mixture to a boil. Reduce the heat to a simmer, cover, and cook for about 10 minutes, or until the pasta is tender. Serve hot.

NUTRITION FACTS (PER 1-CUP SERVING)

Calories: 198   Carbohydrates: 22 g   Fiber: 4.8 g   Protein: 18 g
Fat: 4.6 g   Sat. Fat: 1.7 g   Cholesterol: 36 mg   Sodium: 407 mg   Calcium: 49 mg

---

MEATBALL SOUP

YIELD: 6 SERVINGS

3 cups no-salt-added beef broth

$^3/_4$ cup diced carrots

1$^1/_2$ teaspoons crushed garlic

1 cup low-sodium vegetable juice, such as V-8

$^3/_4$ teaspoon dried thyme

$^3/_4$ teaspoon salt

$^1/_2$ teaspoon ground black pepper

3 ounces whole wheat orzo (about $^1/_2$ cup)

1$^1/_2$ cups sliced fresh mushrooms (about 4 ounces)

$^3/_4$ cup fresh or frozen green peas

3$^1/_2$ cups (lightly packed) chopped fresh spinach

MEATBALLS

8 ounces ground beef or turkey (at least 93% lean)

$^1/_2$ cup whole wheat bread crumbs,* or $^1/_4$ cup quick-cooking oatmeal (1-minute cooking time)

$^1/_4$ cup finely chopped yellow onion

2 teaspoons dried parsley

1 teaspoon crushed garlic

$^1/_4$ teaspoon ground black pepper

---

* To make $^1/_2$ cup bread crumbs, tear about 1 slice of whole wheat bread into pieces, and process into crumbs in a food processor.

1. Place all of the meatball ingredients in a large bowl, and mix well. Shape into 18 meatballs (each about 1 inch in diameter) and set aside.

2. Place the broth, carrots, and garlic in a blender, and purée until smooth. Pour the mixture into a 4-quart pot, and add the vegetable juice, thyme, salt, and pepper. Bring to a boil. Then adjust the heat to maintain a simmer, cover, and cook for 10 minutes.

3. Add the meatballs to the broth mixture, and adjust the heat to maintain a simmer. Cover and cook for 5 minutes.

4. Add the orzo and mushrooms to the pot, cover, and simmer for 8 minutes. Add the peas, and simmer for about 5 minutes, or until the orzo is tender. Add the spinach, and simmer for about 2 minutes, or until wilted. Add a little more broth or vegetable juice, if needed, and serve hot.

NUTRITION FACTS (PER 1-CUP SERVING)

Calories: 161   Carbohydrates: 20   Fiber: 4.4 g   Protein: 13 g

Fat: 3.3 g   Sat. Fat: 1.2 g   Cholesterol: 24 mg   Sodium: 415 mg   Calcium: 52 mg

SEAFOOD STEW WITH FIRE-ROASTED TOMATOES

YIELD: 4 SERVINGS

1/2 cup plus 2 tablespoons finely chopped yellow onion

Water for cooking

2 teaspoons crushed garlic

1 can (14 1/2 ounces) diced fire-roasted tomatoes, undrained

1/2 cup dry white wine

1/4 teaspoon crushed red pepper flakes

2 tablespoons extra-virgin olive oil, divided

1 dozen small (about 2 inches in diameter) fresh clams in the shell

8 ounces medium peeled and deveined raw shrimp

8 ounces scallops

1/4 cup finely chopped fresh parsley

1. Place the onion and 2 tablespoons of water in a large deep nonstick skillet. Cover and cook over medium heat for about 5 minutes, or until the onion softens. Add a little more water during cooking, if needed, but only enough to prevent scorching. Add the garlic and cook for 15 seconds more, or until fragrant.

2. Add the undrained tomatoes, wine, crushed red pepper, and 1 tablespoon of the olive oil to the skillet, and bring to a boil over medium heat. Cover and cook for 3 minutes.

3. Increase the heat to medium-high and add the clams. Cover and cook for 3 minutes. Stir in the shrimp and scallops, cover, and cook for 3 to 4 additional minutes, or until the clam shells have opened and the shrimp and scallops have turned opaque. Discard any clams that have not opened. Stir in the remaining tablespoon of olive oil.

4. Divide the stew among 4 shallow bowls, and top each serving with a tablespoon of the parsley. Serve immediately.

NUTRITION FACTS (PER SERVING)

Calories: 232   Carbohydrates: 13 g   Fiber: 2 g   Protein: 23 g

Fat: 7.8 g   Sat. Fat: 1.2 g   Cholesterol: 113 mg   Sodium: 429 mg   Calcium: 91 mg

---

SHRIMP GAZPACHO

YIELD: 4 SERVINGS

1 1/4 cups low-sodium vegetable juice, such as V-8

2 tablespoons sherry vinegar

2 to 3 tablespoons extra-virgin olive oil

1 tablespoon smoked paprika

2 teaspoons crushed garlic

1/2 teaspoon salt

1/4 teaspoon ground black pepper

1/4 teaspoon crushed red pepper flakes

2 cups chopped fresh tomatoes (about 3 medium)

1 1/2 cups diced peeled cucumber (about 1 large)

1 1/4 cups chopped red or yellow bell pepper (about 1 large)

3/4 cup chopped red or sweet white onion

1 recipe Shrimp Poached in White Wine (page 226), or 2 cups boiled or steamed shrimp, chilled

3 tablespoons chopped fresh parsley or cilantro

1. Place the first 8 ingredients (vegetable juice through crushed red pepper) in a blender or food processor, and process for about 10 seconds or until well blended.

2. Add the tomatoes, cucumber, bell pepper, and onion to the blender, and process for 5 to 10 additional seconds, or until the vegetables are chopped to a medium-fine texture. Allow the mixture to sit for 10 minutes, or cover and chill until ready to serve.

3. To serve, divide the gazpacho among 4 shallow bowls. Arrange one-fourth of the shrimp over each serving, and garnish with a sprinkling of parsley or cilantro.

NUTRITION FACTS (PER 1 1/8-CUP SERVING OF SOUP, PLUS SHRIMP)

Calories: 191   Carbohydrates: 11 g   Fiber: 3.9 g   Protein: 20 g

Fat: 7.7 g   Sat. Fat: 1.1 g   Cholesterol: 137 mg   Sodium: 454 mg   Calcium: 86 mg

---

ORZO AND WHITE BEAN SOUP

YIELD: 8 SERVINGS

1 cup thinly sliced leeks (white and light green parts)

1 cup thinly sliced celery (include some leaves)

2 teaspoons crushed garlic

5 cups no-salt-added chicken or vegetable broth, divided

$^2/_3$ cup whole wheat orzo

1 teaspoon dried thyme or Herbes de Provence

1 teaspoon salt

$^1/_2$ teaspoon ground black pepper

1 cup frozen or fresh green peas

1 can (15 ounces) cannellini beans, drained

1 cup 1-inch pieces fresh asparagus

1 cup (packed) thinly sliced fresh spinach

$1^1/_2$ tablespoons extra-virgin olive oil

2 tablespoons plus 2 teaspoons Basil Pesto (page 282) or ready-made pesto (optional)

1. Place the leeks, celery, garlic, and $^1/_3$ cup of the broth in a 4-quart pot. Cover and cook over medium heat, stirring occasionally, for about 6 minutes or until the vegetables have softened. Add a little more broth if needed, but only enough to prevent scorching.

2. Add the remaining $4^2/_3$ cups broth and the orzo, thyme or other herbs, salt, and pepper to the pot, and bring to a boil. Adjust the heat to maintain a simmer, cover, and cook for 5 minutes.

3. Add the peas, cannellini beans, and asparagus to the pot, and return the soup to a simmer. Cover and cook for about 3 minutes, or until the orzo and asparagus are tender.

4. Add the spinach and olive oil to the pot, and simmer for about one minute to wilt the spinach. Remove the pot from the heat, and allow to sit covered for 3 minutes.

5. Serve hot, topping each serving with a teaspoon of pesto, if desired.

NUTRITION FACTS (PER 1-CUP SERVING)

Calories: 143   Carbohydrates: 22 g   Fiber: 5.4 g   Protein: 7 g

Fat: 3.4 g   Sat. Fat: 0.4 g   Cholesterol: 0 mg   Sodium: 383 mg   Calcium: 51 mg

SLOW-COOKED BLACK BEAN SOUP

YIELD: 9 SERVINGS

2 cups dried black beans (about 12 ounces), soaked for 8 hours or overnight and drained

4 cups water

1 can (10 ounces) diced tomatoes with green chilies, such as Ro-tel, undrained

1 cup chopped yellow onion

$^3/_4$ cup seeded and chopped green bell pepper

2 teaspoons crushed garlic

1 tablespoon chili powder

1 teaspoon ground cumin

1 teaspoon dried oregano

1 teaspoon salt

$^1/_4$ teaspoon ground black pepper

1 tablespoon extra-virgin olive oil

1 to 1$^1/_2$ tablespoons sherry vinegar or red wine vinegar

TOPPINGS

$^3/_4$ cup shredded reduced-fat Monterey Jack cheese or crumbled queso fresco

$^1/_2$ cup plus 1 tablespoon finely chopped red onion

$^1/_2$ cup plus 1 tablespoon finely chopped fresh cilantro or green bell pepper

1. Place the drained beans in a 3$^1/_2$-quart slow cooker, and add the next 10 ingredients (water through black pepper). Cook at high power for 4 to 5 hours or at low power for 8 to 10 hours, until the beans are soft. (If you want to prepare this soup without a slow cooker, see the Variation below.)

2. Add the olive oil and vinegar to the soup, and use a stick blender to blend until smooth, or leave a little texture if desired. Alternatively, working in batches, carefully purée the soup in a standing blender at low speed. (Never fill a blender more than half-full with hot liquids. Vent the top to allow steam to escape, and cover the top loosely with a clean kitchen towel.)

3. Serve hot, topping each serving with 1$^1/_2$ tablespoons of cheese and 1 tablespoon each of onion and cilantro or bell pepper.

VARIATION

❏ **To Prepare on the Stove:** Place the drained beans in a 4-quart pot, and add the next 10 ingredients (water through black pepper). Bring to a boil; then reduce the heat to maintain a simmer. Cover and cook, stirring occasionally, for about 1$^1/_2$ hours, or until the beans are soft and the liquid is thick. Proceed with Steps 2 and 3 as directed.

NUTRITION FACTS (PER 1-CUP SERVING)
Calories: 203   Carbohydrates: 32 g   Fiber: 12 g   Protein: 12 g
Fat: 4.1 g   Sat. Fat: 1.5 g   Cholesterol: 7 mg   Sodium: 430 mg   Calcium: 151 mg

SAVORY LENTIL SOUP

YIELD: 8 SERVINGS

5 cups no-salt-added chicken or vegetable broth, divided

1 cup chopped yellow onion

1 cup chopped carrots

1 cup chopped celery (include some leaves)

$1\frac{1}{2}$ cups dried brown lentils

1 can ($14\frac{1}{2}$-ounces) no-salt-added diced or stewed tomatoes, undrained and crushed

1 tablespoon crushed garlic

1 teaspoon dried thyme

1 teaspoon salt

$\frac{1}{2}$ teaspoon ground black pepper

2 tablespoons extra-virgin olive oil

Lemon juice, red wine vinegar, or balsamic vinegar (optional)

1. Place $\frac{1}{4}$ cup of the broth and all of the onion, carrots, and celery in a 4-quart pot. Cover and cook over medium heat, stirring occasionally, for about 5 minutes, or until the vegetables start to soften.

2. Add the lentils, tomatoes, garlic, thyme, salt, pepper, and remaining $4\frac{3}{4}$ cups broth to the pot, and bring to a boil. Adjust the heat to maintain a simmer, cover, and cook for 45 minutes, or until the lentils are soft and the liquid is thick. Stir the olive oil into the soup.

3. Use a stick blender to purée the soup, leaving it slightly chunky. Alternatively, transfer 3 cups of the soup to a regular blender, carefully purée until it reaches the desired consistency, and stir the soup back into the pot. (Never fill a blender more than half-full with hot liquids. Vent the top to allow steam to escape, and cover the top loosely with a clean kitchen towel.)

4. Taste the soup and add a little more salt, if needed. Serve hot, stirring about $\frac{1}{4}$ teaspoon of lemon juice or vinegar into each serving, if desired.

NUTRITION FACTS (PER 1-CUP SERVING)
Calories: 194   Carbohydrates: 29 g   Fiber: 12.9 g   Protein: 11.5 g
Fat: 3.8 g   Sat. Fat: 0.6 g   Cholesterol: 0 mg   Sodium: 365 mg   Calcium: 37 mg

FASOLADA (GREEK WHITE BEAN SOUP)

YIELD: 9 SERVINGS

2 cups dried white beans (about 12 ounces), such as navy or great northern, soaked for 8 hours or overnight and drained

1$^1/_4$ cups chopped yellow onion

1$^1/_4$ cups diced carrots

1 cup thinly sliced celery

4 cups no-salt-added chicken or vegetable broth

1 cup low-sodium vegetable juice, such as V-8, or tomato juice

1 bay leaf

1 teaspoon crushed garlic

$^3/_4$ teaspoon ground black pepper

3 tablespoons finely chopped fresh parsley

2 tablespoons extra-virgin olive oil

1 teaspoon salt

Lemon juice or red wine vinegar (optional)

1. Place the drained beans in a 4-quart pot and add the next 8 ingredients (onion through black pepper). Bring to a boil; then reduce the heat to maintain a simmer. Cover and cook, stirring occasionally, for about 1$^1/_2$ hours, or until the beans are soft and the liquid is thick. Add a little more broth during cooking if needed. (If you want to prepare this soup in a slow cooker, see the Variation below.)

2. Stir the parsley, olive oil, and salt into the pot. Remove the pot from the heat, cover, and let sit for 5 minutes.

3. Taste the soup and add a little more salt, if needed. Serve hot, stirring a little lemon juice or vinegar (about $^1/_2$ teaspoon) into each serving, if desired.

VARIATION

❏ **To Prepare in a Slow Cooker:** Soak and drain the beans as described in Step 1. Then place the drained beans and the next 8 ingredients (onion through black pepper) in a 4-quart slow cooker, and cook at high power for about 4 hours or at low power for about 8 hours. Do not lift the lid or stir during cooking. Proceed with Steps 2 and 3 as directed above.

NUTRITION FACTS (PER 1-CUP SERVING)

Calories: 203   Carbohydrates: 33 g   Fiber: 8 g   Protein: 12 g

Fat: 3.5 g   Sat. Fat: 0.5 g   Cholesterol: 0 mg   Sodium: 322 mg   Calcium: 127 mg

Sandwiches and Such

The humble sandwich is perhaps the all-time favorite fast food solution. There are several reasons why sandwiches can also be perfect for AGE-less eating. For starters, most sandwich-type breads are quite low in AGEs. In addition, a good selection of savory fillings and spreads are compatible with an AGE-way of life. As a bonus, sandwiches are a great way to satisfy a taste for grilled or roasted foods, since grilled and roasted breads and vegetables are quite low in AGEs compared with meats that are prepared using the same methods.

This chapter offers a tasty selection of sandwiches and sandwich spin-offs such as tacos, pizza, and wraps, all made the AGE-less way. Lower-AGE fillings such as poached chicken, tuna, eggs, and beans are combined with light spreads, lower-fat cheeses, plenty of flavorful veggies, and whole grain breads to create an array of delightfully simple sandwiches. Pair your sandwich with a cup of soup, a side salad, or fruit for a tasty and filling meal.

SPICY EGG SALAD SANDWICHES

YIELD: 4 SERVINGS

6 hard-boiled eggs, peeled and coarsely chopped

$^1/_3$ cup thinly sliced scallions

$^1/_3$ cup finely chopped celery

3 tablespoons nonfat or low-fat plain Greek yogurt or low-fat or light mayonnaise

2 tablespoons spicy or Dijon mustard

8 slices multigrain, dark rye, or pumpernickel bread

$1^1/_4$ cups fresh arugula, watercress, or spinach

1. Place the eggs in a bowl and mash with a fork. Add the scallions, celery, yogurt or mayonnaise, and mustard, and stir to mix. Add a little more yogurt or mayonnaise if the mixture seems too dry.

2. For each sandwich, place a bread slice on a work surface and spread with one-fourth of the egg salad. Top with one-fourth of the arugula, watercress, or spinach. Place a remaining bread slice on top of the sandwich, and cut in halves or quarters to serve.

VARIATIONS

❑ Add $^1/_4$ cup of well-drained chopped pickles (dill or sweet) or olives (black or green) to the egg mixture.

❑ Add 2 teaspoons of finely chopped fresh dill to the egg mixture.

NUTRITION FACTS (PER SANDWICH)

Calories: 296   Carbohydrates: 32 g   Fiber: 6.4 g   Protein: 19 g

Fat: 9 g   Sat. Fat: 2.5 g   Cholesterol: 280 mg   Sodium: 383 mg   Calcium: 69 mg

---

TUSCAN TUNA WRAPS

YIELD: 4 SERVINGS

3 cups mixed baby salad greens

1 can (5 ounces) tuna in water, drained

$^3/_4$ cup chopped marinated artichoke hearts, drained (reserve the marinade)

$^1/_2$ cup shredded reduced-fat mozzarella cheese, or $^1/_4$ cup crumbled reduced-fat feta cheese

2 slices red onion, cut into quarter-rings

4 whole wheat flour tortillas (9-inch rounds)

8 slices plum tomato (about $1^1/_2$ tomatoes)

1. Combine the salad greens, tuna, artichoke hearts, cheese, and onion in a large bowl. Drizzle with 2 tablespoons of the reserved marinade, and toss to mix.

2. For each wrap, place a tortilla on a work surface. Arrange a quarter of the salad mixture over the *bottom half only* of the tortilla, stopping about an inch from the edges. Top the salad mixture with 2 slices of tomato.

3. Fold the sides of the tortilla in about 1 inch, and roll up snugly from the bottom. Cut in half and serve.

NUTRITION FACTS (PER WRAP)

Calories: 277   Carbohydrates: 32 g   Fiber: 5.2 g   Protein: 19 g
Fat: 8.6 g   Sat. Fat: 2.2 g   Cholesterol: 20 mg   Sodium: 479 mg   Calcium: 233 mg

HERBED CHICKEN SALAD SANDWICHES

YIELD: 4 SERVINGS

2 cups chopped Basic or Classic French Poached Chicken (page 224)

$1/_4$ cup finely chopped celery

$1/_4$ cup thinly sliced scallions

1 tablespoon finely chopped fresh dill, or 1 teaspoon dried

3 tablespoons nonfat or low-fat plain Greek yogurt or light sour cream

3 tablespoons low-fat or light mayonnaise

8 slices whole grain bread

1 medium avocado, peeled and sliced

4 Boston or romaine lettuce leaves, or $1^1/_4$ cups mixed baby salad greens

1. Place the chicken, celery, scallions, and dill in a medium-size bowl. Add the yogurt or sour cream and the mayonnaise, and stir to mix. Add a little more yogurt or mayonnaise if the mixture seems too dry.

2. For each sandwich, place a bread slice on a work surface and spread with one-fourth of the chicken salad (about $1/_2$ cup). Top with a quarter of the avocado slices and either a lettuce leaf or a quarter of the salad greens

3. If desired, spread some mayonnaise on one side of a remaining bread slice. Place the slice on top of the sandwich, and cut in halves or quarters to serve.

NUTRITION FACTS (PER SANDWICH)

Calories: 341   Carbohydrates: 36 g   Fiber: 8.9 g   Protein: 30 g
Fat: 8.7 g   Sat. Fat: 1.4 g   Cholesterol: 55 mg   Sodium: 308 mg   Calcium: 38 mg

ROASTED ASPARAGUS PANINI

YIELD: 4 SERVINGS

12 ounces fresh thin asparagus spears

$1/_2$ medium-large red onion, sliced $1/_4$-inch thick

Scant $1/_4$ teaspoon salt

$1/_4$ teaspoon ground black pepper

Cooking spray

8 slices firm whole grain bread

1 tablespoon plus 1 teaspoon Dijon mustard

5 ounces thinly sliced reduced-fat Swiss, mozzarella, or white Cheddar cheese

Olive oil cooking spray

1. Preheat the oven to 450°F. Rinse the asparagus with cool water, snap off the tough ends, and pat dry with paper towels. If necessary, trim the asparagus spears so they are the same length as the bread slices.

2. Coat a large (at least 11 x 17-inch) rimmed baking sheet with cooking spray, and arrange the asparagus in a single layer on the sheet. Top with the onions. Sprinkle with the salt and pepper, and spray lightly with the cooking spray. Roast for about 15 minutes, or until tender and nicely browned, turning with a spatula after 8 minutes.

3. For each sandwich, place a bread slice on a work surface and spread with 1 teaspoon of mustard. Top with one-fourth of the vegetable mixture and one-fourth of the cheese. Then top with one of the remaining bread slices. Spray the top of the sandwich lightly with cooking spray.

4. Coat a sandwich press or tabletop grill (such as a George Foreman Grill) with cooking spray, and lay the sandwich in the grill. (If you don't have a sandwich press or tabletop grill, see the Variation below.) Close the grill and cook for about 5 minutes, or until the bread is toasted and the cheese is melted. Cut the sandwich into halves or quarters and serve hot.

VARIATIONS

❏ **To Prepare in a Skillet**: Coat a nonstick skillet with cooking spray and place the sandwich in the pan. Spray the top of the sandwich lightly with cooking spray, and top it with a flat object that's heavy enough to press the sandwich down, such as a grill press, a smaller skillet, or a plate weighted with a 1-pound food can. Cook over medium heat for 2 to 3 minutes on each side. (When removing the weighted object, be aware that it may be hot and should be handled with a pot holder.) Cut the sandwich into halves or quarters and serve hot.

❏ Substitute 4 medium portabella mushrooms for the asparagus. Scrape out the gills and slice $1/_2$-inch thick before placing on the baking sheet and roasting according to Step 2. Then proceed with Steps 3 and 4.

NUTRITION FACTS (PER SERVING)

Calories: 282   Carbohydrates: 36 g   Fiber: 7.4 g   Protein: 19 g

Fat: 7.1 g   Sat. Fat: 3.2 g   Cholesterol: 19 mg   Sodium: 560 mg   Calcium: 326 mg

PANINI CAPRESE

YIELD: 4 SERVINGS

8 slices firm whole grain bread

5 ounces fresh mozzarella cheese, thinly sliced

12 slices plum tomato (about 2 tomatoes), or $1/4$ cup chopped sun-dried tomatoes (not packed in oil)

12 to 16 fresh spinach leaves

$1/4$ cup Basil Pesto (page 282) or ready-made pesto

Olive oil cooking spray

1. For each sandwich, place a bread slice on a work surface and top with one-fourth of the cheese. Over the cheese, layer about 3 slices of tomato and 3 to 4 leaves of spinach. Spread a remaining bread slice with 1 tablespoon of the pesto and place on the sandwich. Spray the top of the sandwich lightly with cooking spray.

2. Coat a sandwich press or tabletop grill (such as a George Foreman Grill) with cooking spray, and lay the sandwich in the grill. (If you don't have a sandwich press or tabletop grill, see the Variation below.) Close the grill and cook for about 5 minutes, or until the bread is toasted and the cheese is melted. Cut the sandwich in halves or quarters and serve hot.

VARIATION

❏ **To Prepare in a Skillet:** Coat a nonstick skillet with cooking spray and place the sandwich in the pan. Spray the top of the sandwich lightly with cooking spray, and top it with a flat object that's heavy enough to press the sandwich down, such as a grill press, a smaller skillet, or a plate weighted with a 1-pound food can. Cook over medium heat for 2 to 3 minutes on each side. (When removing the weighted object, be aware that it may be hot and should be handled with a pot holder.) Cut the sandwich into halves or quarters and serve hot.

NUTRITION FACTS (PER SANDWICH)

Calories: 336   Carbohydrates: 33 g   Fiber: 7.4 g   Protein: 17 g

Fat: 15 g   Sat. Fat: 3.8 g   Cholesterol: 25 mg   Sodium: 441 mg   Calcium: 239 mg

FLAVORFUL FALAFEL

YIELD: 4 SERVINGS

1 can (15 ounces) chickpeas
or 1$^{1}/_{2}$ cups cooked chickpeas, drained

$^{1}/_{4}$ cup chopped fresh parsley

$^{1}/_{4}$ cup sliced scallions

2 teaspoons ground cumin

$^{1}/_{2}$ teaspoon ground coriander

1$^{1}/_{2}$ teaspoons crushed garlic

$^{1}/_{8}$ to $^{1}/_{4}$ teaspoon cayenne pepper

$^{1}/_{8}$ to $^{1}/_{4}$ teaspoon salt (optional)

Olive oil cooking spray

4 whole grain pitas
(5- or 6-inch rounds), cut in half

SALAD

2 cups shredded lettuce

$^{3}/_{4}$ cup chopped tomato

$^{3}/_{4}$ cup chopped cucumber

SAUCE

$^{1}/_{3}$ cup sesame tahini

3 tablespoons water

2 to 3 tablespoons lemon juice

$^{1}/_{2}$ teaspoon crushed garlic

$^{1}/_{4}$ teaspoon salt

1. Place all of the salad ingredients in a small bowl, and toss to mix. Set aside.

2. To make the sauce, place the tahini in another small bowl, and gradually whisk in the water. Add the remaining sauce ingredients, and whisk until smooth. Set aside.

3. Place the first seven ingredients (chickpeas through cayenne pepper) in a food processor, and process until the mixture is pasty enough to be shaped into patties. The mixture should be thick; do not add any liquid during processing. Taste, and add a little salt if needed.

4. Scoop out a 2$^{1}/_{2}$-tablespoon portion of the chickpea mixture, and shape it into a patty about 2 inches in diameter. Repeat with the remaining mixture to make 8 patties.

5. Coat a large nonstick skillet or griddle with cooking spray and preheat over medium heat until a drop of water sizzles when added. Add the patties to the skillet and spray the tops lightly with cooking spray. Cook uncovered for 2 to 3 minutes per side, or until nicely browned and heated through. Alternatively, arrange the patties on a baking sheet that has been coated with cooking spray, and bake in a 400°F oven for about 8 minutes on each side, or until nicely browned.

6. If desired, warm the pitas by wrapping them in aluminum foil and heating in a 350°F oven for about 10 minutes. Fill each pita half with 1 falafel patty, a scant $^{1}/_{2}$ cup of the salad mixture, and about 1 tablespoon of sauce. Serve immediately.

NUTRITION FACTS (PER 2 PITA HALVES)

Calories: 341   Carbohydrates: 48 g   Fiber: 12 g   Protein: 14 g

Fat: 13.1 g   Sat. Fat: 1.7 g   Cholesterol: 0 mg   Sodium: 445 mg   Calcium: 163 mg

CHIPOTLE CHICKEN TACOS

YIELD: 4 SERVINGS

1 recipe Basic Poached Chicken (page 224)

1 cup Chipotle Sauce (page 284)

8 corn or whole grain flour tortillas (5- or 6-inch rounds)

TOPPINGS

2 cups shredded romaine lettuce

16 thin slices avocado (about 1 medium)

$^1/_2$ cup crumbled queso fresco or shredded reduced-fat Monterey Jack cheese (optional)

1. Place the chicken on a work surface, and use 2 forks to pull the chicken into shreds. Set aside.

2. Pour the sauce into a 10-inch nonstick skillet, and bring to a simmer. Add the shredded chicken to the skillet, and simmer uncovered, stirring occasionally, for about 5 minutes, or until most of the liquid has been absorbed and the mixture is moist but not runny.

3. Warm the tortillas according to package directions. For each taco, place 1 warmed tortilla on a work surface. Fill it with about $^1/_4$ cup of the chicken mixture, and top with $^1/_4$ cup lettuce, 2 avocado slices, and 1 tablespoon of cheese, if desired. Fold in half and serve immediately.

VARIATION

❑ For low-carb tacos, serve the chicken mixture in romaine lettuce leaves instead of tortillas, and top with avocado slices and cheese. Or serve the chicken mixture over a Southwestern-style salad.

NUTRITION FACTS (PER 2 TACOS)

Calories: 309   Carbohydrates: 30 g   Fiber: 7 g   Protein: 24 g

Fat: 9.8 g   Sat. Fat: 1.6 g   Cholesterol: 54 mg   Sodium: 346 mg   Calcium: 80 mg

SPICY SOFT TACOS

Yield: 5 servings

1 can (14$^1/_2$ ounces) Mexican-style diced tomatoes, undrained

1 teaspoon chili powder

1 teaspoon ground cumin

$^1/_2$ teaspoon dried oregano

1 pound ground beef, chicken, or turkey (at least 93% lean)

1 cup chopped yellow onion

$^1/_4$ teaspoon salt (optional)

10 corn or whole grain flour tortillas (5- to 6-inch rounds)

TOPPINGS

2 cups shredded lettuce

1 cup chopped fresh tomato

1. Place the canned tomatoes, chili powder, cumin, and oregano in a blender, and blend until smooth. Set aside.

2. Coat a large nonstick skillet with cooking spray. Add the ground meat and onion and use a spatula to break up the meat. Cover and cook over medium heat, stirring occasionally to crumble, for about 6 minutes, or until the meat is no longer pink.

3. Add the blended tomato mixture to the skillet, and bring to a boil. Adjust the heat to maintain a simmer, and cook covered for 5 minutes. Remove the lid and simmer uncovered for about 5 minutes, or until most of the liquid has evaporated. Stir in the salt, if needed, and set aside to keep warm.

4. Heat the tortillas according to package directions. For each taco, place 1 warmed tortilla on a work surface. Fill it with about $^1/_4$ cup of the meat mixture, and top with about 3 tablespoons of the lettuce and 1$^1/_2$ tablespoons of the chopped tomatoes. Fold in half and serve immediately.

Nutrition Facts (Per 2 Tacos)

Calories: 263   Carbohydrates: 27 g   Fiber: 5.3 g   Protein: 23 g

Fat: 7.8 g   Sat. Fat: 2.7 g   Cholesterol: 57 mg   Sodium: 258 mg   Calcium: 189 mg

---

BLACK BEAN TACOS

YIELD: 4 SERVINGS

1 can (15 ounces) or 1^1/$_2$ cups cooked black beans, drained and coarsely mashed

^{1}/$_4$ cup chunky-style salsa

8 corn tortillas (5- or 6-inch rounds)

^{1}/$_2$ cup shredded reduced-fat Monterey Jack cheese

SALAD

1^1/$_2$ cups shredded romaine lettuce

^{1}/$_2$ cup diced fresh tomato

^{1}/$_3$ cup chopped fresh cilantro

^{1}/$_3$ cup sliced scallions or chopped red onion

1 tablespoon finely chopped pickled jalapeño pepper

1. Place all of the salad ingredients in a small bowl, and toss to mix. Set aside.

2. Place the beans and salsa in a medium skillet. Cook uncovered over medium heat, stirring frequently, for 3 to 4 minutes or until heated through and thick, like refried beans.

3. Arrange the tortillas on a work surface, and spread a scant ^{1}/$_4$ cup of the bean mixture over each tortilla to within ^{1}/$_4$-inch of the edges. Coat a large non-stick skillet or griddle with cooking spray, and place over medium heat. Arrange the tortillas in the skillet or on the griddle and, working in batches if necessary, cook each tortilla for about a minute, or until it is soft and pliable enough to fold in half.

4. Fold each tortilla in half to enclose the filling, and cook for a minute or 2 on each side, or until lightly browned. Open each tortilla slightly and fill with 1 tablespoon of the cheese and about ^{1}/$_4$ cup of the salad mixture. Serve hot.

NUTRITION FACTS (PER 2 TACOS)

Calories: 232   Carbohydrates: 37 g   Fiber: 11 g   Protein: 13 g

Fat: 4.4 g   Sat. Fat: 1.9 g   Cholesterol: 10 mg   Sodium: 481 mg   Calcium: 295 mg

---

VERY VEGGIE SANDWICHES

YIELD: 4 SERVINGS

8 slices multigrain bread

1 cup mashed avocado
(about 1 medium-large)

16 thin slices cucumber
(about $^1/_2$ medium)

4 ounces thinly sliced reduced-fat
mozzarella or Swiss cheese

8 thin slices tomato (about 1 medium)

$^1/_2$ cup shredded carrot

24 to 32 large fresh spinach leaves,
or 4 romaine lettuce leaves

1. For each sandwich, place one bread slice on a work surface and spread with 2 tablespoons of the mashed avocado. Over the avocado, layer 4 slices of cucumber, a quarter of the cheese, 2 slices of tomato, 2 tablespoons of carrot, and a few leaves of spinach or 1 leaf of romaine.

2. Spread a remaining bread slice with 2 more tablespoons of the avocado and place over the sandwich. Cut in half and serve.

NUTRITION FACTS (PER SANDWICH)

Calories: 348   Carbohydrates: 36 g   Fiber: 7.6 g   Protein: 17 g

Fat: 16 g   Sat. Fat: 4 g   Cholesterol: 10 mg   Sodium: 426 mg   Calcium: 276 mg

---

MEDITERRANEAN MUSHROOM WRAPS

YIELD: 4 SERVINGS

8 ounces baby portabella or
white button mushrooms, sliced
(about 3 cups)

$^1/_4$ teaspoon ground black pepper

4 whole grain flour tortillas
(9-inch rounds)

1 cup Classic Hummus (page 260)
or ready-made hummus

8 slices plum tomato
(about 1 $^1/_2$ tomatoes)

3 to 4 thin slices red onion,
separated into rings

$^1/_4$ cup sliced black olives

$^1/_4$ cup crumbled reduced-fat
feta cheese

24 to 32 large fresh spinach leaves

1. Coat a large nonstick skillet with cooking spray, and add the mushrooms and pepper. Cook over medium-high heat, stirring frequently, for about 6 minutes or until the mushrooms are nicely browned. Remove from the heat and set aside.

2. For each wrap, place a tortilla on a work surface. Spoon $1/4$ cup of hummus in an even layer over the *bottom half only* of the tortilla, stopping about an inch from the edges. Over the hummus, layer one-fourth of the tomatoes, mushrooms, onion, olives, feta cheese, and spinach.

3. Fold the sides of the tortilla in about 1 inch, and roll up snugly from the bottom. Cut in half and serve.

NUTRITION FACTS (PER WRAP)

Calories: 298   Carbohydrates: 39 g   Fiber: 8.3 g   Protein: 13 g
Fat: 12.1 g   Sat. Fat: 1.4 g   Cholesterol: 0 mg   Sodium: 562 mg   Calcium: 193 mg

---

GARDEN ARTICHOKE SANDWICHES

YIELD: 4 SERVINGS

8 slices multigrain bread	$1/2$ cup shredded carrot
1 cup Classic Hummus (page 260) or ready-made hummus	4 ounces thinly sliced reduced-fat mozzarella cheese
1 cup sliced marinated artichoke hearts, drained	24 to 32 large fresh spinach leaves, or 4 romaine lettuce leaves

1. For each sandwich, place one bread slice on a work surface and spread with 2 tablespoons of the hummus. Over the hummus, layer $1/4$ cup of artichoke hearts, 2 tablespoons of carrot, a quarter of the cheese, and a few leaves of spinach or 1 leaf of romaine.

2. Spread a remaining bread slice with 2 tablespoons of hummus and place over the sandwich. Cut in half and serve.

NUTRITION FACTS (PER SANDWICH)

Calories: 362   Carbohydrates: 45 g   Fiber: 9 g   Protein: 19 g
Fat: 12 g   Sat. Fat: 3.8 g   Cholesterol: 15 mg   Sodium: 509 mg   Calcium: 249 mg

---

Making Your Own AGE-Less Hummus

Once available only in Middle Eastern restaurants, hummus is now enjoyed by millions of Americans who appreciate a versatile spread and dip that is not only creamy and bursting with flavor, but also high in protein and fiber. Although you can now buy hummus in supermarkets, it's easy to make your own delicious chickpea spread at home. To minimize AGEs, this recipe limits high-fat ingredients, while a tasty blend of seasonings adds classic hummus flavor.

CLASSIC HUMMUS

YIELD: ABOUT 1$^1/_2$ CUPS

1 can (15 ounces) chickpeas
or 1$^1/_2$ cups cooked chickpeas, drained
(reserve the liquid)

2 tablespoons lemon juice

2 tablespoons sesame tahini

1$^1/_2$ tablespoons extra-virgin olive oil

1 teaspoon crushed garlic

$^1/_2$ teaspoon ground cumin

$^1/_8$ teaspoon cayenne pepper

$^1/_8$ to $^1/_4$ teaspoon salt (optional)

1. Place the first 7 ingredients (chickpeas through cayenne pepper) along with 2 tablespoons of the reserved chickpea liquid in a food processor, and process until smooth and creamy. If needed, add more of the reserved liquid to create a soft spreadable consistency. Taste, and add a little salt if desired.

2. Serve immediately, or cover and refrigerate until ready to serve or for up to 3 days. You can also place any leftover hummus in an airtight freezer-proof container and store in the freezer for up to 3 months.

VARIATION

❑ To make Roasted Red Pepper Hummus, add $^1/_3$ cup well-drained chopped roasted red bell pepper along with the other ingredients before processing.

NUTRITION FACTS (PER 2-TABLESPOON SERVING)

Calories: 65   Carbohydrates: 6 g   Fiber: 1.8 g   Protein: 2.3 g

Fat: 3.6 g   Sat. Fat: 0.4 g   Cholesterol: 0 mg   Sodium: 97 mg   Calcium: 26 mg

FLATBREAD PIZZAS WITH ROASTED RED PEPPERS, ONIONS, AND OLIVES

YIELD: 4 SERVINGS

4 whole grain flatbreads (7 x 9-inch rectangles), or 4 whole grain flour tortillas (9-inch rounds)

$1/2$ cup jarred marinara sauce

$1/2$ cup chopped jarred roasted red bell pepper, drained

$1/2$ cup thin slivers yellow onion

$1/3$ cup chopped black olives

1 cup shredded reduced-fat mozzarella cheese

2 tablespoons finely chopped fresh basil, oregano, or thyme

$1/2$ teaspoon crushed red pepper flakes (optional)

1. Preheat the oven to 400°F. Coat 2 large baking sheets with cooking spray, and arrange the flatbreads on the sheets.

2. Bake the bread for 2 minutes. Turn the bread over and top each piece with one-fourth of the sauce, bell pepper, onion, and olives. Return to the oven and bake for 4 minutes.

3. Sprinkle each pizza with $1/4$ cup of the cheese and bake for 1 additional minute, or just until the cheese begins to melt.

4. Remove the pizzas from the oven, and top each one with some of the herbs and crushed red pepper. Serve immediately.

VARIATION

❏ Substitute $1/2$ cup chopped canned artichoke hearts (drained) or cooked spinach for the roasted red pepper.

NUTRITION FACTS (PER PIZZA)

Calories: 215   Carbohydrates: 25 g   Fiber: 4.4 g   Protein: 17 g

Fat: 8.5 g   Sat. Fat: 3 g   Cholesterol: 19 mg   Sodium: 687 mg   Calcium: 301 mg

---

*S*ide Dishes

Choosing smart side dishes is essential to eating the AGE-less way. Fortunately, this is easily accomplished, since vegetables, fruits, and whole grains are naturally low in AGEs. As a bonus, these foods are packed with plenty of anti-aging, anti-inflammatory nutrients.

Of course, side dishes take a turn for the worse when they are deep-fried or drenched with butter, oil, cheese, or other fatty ingredients that add unhealthy amounts of AGEs. That's why "less is more" when it comes to these accompaniments. Vegetables and fruits served raw or lightly cooked retain the most nutrients, color, and flavor. Simple ingredients such as fresh herbs, spices, lemon, and a drizzle of olive oil allow natural flavors to shine through. And wholesome whole grains, nuts, and seeds add great taste, texture, and variety. This chapter embraces these healthful principles to create a delicious array of simple side dishes perfect for AGE-less meals.

CAULIFLOWER COUSCOUS

YIELD: 5 SERVINGS

5 cups fresh cauliflower florets
(about 1 large head)

1/4 teaspoon salt

1/4 teaspoon ground black pepper

Water for cooking

1 tablespoon extra-virgin olive oil

1 teaspoon crushed garlic

1/3 cup finely chopped fresh parsley

1/3 cup thinly sliced scallions

1. Place the cauliflower florets in a food processor, and pulse for several seconds at a time until the cauliflower is ground to a texture that resembles coarse couscous or rice kernels.

2. Coat a large nonstick skillet with cooking spray and add the cauliflower, salt, pepper, and 2 tablespoons of water. Cover and cook over medium heat, stirring occasionally, for about 5 minutes, or just until tender (like al dente pasta). Add a little more water during cooking if needed, but only enough to prevent scorching.

3. Push the cauliflower to one side of the skillet and add the olive oil and garlic. Cook for about 10 seconds or until the garlic smells fragrant. Stir to mix the garlic and olive oil into the cauliflower. Remove from the heat and stir in the parsley and scallions. Serve immediately.

VARIATION

❏ Add 1/4 cup finely chopped walnuts (unroasted) along with the parsley and scallions.

NUTRITION FACTS (PER 2/3-CUP SERVING)
Calories: 54   Carbohydrates: 6 g   Fiber: 2.4 g   Protein: 2.3 g
Fat: 3 g   Sat. Fat: 0.4 g   Cholesterol: 0 mg   Sodium: 152 mg   Calcium: 34 mg

SAUTÉED GREEN BEANS AND MUSHROOMS

YIELD: 4 SERVINGS

1 pound fresh green beans

3 cups sliced fresh mushrooms (about 8 ounces)

$1/_4$ teaspoon salt

Scant $1/_4$ teaspoon ground black pepper

1 teaspoon crushed garlic

$1^1/_2$ teaspoons extra-virgin olive oil

2 to 3 teaspoons finely chopped fresh lemon or other thyme, or $3/_4$ teaspoon dried thyme

1. Rinse the beans and shake off the excess water, but do not dry. Snap off and discard the ends. Leave the beans whole, or if desired, snap into $1^1/_2$-inch pieces.

2. Coat a large deep nonstick skillet with cooking spray. Place the beans in the skillet along with the mushrooms, salt, and pepper. Cover and cook over medium-high heat, stirring occasionally, for about 8 minutes, or just until the beans are tender and the mushrooms are beginning to brown. If necessary, reduce the heat slightly or add a little water during cooking, but only enough to prevent scorching. If there is any liquid left in the skillet, cook uncovered briefly to allow the liquid to evaporate and the mushrooms to lightly brown.

3. Add the garlic to the skillet, and cook for about 30 seconds. Remove the skillet from the heat and toss in the olive oil and thyme. Serve immediately.

NUTRITIONAL FACTS (PER $7/_8$-CUP SERVING)
Calories: 60   Carbohydrates: 9 g   Fiber: 3.4 g   Protein: 3.6 g

Fat: 2.2 g   Sat. Fat: 0.3 g   Cholesterol: 0 mg   Sodium: 154 mg   Calcium: 42 mg

SPINACH WITH CORN AND LEEKS

YIELD: 4 SERVINGS

1 cup thinly sliced leeks, white and light green parts only (about 1 medium)

Water for cooking

$1^1/_2$ cups fresh or frozen whole kernel corn

1 tablespoon extra-virgin olive oil

1 teaspoon crushed garlic

9 cups (moderately packed) sliced fresh spinach (about 9 ounces)

$1/_4$ teaspoon salt

Scant $1/_4$ teaspoon ground black pepper

1. Coat a large deep nonstick skillet with cooking spray. Add the leeks and 2 tablespoons of water, cover, and cook over medium heat for about 4 minutes, or until the leeks start to soften. Add a little water if the skillet becomes too dry, but only enough to prevent scorching.

2. Add the corn and 1 tablespoon of water to the skillet. Cover and cook for an additional minute or 2 to lightly cook the corn or, if frozen, to thaw it and heat it through.

3. Stir the olive oil and garlic into the skillet and cook for 15 seconds, or until the garlic smells fragrant. Stir in the spinach, salt, and pepper, and cook uncovered, tossing often, for a couple of minutes or until the spinach is wilted. Serve immediately.

NUTRITION FACTS (PER $^7/_8$-CUP SERVING)

Calories: 112   Carbohydrates: 18 g   Fiber: 3.6 g   Protein: 4 g

Fat: 4.1 g   Sat. Fat: 0.6 g   Cholesterol: 0 mg   Sodium: 200 mg   Calcium: 79 mg

PAN-SEARED ASPARAGUS

YIELD: 2 SERVINGS

8 ounces fresh thin asparagus spears

$^1/_2$ teaspoon extra-virgin olive oil

$^1/_2$ teaspoon finely chopped fresh dill

Pinch salt

Pinch ground black pepper

2 teaspoons sliced almonds (unroasted) (optional)

1. Rinse the asparagus with cool water and snap off the tough stem ends. Shake off the excess water, but do not pat dry.

2. Coat a large nonstick skillet with cooking spray and arrange the asparagus in the pan. Cover and cook over medium-high heat for 5 to 6 minutes, or until the spears are crisp-tender and beginning to brown in spots. Shake the pan occasionally or use a wooden spoon to roll the spears over so they cook evenly. Add a little water during cooking or reduce the heat slightly if needed, but only enough to prevent scorching.

3. Turn off the heat and drizzle the olive oil over the asparagus. Sprinkle with the dill, salt, pepper, and, if desired, the almonds. Shake the pan to coat the spears with the oil and seasonings, and serve immediately.

NUTRITIONAL FACTS (PER SERVING)

Calories: 29   Carbohydrates: 4 g   Fiber: 2 g   Protein: 2 g

Fat: 1.3 g   Sat. Fat: 0.2 g   Cholesterol: 0 mg   Sodium: 74 mg   Calcium: 29 mg

SMASHED PURPLE POTATOES

YIELD: 4 SERVINGS

1 pound small unpeeled purple potatoes, halved or quartered to make $^3/_4$-inch chunks

$^1/_2$ cup finely chopped red onion

1 tablespoon plus 1 teaspoon extra-virgin olive oil

1 teaspoon crushed garlic

2 teaspoons lemon juice

Scant $^1/_2$ teaspoon salt

Scant $^1/_2$ teaspoon ground black pepper

$^1/_4$ cup finely chopped fresh parsley, or 2 tablespoons finely chopped fresh dill or chives

1. Place a steamer basket in a 6-quart pot, and fill with enough water to reach within $^1/_2$ inch of the bottom of the basket. Arrange the potatoes in the basket, cover, and bring to a boil. Allow the potatoes to steam for 10 to 12 minutes, or until tender when pierced with a fork.

2. Drain the potatoes, reserving the cooking liquid. Return the potatoes to the pot, cover, and set aside to keep warm.

3. Coat a small nonstick skillet with cooking spray, and add the onion and 2 tablespoons of the reserved cooking liquid to the skillet. Cover and cook over medium heat for about 5 minutes, or until the onion is tender. Stir in the olive oil and garlic, and cook for about 10 seconds or just until fragrant.

4. Add the cooked onion mixture to the potatoes, along with $^1/_3$ cup of the reserved cooking liquid. Use a potato masher to mash the potatoes, leaving them fairly coarse and chunky. Stir in the lemon juice, salt, and pepper. If the potatoes seem too dry, stir in a little more of the reserved cooking liquid.

5. Add the herbs to the potato mixture, and toss to mix. Serve immediately.

VARIATION

❑ Substitute small red-skinned new potatoes or small Yukon gold or fingerling potatoes for the purple potatoes, and use yellow onion in place of the red onion.

NUTRITION FACTS (PER $^2/_3$-CUP SERVING)

Calories: 139   Carbohydrates: 21 g   Fiber: 2 g   Protein: 2.6 g

Fat: 4.5 g   Sat. Fat: 0.6 g   Cholesterol: 0 mg   Sodium: 218 mg   Calcium: 18 mg

ZUCCHINI NOODLES

YIELD: 4 SERVINGS

4 medium-large zucchini
(about 8 ounces each)

1 1/2 teaspoons crushed garlic

1/4 teaspoon salt

1/4 teaspoon ground black pepper

1 teaspoon extra-virgin olive oil
(optional)

1. Use a julienne vegetable peeler to shred the zucchini into long, thin spaghetti-like "noodles." Shred only the skin and firm outer portions of the zucchini, stopping when you reach the center seeded portion. Reserve the centers pieces for other uses. (They can be diced and added to salads.) Alternatively, use a vegetable spiral slicer to make the noodles, and use scissors to snip the noodles into 6- to 8-inch strands.

2. Coat a large nonstick skillet with cooking spray, and preheat over medium-high heat until a drop of water sizzles when added. Add the noodles and cook uncovered for about 4 minutes, tossing frequently, until crisp-tender.

3. Add the garlic, salt, and pepper along with the olive oil (if using) to the skillet, and cook for about 20 seconds or until the garlic begins to smell fragrant. Serve as a side dish, or top with spaghetti sauce, meatballs, or any saucy entrée you might serve over pasta.

VARIATIONS

❑ Toss in 2 to 3 teaspoons finely chopped fresh dill or parsley along with the salt and pepper.

❑ Substitute 2 medium carrots for 2 of the zucchini.

NUTRITION FACTS (PER 3/4-CUP SERVING)
Calories: 31   Carbohydrates: 6 g   Fiber: 2.4 g   Protein: 2.1 g
Fat: 0.6 g   Sat. Fat: 0.1 g   Cholesterol: 0 mg   Sodium: 159 mg   Calcium: 30 mg

CARROT-RICE PILAF

YIELD: 6 SERVINGS

2$\frac{1}{4}$ cups no-salt-added vegetable or chicken broth, divided

1 cup uncooked brown rice

2 cups matchstick or julienne-cut carrots (about 5 ounces, or 2$\frac{1}{2}$ medium carrots)

$\frac{1}{4}$ cup thinly sliced scallions

Water for cooking

1 tablespoon extra-virgin olive oil

$\frac{1}{4}$ teaspoon salt

$\frac{1}{4}$ teaspoon ground black pepper

1. Bring the broth to a boil in a 2-quart pot. Stir in the rice, and adjust the heat to maintain a simmer. Cover and cook without stirring for about 45 minutes, or until the broth is absorbed and the rice is tender. Remove from the heat and allow to sit covered for 10 minutes. (If desired, make the rice the day before and refrigerate until needed.)

2. While the rice sits, coat a large deep nonstick skillet with cooking spray, and add the carrots, scallions, and 2 tablespoons of water. Cover and cook over medium heat for about 4 minutes or until crisp-tender. Add a little more water if needed, but only enough to prevent scorching.

3. Add the cooked rice, olive oil, salt, and pepper to the skillet, and toss to mix. Serve immediately.

VARIATIONS

❏ Substitute small broccoli florets for the carrots.

❏ Substitute barley or farro for the brown rice, and cook the grain according to package directions.

NUTRITION FACTS (PER $\frac{3}{4}$-CUP SERVING)

Calories: 155   Carbohydrates: 28 g   Fiber: 2.2 g   Protein: 3.8 g

Fat: 3.2 g   Sat. Fat: 0.5 g   Cholesterol: 0 mg   Sodium: 157 mg   Calcium: 22 mg

BLACK BEANS AND BROWN RICE

YIELD: 5 SERVINGS

1$\frac{1}{2}$ cups plus 2 tablespoons no-salt-added chicken or vegetable broth, divided

$\frac{2}{3}$ cup uncooked brown rice

$\frac{1}{2}$ cup finely chopped yellow onion

1 tablespoon extra-virgin olive oil

$\frac{3}{4}$ teaspoon ground cumin

1 teaspoon crushed garlic

1 can (15 ounces) black beans, drained (reserve the liquid)

1 teaspoon finely chopped pickled jalapeño pepper

$\frac{1}{8}$ teaspoon salt

1. Bring 1$\frac{1}{2}$ cups of the broth to a boil in a 2-quart pot. Stir in the rice and adjust the heat to maintain a simmer. Cover and cook without stirring for about 45 minutes, or until the broth is absorbed and the rice is tender. Remove from the heat and allow to sit covered for 10 minutes. (If desired, make the rice the day before and refrigerate until needed.)

2. While the rice is sitting, place the onion, olive oil, cumin, and the remaining 2 tablespoons of broth in a large nonstick skillet. Cover and cook over medium heat, stirring occasionally, for about 5 minutes, or until the onion softens. Add the garlic and cook for an additional 15 seconds, or until the garlic smells fragrant.

3. Add the cooked rice, beans, jalapeño pepper, salt, and $\frac{1}{4}$ cup of the reserved liquid from the beans to the skillet. Cook uncovered, stirring occasionally, for 3 to 4 minutes, or until the mixture is heated through and most of the liquid has evaporated. Serve immediately.

VARIATION

❑ For a brunch entrée, top each serving with a poached egg and a tablespoon or 2 of Cilantro Salsa (page 282) or ready-made salsa.

NUTRITION FACTS (PER $\frac{3}{4}$ CUP SERVING)

Calories: 165   Carbohydrates: 31 g   Fiber: 6 g   Protein: 6 g

Fat: 3.4 g   Sat. Fat: 0.5 g   Cholesterol: 0 mg   Sodium: 310 mg   Calcium: 39 mg

---

FARRO WITH PEAS AND PECANS

YIELD: 6 SERVINGS

1 cup thinly sliced leek, white and light green parts only (about 1 medium)

Water for cooking

2 cups frozen green peas

2 cups cooked farro*

1 tablespoon extra-virgin olive oil

1 teaspoon crushed garlic

2 teaspoons lemon juice

$1/4$ teaspoon salt

$1/4$ teaspoon ground black pepper

$1/3$ cup chopped pecans (unroasted)

$1/4$ cup finely chopped fresh parsley

---

* To make 2 cups cooked farro, start with $2/3$ cup uncooked farro and prepare according to package directions.

1. Coat a large nonstick skillet with cooking spray, and add the leek and 2 tablespoons of water. Cover and cook over medium heat for about 5 minutes, or until the leek softens. Add a little more water during cooking if needed, but only enough to prevent scorching.

2. Add the peas to the skillet, cover, and cook for about 3 minutes or just until thawed. Add a little water if the skillet seems too dry. Add the farro, olive oil, and garlic, and cook uncovered for about a minute to heat through.

3. Remove the skillet from the heat, and add the lemon juice, salt, and pepper, tossing to mix. Add the pecans and parsley, and toss again. Serve immediately.

NUTRITIONAL FACTS (PER $3/4$-CUP SERVING)

Calories: 195   Carbohydrates: 26 g   Fiber: 6 g   Protein: 6 g

Fat: 7.3 g   Sat. Fat: 0.7 g   Cholesterol: 0 mg   Sodium: 150 mg   Calcium: 35 mg

ROASTED BEET SALAD

YIELD: 4 SERVINGS

1 pound fresh beets
(about 3 large or 6 medium)

8 cups mixed baby salad greens

$1/4$ cup chopped walnuts
(unroasted)

$1/4$ cup crumbled reduced-fat
blue cheese or goat cheese

DRESSING

2 tablespoons extra-virgin olive oil

2 tablespoons balsamic vinegar

2 tablespoons orange juice

1 teaspoon Dijon mustard

$1/4$ teaspoon salt

$1/4$ teaspoon ground black pepper

1. Preheat the oven to 400°F. Leave the rootlets and 1-inch of the stems on the beets and rinse well.

2. Arrange the beets on a large piece of aluminum foil and fold up the sides to make a sealed packet. Place the packet on a baking sheet and bake for about 45 minutes (for small beets) or $1^1/4$ hours (for large beets), or until the beets are easily pierced with a wooden toothpick. Open the foil and allow the beets to cool to room temperature.

3. Peel the beets (the skins should slip off easily). Then slice or cut into $3/4$-inch pieces. You should have about 2 cups. Set aside.

4. Place all of the dressing ingredients in a small bowl, and whisk to combine.

5. Place the salad greens in a large bowl. Add $1/4$ cup of the dressing, and toss to mix.

6. To assemble the salads, divide the dressed greens among 4 salad plates. Top each salad with one-fourth of the beets, and drizzle the beets with 1 teaspoon of the remaining dressing. Sprinkle one-fourth of the walnuts and cheese (about 1 tablespoon each) over every salad. Serve immediately.

NUTRITION FACTS (PER SERVING)
Calories: 180   Carbohydrates: 13 g   Fiber: 2.9 g   Protein: 5 g
Fat: 12.9 g   Sat. Fat: 2.3 g   Cholesterol: 4 mg   Sodium: 342 mg   Calcium: 72 mg

---

BRUSSELS SPROUT SALAD

YIELD: 4 SERVINGS

8 ounces fresh Brussels sprouts
(about 12 medium)

6 cups mixed baby salad greens

3 tablespoons dried cranberries

3 tablespoons sliced almonds
(unroasted)

2 tablespoons crumbled reduced-fat
blue cheese

DRESSING

2 tablespoons extra-virgin olive oil

1 tablespoon lemon juice

1 tablespoon orange juice

1 teaspoon Dijon mustard

$1/4$ teaspoon salt

$1/4$ teaspoon ground black pepper

1. Rinse the Brussels sprouts with cool water, and shake off any excess water. Remove the tough outer leaves and slice very thinly, discarding the tough stem end. Separate the slices into shreds. There should be about 3 cups.

2. Combine the salad greens and shredded Brussels sprouts in a large bowl.

3. Place all of the dressing ingredients in a small bowl, and whisk to combine. Pour the dressing over the salad, and toss to mix.

4. Divide the salad among 4 salad plates, and top each with one-fourth of the cranberries, almonds, and cheese. Serve immediately.

NUTRITION FACTS (PER SERVING)

Calories: 149   Carbohydrates: 13 g   Fiber: 4 g   Protein: 4.5 g
Fat: 9.7 g   Sat. Fat: 1.6 g   Cholesterol: 0 mg   Sodium: 245 mg   Calcium: 68 mg

---

COLORFUL CHOPPED SALAD

YIELD: 4 SERVINGS

6 cups thinly sliced romaine lettuce
or spinach

$3/4$ cup cauliflower florets chopped
into $1/4$-inch pieces

$3/4$ cup broccoli florets chopped into
$1/4$-inch pieces

$1/2$ cup julienne-cut carrots

$1/2$ cup thinly sliced scallions

$1/4$ cup dried cranberries
or golden raisins

$1/4$ cup chopped pecans, walnuts, or
pumpkin seeds (unroasted)

$1/4$ cup plus 2 tablespoons bottled
light olive oil vinaigrette or
light balsamic vinaigrette

3 tablespoons crumbled reduced-fat
feta, blue, or goat cheese

1. Place all of the ingredients except for the dressing and cheese in a large bowl, and toss to mix.

2. Drizzle the dressing over the salad, and toss to mix.

3. Divide the salad among four salad plates. Sprinkle one-fourth of the cheese over each salad, and serve immediately.

NUTRITION FACTS (PER SERVING)
Calories: 163   Carbohydrates: 16 g   Fiber: 4.3 g   Protein: 4.1 g

Fat: 10.6 g   Sat. Fat: 1.2 g   Cholesterol: 0 mg   Sodium: 298 mg   Calcium: 55 mg

---

KALE SALAD WITH CORN AND TOMATOES

YIELD: 4 SERVINGS

6 cups thinly sliced fresh kale (use baby kale or tender leaves, with any tough stems removed)

$2/3$ cup frozen (thawed) or fresh whole kernel corn

$2/3$ cup diced grape tomatoes

$1/4$ cup thinly bias-sliced scallions

3 tablespoons pumpkin seeds (unroasted), crumbled queso fresco, or shredded reduced-fat Monterey Jack cheese (optional)

DRESSING

2 tablespoons extra-virgin olive oil

1 tablespoon lime juice

1 tablespoon orange juice

1 to $1\frac{1}{2}$ teaspoons very finely chopped seeded pickled jalapeño pepper

Scant $1/2$ teaspoon salt

$1/8$ teaspoon ground black pepper

1. Place the kale, corn, tomatoes, and scallions in a large bowl, and toss to mix.

2. Place all of the dressing ingredients in a small bowl, and whisk to combine. Pour the dressing over the salad, and toss to mix.

3. Divide the salad among 4 salad plates, and top with some of the pumpkin seeds or cheese, if using. Serve immediately.

NUTRITION FACTS (PER 1 $2/3$-CUP SERVING)
Calories: 138   Carbohydrates: 16 g   Fiber 4.4 g   Protein 4 g

Fat 7.8 g   Sat. Fat 1.1 g   Cholesterol: 0 mg   Sodium: 281 mg   Calcium: 140 mg

---

ORANGE-AVOCADO SALAD

YIELD: 4 SERVINGS

2 medium-large seedless oranges
(such as navel oranges)

8 cups mixed baby salad greens

1 cup diced avocado (about 1 large)

3 thin slices red onion,
cut into quarter-rings

$1/3$ cup shredded reduced-fat Monterey
Jack or crumbled queso fresco

DRESSING

2 tablespoons extra-virgin olive oil

1 tablespoon white wine vinegar

1 tablespoon orange juice

$1/4$ teaspoon salt

$1/4$ teaspoon ground black pepper

1. Using a sharp knife, peel the oranges, cutting all the way down to the flesh. Dice the peeled oranges to make 1 cup of $3/4$-inch pieces. Use the scraps to squeeze out 1 tablespoon of juice for the dressing. Set aside.

2. Place all of the dressing ingredients in a small bowl, and whisk to combine.

3. Place the salad greens in a large bowl, and pour 3 tablespoons of the dressing over the salad greens. Toss to mix.

4. To assemble the salads, divide the salad greens among 4 salad plates. Top each serving with one-fourth of the oranges, avocado, and onion. Drizzle $3/4$ teaspoon of the remaining dressing over each salad, and top with a sprinkling of cheese. Serve immediately.

NUTRITION FACTS (PER SERVING)

Calories: 176   Carbohydrates: 11 g   Fiber: 4.1 g   Protein: 4.4 g
Fat: 14.3 g   Sat. Fat: 2.9 g   Cholesterol: 7 mg   Sodium: 237 mg   Calcium: 99 mg

---

CUCUMBER AND TOMATO SALAD

YIELD: 6 SERVINGS

1 medium-large hothouse
(English) cucumber

4 slices red onion, cut into quarter-rings

2 cups halved grape tomatoes

3 tablespoons finely chopped fresh basil

1 tablespoon extra-virgin olive oil

DRESSING

2 tablespoons red wine vinegar

1 teaspoon sugar

$1/2$ teaspoon salt

$1/4$ teaspoon ground black pepper

1. Cut the cucumber in half lengthwise, and use the small end of a melon baller or a spoon to scrape out and discard the seeds. Thinly slice the cucumber (slightly less than $1/4$-inch thick). There should be about 2 cups. Place the cucumber and onion in a large bowl.

2. Place all of the dressing ingredients in a small bowl, and stir to combine. Pour the dressing over the cucumber mixture, and toss to mix.

3. Cover the salad and chill for at least 2 hours. About 30 minutes before serving, stir in the tomatoes, basil, and olive oil.

NUTRITION FACTS (PER $2/3$-CUP SERVING)
Calories: 50   Carbohydrates: 7 g   Fiber: 1.5 g   Protein: 1.1 g
Fat: 2.5 g   Sat. Fat: 0.4 g   Cholesterol: 0 mg   Sodium: 173 mg   Calcium: 15 mg

GARDEN FRESH TABBOULEH

YIELD: 8 SERVINGS

1 cup uncooked bulgur wheat

$1^1/_2$ cups chopped fresh tomatoes (about 2 medium)

$1^1/_2$ cups chopped peeled and seeded cucumber (about $1^1/_2$ medium)

1 cup finely chopped fresh parsley (or more to taste)

$3/_4$ cup sliced scallions

$1/_3$ cup finely chopped fresh mint

DRESSING

3 tablespoons extra-virgin olive oil

3 tablespoons lemon juice

1 teaspoon crushed garlic

$3/_4$ teaspoon salt

$1/_2$ teaspoon ground black pepper

1. Prepare the bulgur wheat according to package directions and allow to cool.

2. Place the bulgur wheat, tomatoes, cucumber, parsley, scallions, and mint in a large bowl, and toss to mix.

3. Place all of the dressing ingredients in a small bowl, and whisk to combine. Pour the dressing over the salad, and toss to mix.

4. Cover the salad and chill for at least 20 minutes before serving.

NUTRITION FACTS (PER $7/_8$-CUP SERVING)
Calories: 135   Carbohydrates: 17 g   Fiber: 4.4 g   Protein: 3.1 g
Fat: 6.1 g   Sat. Fat: 1 g   Cholesterol: 0 mg   Sodium: 228 mg   Calcium: 36 mg

CARROT SALAD
WITH PARSLEY AND SPRING ONIONS

YIELD: 6 SERVINGS

4 cups julienne-cut or matchstick carrots (about 10 ounces, or 5 medium carrots)

1 cup finely chopped fresh parsley

$^3/_4$ cup sliced scallions

DRESSING

2 tablespoons extra-virgin olive oil

1 tablespoon white wine vinegar

$^1/_4$ teaspoon salt

$^1/_4$ teaspoon ground black pepper

1. Place the carrots, parsley, and scallions in a medium-size bowl, and toss to mix.

2. Place all of the dressing ingredients in a small bowl, and whisk to combine. Pour the dressing over the salad, and toss to mix.

3. Set the salad aside for 15 minutes, or cover and chill until ready to serve.

NUTRITION FACTS (PER $^3/_4$-CUP SERVING)

Calories: 80   Carbohydrates: 9 g   Fiber: 2.9 g   Protein: 1.3 g
Fat: 4.7 g   Sat. Fat: 0.6 g   Cholesterol: 0 mg   Sodium: 129 mg   Calcium: 43 mg

SOUTHWEST CABBAGE SALAD

YIELD: 6 SERVINGS

5 cups thinly sliced green cabbage (about $^1/_2$ medium head cabbage)

1 cup frozen (thawed) or fresh whole kernel corn

$^1/_2$ cup thinly sliced scallions

$^1/_4$ cup plus 2 tablespoons thin slivers red or yellow bell pepper

2 to 3 tablespoons finely chopped fresh cilantro

DRESSING

2 tablespoons extra-virgin olive oil

2 tablespoons white wine vinegar

2 tablespoons orange juice

2 teaspoons sugar

$^1/_2$ teaspoon ground black pepper

$^1/_2$ teaspoon salt

$^1/_2$ to $^3/_4$ teaspoon finely chopped pickled jalapeño pepper

1. Place the cabbage, corn, scallions, bell pepper, and cilantro in a large bowl, and toss to mix.

2. Place all of the dressing ingredients in a small bowl, and whisk to combine. Pour the dressing over the salad, and toss to mix.

3. Cover the salad and chill for at least 1 hour before serving.

NUTRITION FACTS (PER $^3/_4$-CUP SERVING)

Calories: 96   Carbohydrates: 13 g   Fiber: 2.9 g   Protein: 1.9 g
Fat: 4.8 g   Sat. Fat: 0.7 g   Cholesterol: 0 mg   Sodium: 191 mg   Calcium: 37 mg

GREEN BEAN AND POTATO SALAD

YIELD: 6 SERVINGS

2 cups unpeeled red-skinned new potatoes or golden fingerling potatoes cut into $^3/_4$-inch pieces (about 10 ounces)

3 cups 1-inch pieces fresh green beans (about 12 ounces)

$^1/_3$ cup thin slivers red onion

DRESSING

2 tablespoons extra-virgin olive oil

1 tablespoon white wine vinegar

1 tablespoon lemon juice

2 teaspoons Dijon mustard

$^3/_4$ teaspoon crushed garlic

$^1/_2$ teaspoon salt

$^1/_2$ teaspoon ground black pepper

1. Place a steamer basket in a 6-quart pot, and fill with enough water to reach within $^1/_2$ inch of the bottom of the basket. Arrange the potatoes in the basket, cover, and bring to a boil. Allow the potatoes to steam for 5 minutes. Add the green beans and steam for 5 additional minutes, or until the potatoes are easily pierced with a fork and the green beans are crisp-tender. Transfer the vegetables to a large bowl, and set aside.

2. Place all of the dressing ingredients in a small bowl, and whisk to combine. Pour the dressing over the warm vegetables, and toss to mix. Add the onion, and toss again.

3. Allow the salad to sit for 15 minutes before serving, and serve warm. Alternatively, cover and chill before serving.

NUTRITION FACTS (PER $^3/_4$-CUP SERVING)

Calories: 96   Carbohydrates: 12 g   Fiber: 2 g   Protein: 2 g
Fat: 4.6 g   Sat. Fat: 0.6 g   Cholesterol: 0 mg   Sodium: 217 mg   Calcium: 19 mg

QUINOA SALAD WITH BROCCOLI AND CARROTS

YIELD: 6 SERVINGS

1 cup uncooked quinoa

1 $^3/_4$ cups water

1 $^1/_2$ cups broccoli florets chopped into $^1/_4$- to $^1/_2$-inch pieces

$^3/_4$ cup julienne-cut carrots

$^1/_2$ cup thinly sliced scallions

$^1/_3$ cup chopped pecans or cashews (unroasted) (optional)

DRESSING

3 tablespoons extra-virgin olive oil

1 $^1/_2$ tablespoons white wine vinegar

1 $^1/_2$ tablespoons lemon juice

1 teaspoon crushed garlic

Scant $^1/_2$ teaspoon salt

Scant $^1/_2$ teaspoon ground black pepper

1. Place the quinoa in a wire strainer, and rinse well with cool running water. Place the 1 $^3/_4$ cups water in a 2-quart pot, and bring to a boil. Stir in the quinoa and reduce the heat to maintain a simmer. Cover and cook without stirring for 12 minutes, or until the water is absorbed. Turn off the heat and allow the covered pot to sit for 5 minutes. Chill the quinoa before proceeding with the recipe.

2. Place the chilled quinoa, broccoli, carrots, scallions, and nuts (if using) in a large bowl, and toss to mix.

3. Place all of the dressing ingredients in a small bowl, and whisk to combine. Pour the dressing over the salad, and toss to mix.

4. Cover the salad and chill for at least 1 hour before serving.

VARIATION

❑ Substitute barley or farro for the quinoa, and cook the grain according to package directions.

NUTRITION FACTS (PER $^7/_8$-CUP SERVING)

Calories: 182   Carbohydrates: 22 g   Fiber: 3.3 g   Protein: 5 g
Fat: 8.6 g   Sat. Fat: 1.2 g   Cholesterol: 0 mg   Sodium: 215 mg   Calcium: 36 mg

---

Sauces and Marinades

People often fear that cooking with less heat and more water will result in dishes that are flat and flavorless. This is far from true—once you learn the secrets of AGE-less cooking. Boosting taste and visual appeal with sauces, salsas, and marinades is one of those secrets.

Almost every culture has its own piquant sauces or salsas that are perfect for adding flavor to meats, poultry, and seafood. Intensely flavored sauces are especially well suited to complement the mildness of steamed and poached dishes. This collection includes a number of recipes for sauces that can be served with poached or steamed foods such as fish, chicken, or eggs. Some can also be tossed with vegetables, pasta, or rice for a vibrant spin on AGE-less style.

You can also enhance flavor with marinades. Just as important, when these tasty liquids are prepared with acidic ingredients such as lemon juice, wine, vinegar, and tomato juice, they serve the practical function of reducing AGE formation. Marinating is a must before grilling, since it can prevent AGE formation by up to 50 percent, but this technique can also lend flavor to foods that will be sautéed or braised. The following pages present several zesty marinades as well as some practical tips for using these versatile liquids to make your AGE-less dishes as tantalizing as they are healthy.

SAUCES

CHIMICHURRI SAUCE

YIELD: ABOUT $^3/_4$ CUP

$^1/_2$ cup (packed) finely chopped fresh parsley

1 tablespoon finely chopped fresh oregano, or 1 teaspoon dried

$^1/_4$ cup extra-virgin olive oil

$^1/_4$ cup lemon juice, white wine vinegar, or red wine vinegar

1 tablespoon water

1 teaspoon crushed garlic

$^1/_2$ teaspoon salt

$^1/_4$ teaspoon ground black pepper

$^1/_4$ teaspoon crushed red pepper flakes

1. Place the parsley and oregano in a small bowl, and stir to combine. Stir in the remaining ingredients.

2. Allow the sauce to stand for 20 minutes before serving, or cover and refrigerate for up to 2 days. If chilled, return the sauce to room temperature and stir well before serving. Spoon over steamed or poached fish, poultry, or meat.

NUTRITION FACTS (PER 1-TABLESPOON SERVING)

Calories: 42   Carbohydrates: 1 g   Fiber: 0.1 g   Protein: 0.2 g

Fat: 4.5 g   Sat. Fat: 0.6 g   Cholesterol: 0 mg   Sodium: 97 mg   Calcium: 6 mg

LEMON-PARSLEY SAUCE

YIELD: ABOUT $^7/_8$ CUP

1 teaspoon crushed garlic

$^1/_2$ teaspoon salt

$^1/_4$ teaspoon ground black pepper

$^1/_4$ teaspoon crushed red pepper flakes

$^1/_2$ teaspoon freshly grated lemon zest

$^1/_4$ cup lemon juice

1 tablespoon water

$^1/_4$ cup plus 2 tablespoons extra-virgin olive oil

$^1/_2$ cup (packed) finely chopped fresh parsley

1 tablespoon capers, drained

1. Place the first 5 ingredients (garlic through lemon zest) in a small bowl, and mash the mixture into a paste. Whisk in the lemon juice and water.

2. Add the olive oil to the garlic mixture in a thin stream, whisking constantly until blended. Stir in the parsley and capers

3. Allow the sauce to stand for 20 minutes before serving, or cover and refrigerate for up to 2 days. If chilled, return the sauce to room temperature and stir well before using. Spoon a small amount over a portion of poached or steamed fish, poultry, or meat.

NUTRITION FACTS (PER 1-TABLESPOON SERVING)

Calories: 54   Carbohydrates: 1 g   Fiber: 0.1 g   Protein: 0.1 g

Fat: 5.8 g   Sat. Fat: 0.8 g   Cholesterol: 0 mg   Sodium: 101 mg   Calcium: 4 mg

---

LEMON-DILL SAUCE

YIELD: ABOUT $1/2$ CUP

1 cup (moderately packed) fresh dill leaves

$1/2$ cup (moderately packed) fresh parsley leaves

3 tablespoons extra-virgin olive oil

2 tablespoons lemon juice

1 tablespoon Dijon mustard

1 teaspoon crushed garlic

$1/4$ teaspoon salt

$1/4$ teaspoon ground black pepper

1. Place all of the ingredients in a food processor, and process to a pesto-like consistency.

2. Serve immediately, or refrigerate for up to 2 days. If chilled, return the sauce to room temperature and stir well before serving. Spoon over poached or steamed fish or chicken; or toss with steamed carrots, cauliflower, potatoes, asparagus, or other vegetables.

NUTRITION FACTS (PER 1-TABLESPOON SERVING)

Calories: 51   Carbohydrates: 1 g   Fiber: 0.2 g   Protein: 0.3 g

Fat: 5.3 g   Sat. Fat: 0.7 g   Cholesterol: 0 mg   Sodium: 122 mg   Calcium 11 mg

---

BASIL PESTO

YIELD: ABOUT 1 CUP

2 cups (packed) fresh basil leaves

$1/4$ cup plus 2 tablespoons chopped walnuts (unroasted)

$1/4$ cup extra-virgin olive oil

2 tablespoons grated Parmesan cheese

1 to $1^1/2$ teaspoons crushed fresh garlic

$1/4$ teaspoon salt

$1/4$ teaspoon ground black pepper

1. Rinse the basil with cool water. Shake off the excess water, but do not pat dry. Place the basil and the remaining ingredients in a food processor. Process, stopping periodically to scrape down the sides, until the mixture forms a thick sauce consistency. Mix in a little water, a teaspoon at a time, if the mixture seems too thick.

2. Serve immediately, cover and refrigerate for 3 days, or freeze for several months. If frozen or chilled, bring the sauce to room temperature and stir well before using. Spoon over poached or steamed fish or chicken, or toss with pasta, cooked grains, or steamed vegetables.

NUTRITION FACTS (PER 1-TABLESPOON SERVING)
Calories: 49   Carbohydrates: 0.6 g   Fiber: 0.2 g   Protein: 0.8 g

Fat: 5.1 g   Sat. Fat: 0.7 g   Cholesterol: 1 mg   Sodium: 46 mg   Calcium: 19 mg

CILANTRO SALSA

YIELD: $1^1/2$ CUPS

1 cup (moderately packed) chopped fresh cilantro leaves

1 cup chopped fresh tomato

$1/3$ cup finely chopped yellow or red onion

1 to 2 teaspoons finely chopped seeded fresh or pickled jalapeño pepper*

2 teaspoons extra-virgin olive oil

1 teaspoon lime juice

1 teaspoon red wine vinegar

$1/4$ teaspoon salt

$1/4$ teaspoon ground black pepper

*Wear protective gloves when handling fresh hot peppers.

1. Place the cilantro, tomato, onion, and jalapeño pepper in a small bowl, and stir to combine. Set aside.

2. Place the olive oil, lime juice, vinegar, salt, and pepper in a small bowl, and whisk to combine.

3. Pour the olive oil mixture over the cilantro mixture, and toss to mix. Allow the salsa to sit for 10 minutes before serving, or cover and refrigerate for up to several hours. Serve over omelets or poached or steamed chicken or fish.

NUTRITION FACTS (PER ¹/₄-CUP SERVING)
Calories: 24   Carbohydrates: 2 g   Fiber: 0.6 g   Protein: 0.4 g
Fat: 1.7 g   Sat. Fat: 0.2 g   Cholesterol: 0 mg   Sodium: 100 mg   Calcium: 7 mg

TOMATO AND CAPER SALSA

YIELD: ABOUT 1¹/₄ CUPS

1 cup chopped seeded plum tomato (about 3 medium)

¹/₄ cup finely chopped red onion

¹/₄ cup finely chopped fresh parsley or basil

1¹/₂ to 2 tablespoons capers, drained

¹/₄ teaspoon ground black pepper

1. Place all of the ingredients in a small bowl, and stir to mix.

2. Allow the sauce to sit for 10 to 30 minutes before serving, or cover and refrigerate for up to several hours. Spoon over omelets or over poached or steamed chicken or fish.

NUTRITION FACTS (PER ¹/₄-CUP SERVING)
Calories: 12   Carbohydrates: 3 g   Fiber: 0.7 g   Protein: 0.5 g
Fat: 0.2 g   Sat. Fat: 0 g   Cholesterol: 0 mg   Sodium: 73 mg   Calcium: 8 mg

CHIPOTLE SAUCE

YIELD: ABOUT 2 CUPS

1 can (4 ounces) chipotle chile peppers in adobo sauce

1 can (14$^{1}/_{2}$ ounces) no-salt-added diced tomatoes, undrained

5 ounces fresh tomatillos, husked, rinsed, and coarsely chopped (about 1 cup)

$^{1}/_{4}$ cup chopped yellow onion

2 to 3 tablespoons chopped fresh cilantro leaves

1$^{1}/_{2}$ teaspoons chopped fresh oregano, or $^{1}/_{2}$ teaspoon dried

1 tablespoon extra-virgin olive oil

1 teaspoon crushed garlic

$^{1}/_{2}$ teaspoon salt

$^{1}/_{4}$ teaspoon ground black pepper

1. Drain the sauce from the canned chile peppers into a blender. Wearing protective gloves, cut open the chiles and remove and discard all or part of the seeds along with the inner membranes (this tones down the heat). Add the chiles to the blender, and blend until smooth. Transfer the mixture to a small container and set aside.

2. Place all of the remaining ingredients in the blender along with 2 tablespoons of the chile purée. Blend until smooth. (Reserve the remaining purée for another use. Stored in the freezer, it will remain fresh for months.)

3. Pour the tomato mixture into a 10-inch nonstick skillet. Bring to a boil, then adjust the heat to maintain a simmer. Cover and cook for 15 minutes. Remove the lid and simmer uncovered, stirring occasionally, for about 10 minutes, or until the mixture is reduced to about 2 cups. The sauce should have the consistency of marinara sauce.

4. Spoon the hot sauce over eggs, meats, or poultry, or toss with shredded poached chicken to make tacos. Any leftover sauce can be frozen for several months.

NUTRITION FACTS (PER 2-TABLESPOON SERVING)

Calories: 19   Carbohydrates: 2 g   Fiber: 0.6 g   Protein: 0.4 g

Fat: 1 g   Sat. Fat: 0.1 g   Cholesterol: 0 mg   Sodium: 138 mg   Calcium: 10 mg

---

MARINADES

LEMON-CAPER MARINADE

YIELD: ABOUT $^2/_3$ CUP (ENOUGH FOR 1 POUND OF MEAT)

$^1/_3$ cup lemon juice

$^1/_4$ cup water

$1^1/_2$ tablespoons chopped fresh
rosemary or thyme, or
$1^1/_2$ teaspoons dried

$1^1/_2$ tablespoons extra-virgin olive oil

$1^1/_2$ tablespoons capers, drained

1 tablespoon crushed garlic

$^3/_4$ teaspoon salt

$^3/_4$ teaspoon ground black pepper

1. Place all of the ingredients in a small bowl, and stir to blend.

2. Place the food and marinade in a shallow non-reactive container (such as glass, enamel, or ceramic), and turn the food to coat. Marinate meat and poultry in the refrigerator for at least 1 hour or up to 24 hours, turning occasionally. Marinate seafood for no longer than 1 hour, as the acid will start to "cook" the seafood.

3. Remove the food from the marinade, discarding the marinade or boiling it for reuse as a sauce. (See page 286.) Cook the meat as directed in the recipe of your choice.

NUTRITION FACTS (PER $2^1/_2$-TABLESPOON SERVING)

Calories: 55   Carbohydrates: 3 g   Fiber: 0.4 g   Protein: 0.3 g
Fat: 5.2 g   Sat. Fat: 0.8 g   Cholesterol: 0 mg   Sodium: 532 mg   Calcium: 11 mg

---

ZESTY HERB MARINADE

YIELD: ABOUT $^2/_3$ CUP (ENOUGH FOR 1 POUND OF MEAT)

$^1/_3$ cup white or red wine vinegar

$^1/_4$ cup water

$1^1/_2$ tablespoons Dijon mustard

$1^1/_2$ tablespoons chopped fresh thyme
or oregano, or $1^1/_2$ teaspoons dried

$1^1/_2$ tablespoons extra-virgin
olive oil

1 tablespoon crushed garlic

$^3/_4$ teaspoon salt

$^3/_4$ teaspoon ground black pepper

Tips for AGE-Less Marinades

Throughout this book, we've explained that marinades not only add flavor to food, but—when prepared with acidic ingredients such as lemon juice and wine—also reduce AGE formation. That's why this chapter offers recipes for several tasty marinades

The following tips guide you in successfully using marinades to enhance your meals. And because you may not always have time to prepare a savory solution from scratch, we begin by helping you choose the best commercial products for your AGE-less cooking.

❑ When buying commercial marinades, choose low-sugar, low-oil products made with lemon or lime juice, wine, or vinegar, and seasoned with plenty of herbs and spices. Avoid thick, sweet marinades, which can burn and char easily, increasing AGE formation. Bottled low-calorie vinaigrette salad dressings such as light balsamic or light Italian can be good options.

❑ To increase the food's absorption of the marinade and speed cooking time, cut the meat into chunks for kebabs, or "butterfly" it to create a thinner cut of meat. The larger surface area permits more of the solution to penetrate the food. To butterfly a boneless, skinless chicken breast, cut the breast horizontally, slicing almost all the way through the meat. Then open it like a book to form a large flat piece. This technique can also be used with cuts of pork, beef, and lamb.

❑ Marinate foods in a shallow non-reactive container (such as glass, enamel, or ceramic), as certain metals can react with acidic foods, changing the color and flavor of the dish. Marinate your food in the refrigerator to prevent bacterial growth, and turn the food occasionally to ensure that all sides soak up some of the marinade.

❑ Marinate meats and poultry for at least one hour or up to twenty-four hours. Marinate seafood for no longer than one hour, as the acid will start to "cook" the seafood if the two remain in contact for too long.

❑ While simply marinating a food can add flavor, your marinade can also be used to make a tasty sauce to drizzle over the cooked dish. Simply drain the used marinade into a small pot and bring it to a boil for several minutes, until it is reduced by about half. For food safety reasons, you should never consume a marinade that has been in contact with meat, poultry, or seafood without first keeping it at a rolling boil for several minutes.

1. Place all of the ingredients in a small bowl, and stir to blend. Use red wine vinegar for beef and lamb, and white wine vinegar for chicken or seafood.

2. Place the food and marinade in a shallow non-reactive container (such as glass, enamel, or ceramic), and turn the food to coat. Marinate meat and poultry in the refrigerator for at least 1 hour or up to 24 hours, turning occasionally. Seafood should not be marinated for longer than 1 hour, as the acid will start to "cook" the seafood.

3. Remove the food from the marinade, discarding the marinade or boiling it for reuse as a sauce. (See page 286.) Cook the meat as directed in the recipe of your choice.

NUTRITION FACTS (PER 2^1/$_2$-TABLESPOON SERVING)
Calories: 56   Carbohydrates: 2 g   Fiber: 0.3 g   Protein: 0.2 g
Fat: 5.1 g   Sat. Fat: 0.7 g   Cholesterol: 0 mg   Sodium: 571 mg   Calcium: 10 mg

---

LEMON-PEPPER MARINADE

YIELD: ABOUT ^{1}/$_2$ CUP (ENOUGH FOR 1 POUND OF MEAT)

^{1}/$_4$ cup lemon juice

^{1}/$_4$ cup dry white wine

1^1/$_2$ tablespoons extra-virgin olive oil

1 tablespoon crushed garlic

2 teaspoons finely grated lemon zest

1 teaspoon ground black pepper

^{3}/$_4$ teaspoon salt

1. Place all of the ingredients in a small bowl, and stir to blend.

2. Place the food and marinade in a shallow non-reactive container (such as glass, enamel, or ceramic), and turn the food to coat. Marinate meat and poultry in the refrigerator for at least 1 hour or up to 24 hours, turning occasionally. Marinate seafood for no longer than 1 hour, as the acid will start to "cook" the seafood.

3. Remove the food from the marinade, discarding the marinade or boiling it for reuse as a sauce. (See page 286.) Cook the meat as directed in the recipe of your choice.

NUTRITION FACTS (PER 2-TABLESPOON SERVING)
Calories: 65   Carbohydrates: 2 g   Fiber: 0.3 g   Protein: 0.2 g
Fat: 5.1 g   Sat. Fat: 0.7 g   Cholesterol: 0 mg   Sodium: 437 mg   Calcium: 9 mg

---

MOJO MARINADE

YIELD: ABOUT $^2/_3$ CUP
(ENOUGH FOR 1 POUND OF MEAT)

$^1/_4$ cup plus 2 tablespoons orange juice

$^1/_4$ cup lime juice

$^1/_4$ cup chopped fresh oregano, or 1 tablespoon plus 1 teaspoon dried

1$^1/_2$ tablespoons extra-virgin olive oil

1 tablespoon crushed garlic

1 tablespoon finely chopped seeded fresh or pickled jalapeño pepper*

1 teaspoon ground cumin

$^3/_4$ teaspoon salt

$^3/_4$ teaspoon ground black pepper

---

* Wear protective gloves when handling fresh hot peppers.

1. Place all of the ingredients in a small bowl, and stir to blend.

2. Place the food and marinade in a shallow non-reactive container (such as glass, enamel, or ceramic), and turn the food to coat. Marinate meat and poultry in the refrigerator for at least 1 hour or up to 24 hours, turning occasionally. Marinate seafood for no longer than 1 hour, as the acid will start to "cook" the seafood.

3. Remove the food from the marinade, discarding the marinade or boiling it for reuse as a sauce. (See page 286.) Cook the meat as directed in the recipe of your choice.

NUTRITION FACTS (PER 2$^1/_2$-TABLESPOON SERVING)
Calories: 71   Carbohydrates: 6 g   Fiber: 0.7 g   Protein: 0.7 g
Fat: 5.3 g   Sat. Fat: 0.8 g   Cholesterol: 0 mg   Sodium: 437 mg   Calcium: 57 mg

---

AGE-*LESS* TIP—USING MARINADES TO
BOOST FLAVOR AND LIMIT AGES

Marinades not only add flavor to food, but, when prepared with acidic ingredients, they also reduce the formation of AGEs during cooking. Lemon, orange, and lime juice; vinegar; and wine are all great acidic marinade ingredients. Add a bit of olive oil and plenty of herbs and spices, and you'll have a wonderful marinade for use in your AGE-less meals.

$\mathcal{S}$weets and Treats

If you enjoy a sweet treat, you will be happy to know that eating the AGE-less way does not mean doing without. But you have to be smart about your indulgences. It goes without saying that rich desserts are packed with AGEs due to high amounts of both fats and sugars. So if you have a dessert that's loaded with cream, butter, sugar, and the like, be sure to enjoy just a few bites.

Fresh fruit is by far the best choice for satisfying a sweet tooth. Indulge often in tree-ripened organic fruit—it is so luscious that it requires no added sugar. When you want something a bit more elaborate, enjoy one of the AGE-less treats presented in this chapter. These recipes feature wholesome ingredients like fresh or frozen fruits, yogurt, nuts, and chocolate. They also use modest amounts of sugar and fat, making them a good choice whenever you want to minimize AGEs and maximize satisfaction.

BERRIES ZABAGLIONE

YIELD: 4 SERVINGS

3 cups mixed fresh berries, such as raspberries, blueberries, and sliced strawberries

SAUCE

4 large egg yolks

$1/4$ cup sugar

$1/2$ cup minus 1 tablespoon medium-dry Marsala or sherry wine

1. Fill a 2-quart pot with about 3 inches of water and bring to a simmer.

2. While the water is heating , place the egg yolks and sugar in a 2- or 3-quart stainless steel bowl that can sit in the 2-quart pot, extending a few inches into the pot. (If you have a double boiler, you can use that instead of the bowl and pot.) Whisk the eggs and sugar for a couple of minutes, or until pale yellow. Slowly whisk in the Marsala or sherry.

3. Rest the bowl over the simmering pot of water without allowing the bottom of the bowl to touch the water. Whisk constantly for about 6 minutes, or until the mixture triples in volume and thickens to a custard-like consistency. As you whisk, be sure to clear the bottom of the bowl so that the eggs do not scramble, and adjust the heat as needed to keep the water in the pot simmering.

4. To serve, divide the fruit among four 8-ounce wine glasses or dessert dishes, and top each portion with one-fourth of the warm sauce (about $1/3$ cup). (The sauce can be made up to 8 hours before serving, refrigerated, and allowed to reach room temperature before serving.) Serve immediately.

NUTRITION FACTS (PER SERVING)

Calories: 172   Carbohydrates: 25 g   Fiber: 3.7 g   Protein: 3.6 g

Fat: 5 g   Sat. Fat: 1.7 g   Cholesterol: 184 mg   Sodium: 11 mg   Calcium: 41 mg

CINNAMON ROASTED PEARS

Yield: 4 servings

1 tablespoon plus 1 teaspoon turbinado sugar or light brown sugar	2 large ripe but firm pears (about 8 ounces each)
$1/2$ teaspoon ground cinnamon	2 teaspoons frozen (thawed) orange juice concentrate or maple syrup

1. Preheat the oven to 400°F. Coat an 8 x 8-inch pan with cooking spray, and set aside.

2. Place the sugar and cinnamon in a small bowl, and stir to combine. Set aside.

3. Cut the pears in half lengthwise and scoop out the fibrous cores. Trim a small slice from the bottom of each pear half so that the pears will sit firmly on the pan. Arrange the pears on the pan cored-side-down.

4. Bake uncovered for 10 minutes. Turn the pears over. Spread $1/2$ teaspoon of the juice concentrate or maple syrup on each half, and sprinkle with one-fourth of the sugar mixture (about 1 teaspoon). Continue to bake uncovered for about 10 additional minutes, or until the pears are easily pierced with a sharp knife. Serve warm.

VARIATION

❏ Top each pear half with a small scoop (about $1/3$ cup) of light vanilla ice cream or frozen yogurt and a sprinkling (about $1^1/2$ teaspoons) of chopped walnuts (unroasted).

Nutritional Facts (Per Serving)

Calories: 83   Carbohydrates: 22 g   Fiber: 3.5 g   Protein: 0.4 g
Fat: 0.1 g   Sat. Fat: 0 g   Cholesterol: 0 mg   Sodium: 1 mg   Calcium: 14 mg

---

AGE-*LESS* TIP—SATISFYING YOUR TASTE FOR ROASTED AND GRILLED FOODS

Although it's best to avoid roasting and grilling meat and other high-AGE foods, you can satisfy your taste for grilled and roasted foods by using these cooking techniques with fruits and vegetables. True, the AGE count will increase, but it will still be extremely low compared with that of roasted or grilled meats.

ROASTED PEACHES WITH RICOTTA AND HONEY

YIELD: 4 SERVINGS

1 tablespoon plus 1 teaspoon light brown sugar or turbinado sugar

$1/4$ teaspoon ground ginger

2 large ripe but firm peaches (about 8 ounces each)

$1/4$ cup part-skim ricotta cheese

1 tablespoon plus 1 teaspoon honey

1 tablespoon plus 1 teaspoon sliced almonds (unroasted)

1. Preheat the oven to 400°F. Coat an 8 x 8-inch pan with cooking spray, and set aside.

2. Place the brown sugar and ginger in a small dish, and stir to combine. Set aside.

3. Cut the peaches in half lengthwise and discard the pits. Trim a small slice from the bottom of each peach half so the peaches will sit firmly on the pan. Arrange the peaches on the pan, pitted-side-down

4. Bake uncovered for 6 minutes. Turn the peaches over, and sprinkle one-fourth of the brown sugar mixture (about 1 teaspoon) over each peach half. Continue to bake for an additional 6 to 8 minutes, or until the peaches are easily pierced with a sharp knife.

5. For each serving, place one peach half pitted-side-up in a dessert dish. Place 1 tablespoon of ricotta cheese in the center of each peach, drizzle with 1 teaspoon of honey, and top with 1 teaspoon of almonds. Serve warm.

NUTRITIONAL FACTS (PER SERVING)

Calories: 109   Carbohydrates: 21 g   Fiber: 2 g   Protein: 3.2 g

Fat: 2.4 g   Sat. Fat: 1 g   Cholesterol: 5 mg   Sodium: 21 mg   Calcium: 58 mg

CHOCOLATE COVERED STRAWBERRIES

YIELD: 12 PIECES

4 ounces dark chocolate, chopped

12 medium-large fresh strawberries, rinsed and patted dry

$^1/_4$ cup sliced almonds or finely chopped walnuts or hazelnuts (unroasted)

1. Line a large baking sheet with waxed paper and set aside.

2. Fill a 1-quart pot one-third full with water, and bring to a boil. Reduce the heat to maintain a simmer. Place the chocolate in a 2-cup heatproof glass measuring cup. Place the cup in the simmering water, and stir the chocolate frequently for several minutes until it has completely melted.

3. Insert a toothpick into the stem of a strawberry, and dip the berry into the melted chocolate to coat the lower three-fourths of the fruit. Hold the berry by the toothpick over a plate, and rotate while sprinkling the chocolate with a teaspoon of nuts. If necessary, lightly press the nuts into the chocolate to make them stick. Place the berry on the lined baking sheet. Repeat with the remaining berries.

4. Chill for at least 1 hour. Serve or transfer to a covered container and refrigerate for up to 12 hours before serving.

NUTRITION FACTS (PER STRAWBERRY)

Calories: 63 Carbohydrates: 6 g Fiber: 0.9 g Protein: 1.3 g

Fat: 4.9 g Sat. Fat: 2.2 g Cholesterol: 0 mg Sodium: 2 mg Calcium: 13 mg

---

AGE-*LESS* TIP—
INCLUDING NUTS IN YOUR AGE-LESS DIET

Although high in AGEs, nuts are packed with healthy nutrients such as fiber, folate, magnesium, and potassium. To make them part of your AGE-less diet, use them in moderation and avoid roasting or toasting them, as dry heat can double their AGE content.

POACHED PLUMS

Yield: 4 servings

4 medium-large ripe but firm red or purple plums (about 4 ounces each)

$^3/_4$ cup white wine

$^3/_4$ cup orange juice

3 tablespoons sugar

$1^1/_2$ tablespoons sliced almonds (unroasted) (optional)

2 teaspoons finely chopped crystallized ginger (optional)

1. Cut the plums in half lengthwise and discard the pits.

2. Place the wine and orange juice in a large nonstick skillet. Add the plums, cover, and bring to a boil over medium heat.

3. Adjust the heat to maintain a simmer and cook for 4 minutes. Turn the plums over and cook for 4 additional minutes, or until the plums are easily pierced with a sharp knife. Using a slotted spoon, transfer the plums to a dish, cover to keep warm, and set aside.

4. Add the sugar to the liquid in the skillet, and bring to a boil over medium heat. Cook uncovered for about 5 minutes, or until the liquid is syrupy and reduced to about $^1/_3$ cup in volume.

5. To serve, arrange 2 plum halves, cut-side-up, in each of 4 dessert dishes, and pour one-fourth of the sauce over each serving. Top with a sprinkling of almonds and ginger, if desired, and serve warm.

VARIATION

❏ To reduce calories and carbohydrates, substitute low-calorie sweetener for the sugar in the syrup. You will save 35 calories and 9 grams of carbohydrates per serving.

Nutritional Facts (Per Serving)

Calories: 127   Carbohydrates: 24 g   Fiber: 1 g   Protein: 0.6 g

Fat: 0.2 g   Sat. Fat: 0 g   Cholesterol: 0 mg   Sodium: 3 mg   Calcium: 9 mg

---

STEAMED APPLES

YIELD: 4 SERVINGS

3 cups sliced peeled apples (about 4 medium)	1 tablespoon honey or light brown sugar
1 tablespoon water	$1/4$ teaspoon ground cinnamon

1. Place the apples and water in a 2-quart pot. Cover and cook over medium heat for about 5 minutes or until crisp-tender. Add a little water during cooking if needed, but only enough to prevent scorching.

2. Stir the honey or brown sugar and the cinnamon into the apples, cover, and remove the pot from the heat. Allow to sit for 20 minutes so that the apples continue to soften. Serve warm or chilled.

VARIATIONS

❑ Spoon the warm apples over a scoop of vanilla ice cream or frozen vanilla yogurt.

❑ For a breakfast treat, chill the apples, spoon them over Greek-style yogurt, and top with a sprinkling of walnuts (unroasted).

NUTRITION FACTS (PER $1/2$-CUP SERVING)

Calories: 56   Carbohydrates: 15 g   Fiber: 1.5 g   Protein: 0.3 g
Fat: 0.1 g   Sat. Fat: 0 g   Cholesterol: 0 mg   Sodium: 0 mg   Calcium: 6 mg

---

AGE-*LESS* TIP—
SATISFYING YOUR SWEET TOOTH WITH FRUIT

Desserts that are high in fat and sugar are packed with AGEs. So satisfy your sweet tooth with tree-ripened organic fruit. Whether enjoyed raw or cooked, fruit will give you the luscious sweetness you crave without providing the fat, calories, sugar, and AGEs that you want to avoid.

KEY LIME PANNA COTTA

YIELD: 6 SERVINGS

$^1/_2$ cup orange juice, divided

$1^1/_4$ teaspoons unflavored gelatin

$^1/_2$ cup sugar

2 cups whole milk plain Greek-style yogurt

2 tablespoons key lime juice

TOPPING

$1^1/_2$ cups fresh strawberry slices, raspberries, or mixed berries

1 tablespoon sugar

1. Place $^1/_4$ cup of the orange juice in a 1-quart heatproof bowl. Sprinkle the gelatin over the top, and set aside for 10 minutes.

2. Place the remaining $^1/_4$ cup of juice in a small pot, and bring to a boil over medium heat. (Alternatively, microwave at high power for about 30 seconds to bring to a boil.) Add the hot juice to the gelatin mixture and whisk for 1 minute, or until the gelatin is completely dissolved.

3. Add the sugar to the orange juice mixture, and whisk for 1 minute, or until completely dissolved. Set aside for 10 minutes to cool slightly.

4. Add the yogurt to the juice mixture, and whisk until smooth. Whisk in the lime juice.

5. Spray the bottoms of six custard cups lightly with nonstick cooking spray, and divide the mixture among the cups. Cover and chill for at least 8 hours to set. Alternatively, divide the mixture among six 8-ounce wine glasses. (Do not spray the glasses with cooking spray.)

6. To make the topping, place the berries and sugar in a medium-size bowl, and toss to combine. Allow the topping to sit for 20 minutes.

7. When ready to serve, run a knife around the edges of the panna cottas, and invert each one onto a dessert plate. Top each serving with $^1/_4$ cup of the berries, and serve immediately. If you have placed the panna cotta in wine glasses, do not invert. Instead, simply spoon the berries atop the panna cotta and serve.

VARIATION

❏ To reduce calories and carbohydrates, substitute low-calorie sweetener for the sugar in the panna cotta and topping. You will save 67 calories and 17 grams of carbohydrates per serving.

NUTRITION FACTS (PER SERVING)

Calories: 163   Carbohydrates: 28 g   Fiber: 1 g   Protein: 7.3 g

Fat: 3.1 g   Sat. Fat: 2 g   Cholesterol: 15 mg   Sodium: 35 mg   Calcium: 88 mg

---

PINEAPPLE GELATO

YIELD: 5 SERVINGS

$^3/_4$ cup nonfat or low-fat Greek-style plain or vanilla yogurt

$^1/_3$ cup sugar

4 cups frozen pineapple chunks

$^1/_4$ cup chopped almonds (unroasted) (optional)

1. Place the yogurt and sugar in a small bowl, and stir to mix. Set aside for 5 minutes to allow the sugar to dissolve.

2. Place the frozen pineapple in a food processor, and process for about one minute, or until finely ground with a granita-like appearance.

3. Add the yogurt mixture and the almonds, if using, to the food processor, and process, scraping down the sides as needed, for a minute or 2, or until smooth and creamy. Add a little more yogurt if needed for the desired consistency.

4. Divide the mixture among five chilled 8-ounce wine glasses or dessert dishes, and serve immediately.

VARIATIONS

❏ Replace the pineapple with other frozen fruits, such as strawberries, peaches, plums, or mandarin oranges.

❏ To reduce calories and carbohydrates, substitute low-calorie sweetener for the sugar. You will save 48 calories and 12 grams of carbohydrates per serving.

NUTRITION FACTS (PER $^2/_3$-CUP SERVING)

Calories: 144   Carbohydrates: 32 g   Fiber: 1.8 g   Protein: 5 g

Fat: 0.3 g   Sat. Fat: 0.1 g   Cholesterol: 2 mg   Sodium: 18 mg   Calcium: 67 mg

AGE-*LESS* TIP—
CHOOSING AND USING YOGURT

Low in AGEs and high in nutrients, yogurt can be part of a healthy AGE-less diet. Whenever possible, choose nonfat or reduced-fat yogurt, and save full-fat products for those recipes that require a creamier texture.

CHERRY-VANILLA SUNDAES

YIELD: 4 SERVINGS

$1\frac{1}{2}$ cups fresh or frozen dark sweet
pitted cherries, coarsely chopped

$1\frac{1}{2}$ tablespoons orange juice

$1\frac{1}{2}$ tablespoons sugar

2 cups light vanilla ice cream
or frozen yogurt

$\frac{1}{4}$ cup chopped walnuts or pecans
(unroasted)

1. Place the cherries, orange juice, and sugar in a 1-quart pot. Cover and cook over medium heat for about 4 minutes, or until the cherries soften and release their juices. Remove the lid and cook for 5 additional minutes, or until the mixture is syrupy and reduced to $\frac{1}{2}$ cup to $\frac{2}{3}$ cup in volume.

2. Place $\frac{1}{2}$ cup of ice cream in each of four 8-ounce wine glasses. Top with one-fourth of the sauce and 1 tablespoon of the nuts, and serve immediately.

VARIATIONS

❑ Substitute blueberries for the cherries.

❑ To reduce calories and carbohydrates, substitute low-calorie sweetener for the sugar in the cherry mixture, and use light sugar-free ice cream instead of the light ice cream. You will save 28 calories and 7 grams of carbohydrates per serving.

NUTRITIONAL FACTS (PER SERVING)
Calories: 215   Carbohydrates: 34 g   Fiber: 2.7 g   Protein: 4.7 g
Fat: 6.9 g   Sat. Fat: 1.5 g   Cholesterol: 10 mg   Sodium: 60 mg   Calcium: 115 mg

BROILED PINEAPPLE À LA MODE

YIELD: 4 SERVINGS

4 rings fresh pineapple, each
about $\frac{3}{8}$-inch thick

1 tablespoon plus 1 teaspoon turbinado
sugar or light brown sugar, divided

$\frac{1}{2}$ teaspoon ground ginger

2 cups light vanilla ice cream
or frozen yogurt

2 tablespoons sliced almonds

1. Preheat the oven broiler. Line a small baking sheet with aluminum foil, and spray with nonstick cooking spray. Set aside.

2. Place 1 tablespoon of the sugar and all of the ginger in a small dish, and stir to mix. Set aside.

3. Arrange the pineapple rings on the baking sheet and broil for about 5 minutes, or until the pineapple starts to soften. Turn the pineapple over, and sprinkle $^3/_4$ teaspoon of the sugar mixture over each ring. Broil for 4 additional minutes, or until the pineapple is easily pierced with a fork and the top is bubbly and lightly browned.

4. Transfer each pineapple ring to a serving dish and top with a scoop of ice cream or frozen yogurt, $1^1/_2$ teaspoons of almonds, and $^1/_4$ teaspoon of the remaining sugar. Serve immediately.

VARIATION

❏ To reduce calories and carbohydrates, substitute light sugar-free ice cream for the light ice cream, and save 20 calories and 4 grams of carbohydrates per serving.

NUTRITIONAL FACTS (PER SERVING)
Calories: 175   Carbohydrates: 32 g   Fiber: 2 g   Protein: 3.8 g
Fat: 3.5 g   Sat. Fat: 1.1 g   Cholesterol: 10 mg   Sodium: 60 mg   Calcium: 114 mg

---

SIMPLY GRAPE SORBET

YIELD: 5 SERVINGS
4 cups red grapes, frozen

1. Place the frozen grapes in a food processor and process for about a minute, or until finely ground with a granita-like appearance. Continue to process, scraping down the sides as needed, for another minute or 2, or until the mixture is smooth. If the mixture is too icy, mix in about $^1/_4$ cup of fresh (unfrozen) grapes or a few tablespoons of fruit juice to smooth out the consistency.

2. Divide the mixture among five chilled 8-ounce dessert dishes or wine glasses, and serve immediately.

NUTRITION FACTS (PER $^1/_2$-CUP SERVING)
Calories: 91   Carbohydrates: 23 g   Fiber: 1.5 g   Protein: 0.8 g
Fat: 0.7 g   Sat. Fat: 1.5 g   Cholesterol: 0 mg   Sodium: 3 mg   Calcium: 14 mg

---

BLACKBERRY GRANITA

YIELD: 6 SERVINGS

3 cups fresh or frozen (thawed and undrained) blackberries

1 1/4 cups pomegranate or purple grape juice

1/4 cup plus 2 tablespoons sugar

1. Place all of the ingredients in a blender, and process until smooth. Pour the mixture into a wire strainer, and use a wooden spoon to push the mixture through the strainer into a bowl. Discard the seeds.

2. Pour the strained blackberry mixture into a 9 x 9-inch pan, and freeze for about 1 hour or until frozen and icy around the edges.

3. Using a fork, scrape the icy edges into light shavings, and stir the ice crystals into the center portion of the fruit mixture. Press out any lumps with the fork. Return the pan to the freezer and repeat the scraping process about every 45 minutes for around 3 hours, or until the mixture is icy and granular.

4. Cover the pan with aluminum foil until ready to use. To serve, scrape the granita with a fork to loosen the crystals, and lightly spoon into chilled dessert dishes or wine glasses.

VARIATION

❏ To reduce calories and carbohydrates, substitute low-calorie sweetener for the sugar. You will save 45 calories and 12 grams of carbohydrates per serving. The sugar-free mixture will freeze a little more quickly than the sugar-sweetened mixture, so you may need to repeat the scraping process every 30 to 40 minutes instead of every 45 minutes.

NUTRITIONAL FACTS (PER 3/4-CUP SERVING)

Calories: 85   Carbohydrates: 21 g   Fiber: 2 g   Protein: 1 g
Fat: 0.4 g   Sat. Fat: 0 g   Cholesterol: 0 mg   Sodium: 8 mg   Calcium: 21 mg

CAPPUCCINO GRANITA

YIELD: 4 SERVINGS

1/2 cup hot strong black coffee

1/4 cup plus 2 tablespoons turbinado
sugar or light brown sugar

1/4 teaspoon ground cinnamon

1 cup whole milk

1. Place the coffee and sugar in a bowl, and stir to dissolve the sugar. Stir in the cinnamon, and then the milk.

2. Pour the mixture into an 8 x 8-inch pan and freeze for about 45 minutes, or until icy around the edges.

3. Using a fork, scrape the icy edges into light shavings, and stir the ice crystals into the center portion of the coffee mixture. Press out any lumps with the fork. Return the pan to the freezer and repeat the scraping process about every 45 minutes for around 3 hours, or until the mixture is icy and granular.

4. Cover the pan with aluminum foil until ready to use. To serve, scrape the granita with a fork to loosen the crystals, and lightly spoon into chilled dessert dishes or wine glasses and serve.

VARIATION

❑ To reduce calories and carbohydrates, substitute low-calorie sweetener for the sugar. You will save 45 calories and 12 grams of carbohydrates per serving. The sugar-free mixture will freeze a little more quickly than the sugar-sweetened mixture, so you may need to repeat the scraping process every 30 to 40 minutes instead of every 45 minutes.

NUTRITION FACTS (PER 3/4-CUP SERVING)

Calories: 106   Carbohydrates: 22 g   Fiber: 0 g   Protein: 2 g

Fat: 2.3 g   Sat. Fat: 1.3 g   Cholesterol: 9 mg   Sodium: 32 mg   Calcium: 77 mg

---

Organizations & Websites

Throughout this book, we discuss the importance of choosing health-ful foods—foods that not only help keep AGEs under control but also provide good nutrition without harmful contaminants. Below, you will find a number of organizations and websites that can assist you in this task by guiding you to safe produce, low-mercury sustainable seafood, and other wholesome foods, and by instructing you in sound food storage and preparation practices.

Environmental Working Group (EWG)

Website: www.ewg.org

EWG's mission is to empower people to live healthier lives in a healthier environment. Its website offers the "Dirty Dozen Plus" and "Clean Fifteen" lists that highlight pesticide levels in foods so that you can make informed purchases of produce. Click on the "Consumer Guides" tab to find updated versions of these lists as well as other helpful information.

FishWatch

Website: www.fishwatch.gov

Maintained by the National Oceanic and Atmospheric Administration (NOAA) Fisheries, FishWatch provides information about the sustainability of United States seafood, including both wild and farmed species; guidelines for minimizing the risks posed by mercury; instructions for buying and handling seafood; and more.

FoodSafety.gov

U.S. Department of Health and Human Services
200 Independence Avenue, SW
Washington, DC 20201
Website: www.foodsafety.gov

Table of Safe Cooking Temperatures: www.foodsafety.gov/keep/
charts/mintemp.html

*FoodSafety.gov is the gateway to food safety information provided by United
States government agencies. It offers information on safe minimum cooking
temperatures, food storage, food-borne illnesses, and recalls of tainted foods.*

Monterey Bay Aquarium Seafood Watch

886 Cannery Row
Monterey, CA 93940
Website: www.seafoodwatch.org

*The Monterey Bay Aquarium's Seafood Watch program helps consumers and
businesses choose seafood that is fished or farmed in ways that protect sea life
and habitats. Click on "Seafood Recommendations/Consumer Guides" to discover
which seafood in your area is considered "Best Choices" or "Good Alternatives,"
and which seafood to "Avoid."*

Natural Resources Defense Council (NRDC)

1152 15th Street NW, Suite 300
Washington, DC 20005
Phone: 202-289-6868
Website: www.nrdc.org
Seafood Buying Guide: www.nrdc.org/stories/smart-seafood-buying-guide

*The NRDC works in many areas to safeguard the earth and its inhabitants. Its
site offers tips for reducing exposure to pesticides and other chemicals in foods,
and for choosing foods that are environmentally sustainable. The NRDC's Smart
Seafood Buying Guide lets you know which fish have the least mercury and which
have moderate, high, or very high mercury levels.*

USDA National Organic Program (NOP)

1400 Independence Avenue, SW
Room 2642-South, Ag Stop 0268
Washington, DC 20250-0268
Phone: 202-720-3252
Website: www.ams.usda.gov/ about-ams/programs-offices/national-
organic-program

*Housed within the United States Department of Agriculture (USDA) Agricul-
tural Marketing Service, the NOP develops regulations and guidance on organic
standards for agricultural products. Its website provides information on organic
labeling, the USDA organic seal, organic rules and regulations, and more.*

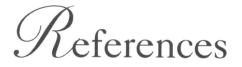
References

Chapter 1: The Missing Link

1. Stevens VJ, Vlassara H, Abati A, Cerami A. Nonenzymatic glycosylation of hemoglobin. *J Biol Chem.* 10;252(9):2998–3002, 1977.

2. Brownlee M, Cerami A, Vlassara H. Advanced glycosylation end products in tissue and the biochemical basis of diabetic complications. *N Engl J Med.* 19;318(20):1315–21. PMID:3283558, 1988.

3. Baynes JW, Thorpe SR. Role of oxidative stress in diabetic complications: a new perspective on an old paradigm. *Diabetes.* J48(1):1–9, 1999. Review. PMID: 9892215.

4. Monnier VM, Cerami A. Nonenzymatic browning in vivo: possible process for aging of long-lived proteins. *Science.* 30;211(4481):491–3,1981. PMID: 6779377.

5. Koenig RJ, Peterson CM, Jones RL, Saudek C, Lehrman M, Cerami A. Correlation of glucose regulation and hemoglobin AIc in diabetes mellitus. *N Engl J Med.* 19;295(8): 417–20, 1976.

6. Brownlee M, Vlassara H, Cerami A. Nonenzymatic glycosylation in the pathogenesis of diabetic complications. *Ann Int Med.* 101:527–537, 1984.

7. Brownlee M, Vlassara H, Cerami A. Measurement of glycosylated amino acids and peptides from urine of diabetic patients using affinity chromatography. *Diabetes.* 29:1044–1047, 1980.

8. Vlassara H, Brownlee M, et al. Cachectin/TNF and IL-1 induced by glucose-modified proteins: role in normal tissue remodeling. *Science.* 240(4858):1546–1548, 1988.

9. Brownlee M, Vlassara H, et al. Aminoguanidine prevents diabetes-induced arterial wall protein cross-linking. *Science.* 232(4758):1629–1632, 1986.

10. Skyler JS, Bergenstal R, Bonow RO, Buse J, Deedwania P, Gale EA, Howard BV, Kirkman MS, Kosiborod M, Reaven P, Sherwin RS; American Diabetes Association; American College of Cardiology Foundation; American Heart Association. Intensive glycemic control and the prevention of cardiovascular events: implications of the ACCORD, ADVANCE, and VA Diabetes Trials: a position statement of the American Diabetes Association and a Scientific Statement of the American College of Cardiology

Foundation and the American Heart Association. *J Am Coll Cardiol*. 2009 Jan 20;53(3): 298–304. doi: 10.1016/j.jacc.2008.10.008.

11. ACCORD Study Group, Cushman WC, Evans GW, Byington RP, Goff DC Jr, Grimm RH Jr, Cutler JA, Simons-Morton DG, Basile JN, Corson MA, Probstfield JL, Katz L, Peterson KA, Friedewald WT, Buse JB, Bigger JT, Gerstein HC, Ismail-Beigi F. Effects of intensive blood-pressure control in type 2 diabetes mellitus. *N Engl J Med*. Apr 29;362(17):1575-85, 2010. doi: 10.1056/NEJMoa1001286. Epub 2010 Mar 14.

12. Fox CS, Pencina MJ, Meigs JB, Vasan RS, Levitzky YS, D'Agostino RB Sr. Trends in the incidence of type 2 diabetes mellitus from the 1970s to the 1990s: the Framingham Heart Study. *Circulation*. 113(25):2914–8, 2006. Epub 2006 Jun 19.

13. Amos AF, McCarty DJ, Zimmet P. The rising global burden of diabetes and its complications: estimates and projections to the year 2010. *Diabet Med*. 14 Suppl 5:S1–85, 1997.

14. Maillard, LC. Action des acides anines sur les sucres: formation des melanoides par voie methodique. *C.R.Acad Sci*. 154:1653-1671, 1912.

15. Finot, PA. Historical perspective of the Maillard reaction in food science. *Ann N Y Acad Sci*. 1043:p. 1–8, 2005.

16. Makita Z, Vlassara H, Cerami A, Bucala R. Immunochemical detection of advanced glycosylation endproducts in vivo. *J Biol Chem*. 267:5133–5138, 1992.

17. Mitsuhashi T, Vlassara H, Founds HW, Li YM. Standardizing the immunological measurement of advanced glycation endproducts using normal human serum. *Journal of Immunological Methods*. 207:79–88, 1997.

18. Koschinsky T, He C, Mitsuhashi T, Bucala R, Liu C, Buenting C, Heitmann K, Vlassara H. Orally absorbed reactive glycation products (glycotoxins): an environmental risk factor in diabetic nephropathy. *Proc Natl Acad Sci USA*. 94(12):6474–9, 1997.

19. Vlassara H, Striker G. AGE restriction in diabetes mellitus: a paradigm shift. *Nature Reviews Endocrinology*. 7(9): 526–39, 2011.

20. Goldberg T, Cai W, Peppa M, Dardaine V, Baliga BS, Uribarri J, Vlassara H. Advanced glycoxidation end products in commonly consumed foods. *J Am Diet Assoc*. 104(8):1287–91, 2004.

21. Uribarri J, Woodruff S, Goodman S, Cai W, Chen X, Pyzik R, Yong A, Striker GE, Vlassara H. Advanced glycation end products in foods and a practical guide to their reduction in the diet. *J Am Dietetic Assoc*. 110(6):911–16.e12, 2010.

22. Vlassara H, Cai W, Crandall J, Goldberg T, Oberstein R, Dardaine V, Peppa M, Rayfield EJ. Inflammatory mediators are induced by dietary glycotoxins, a major risk factor for diabetic angiopathy. *Proc Natl Acad Sci USA*. 99:15596–15601, 2002.

23. Vlassara H, Cai W, Goodman S, Pyzik R, Yong A, Chen X, Zhu L, Neade T, Beeri M, Ferrucci L, Striker GE, Uribarri J. Protection against loss of innate defenses in adulthood by low AGE intake; role of a new anti-Inflammatory AGE-receptor-1. *J Clin Endocrin Metab*. 94(11):4483–91, 2009.

Chapter 2: The Science of AGEs

1. Cerami C, Founds H, Nicholl I, Mitsuhashi T, Giordano D, Vanpatten S, Lee A, Al-Abed Y, Vlassara H, Bucala R, Cerami A. Tobacco smoke is a source of toxic reactive glycation products. *Proc Natl Acad Sci USA*. 94(25): 13915–13920, 1997.

2. Monnier VM, Cerami A. Nonenzymatic browning in vivo: possible process for aging of long-lived proteins. *Science*. 211(4481): 491–493, 1981.

3. Cai W, Gao GD, Zhu L, Peppa M, Vlassara H. Oxidative stress-inducing carbonyl compounds from common foods: Novel mediators of cellular dysfunction. *Mol Med*. 8:337–346, 2002.

4. Brownlee M. Biochemistry and molecular cell biology of diabetic complications. *Nature*. 414(6865): 813–820, 2001.

5. Finot, PA. Historical perspective of the Maillard reaction in food science. *Ann N Y Acad Sci*. 1043: 1–8, 2005.

6. Baynes JW, Thorpe SR. Role of oxidative stress in diabetic complications: a new perspective on an old paradigm. *Diabetes*. 48(1): 1–9, 1999.

7. Makita Z, Radoff S, Rayfield EJ, Yang Z, Skolnik E, Delaney V, Friedman EA, Cerami A, Vlassara H. Advanced glycosylation endproducts in patients with diabetic nephropathy. *N Engl J Med*. 325:836–842, 1991.

8. Vlassara H, Striker GE. AGE restriction in diabetes mellitus: a paradigm shift. *Nat Rev Endocrinol*. 2011 May 24;7(9): 526–39. doi: 10.1038/nrendo.2011.74. Review. PMID: 21610689.

9. Maillard, LC. Action des acides anines sur les sucres: formation des melanoidines par voie methodique. *CR Acad Sci*. 154:1653–1671, 1912.

10. O'Brien J, Morrissey PA. Nutritional and toxicological aspects of the Maillard browning reaction in foods. *Crit Rev Food Sci Nutr*. 28(3): 211–248, 1989.

11. Chuyen NV, et al. Toxicity of the AGEs generated from the Maillard reaction: on the relationship of food-AGEs and biological-AGEs. *Mol Nutr Food Res*. 50(12): 1140–1149, 2006.

12. Bengmark S. Advanced glycation and lipoxidation end products–amplifiers of inflammation: the role of food. *JPEN J Parenter Enteral Nutr*. 31(5): 430–440, 2007.

13. Vlassara H, Brownlee M, Cerami A. High affinity receptor mediated uptake and degradation of glucose modified proteins: a potential mechanism for the removal of senescent macromolecules. *Proc Natl Acad Sci USA*. 82:5588 5592, 1985.

14. Vlassara H, Valinsky J, Brownlee M, Cerami C, Nishimoto S, Cerami A. Advanced glycosylation endproducts on erythrocyte cell surface induce receptor-mediated phagocytosis by macrophages: a model for turnover of aging cells. *J Exp Med*. 166: 539–549, 1987.

15. Vlassara H, Brownlee M, Manogue KR, Dinarello C, and Pasagian A. Cachectin/TNF and IL-1 induced by glucose-modified proteins: role in normal tissue remodeling. *Science*. 240: 1546–1548, 1988.

16. Kirstein M, Brett J, Radoff S, Stern D, Vlassara H. Advanced protein glycosylation induces transendothelial human chemotaxis and secretion of platelet-derived growth factor: role in vascular disease of diabetes and aging. *Proc Natl Acad Sci USA.* 87: 9010–9014, 1990.

17. Koschinsky T, He CJ, Mitsuhashi T, Bucala R, Liu C, Buenting C, Heitmann K, Vlassara H. Orally absorbed reactive glycation products (glycotoxins): an environmental risk factor in diabetic nephropathy. *Proc Natl Acad Sci USA.* 94(12): 6474–6479, 1997.

18. Vlassara H, Cai W, Goodman S, Pyzik R, Yong A, Chen X, Zhu L, Neade T, Beeri M, Ferrucci L, Striker GE, Uribarri J. Protection against loss of innate defenses in adulthood by low AGE intake; role of a new anti-inflammatory AGE-receptor-1. *J Clin Endocrin Metab.* 94(11):4483–91, 2009.

19. Cai W, Ramdas M, Zhu L, Chen X, Striker G, Vlassara H. Oral advanced glycation endproducts (AGEs) promote insulin resistance and diabetes by depleting the antioxidant defenses AGE receptor-1 and sirtuin 1. *Proc Natl Acad Sci USA.* 109(39): 15888–93, 2012.

20. Guarente L. Franklin H. Epstein Lecture: Sirtuins, aging, and medicine. *N Engl J Med.* 364(23): 2235–2244, 2011.

21. Uribarri J, Cai W, Vlassara H. Suppression of native defense mechanisms, SIRT1 and PPARy, by dietary glycoxidants precedes disease in adult humans; relevance to lifestyle-engendered chronic diseases. *Amino Acids.* 46(2):301–9, 2014. PMID: 23636469.

22. Cerami A, Vlassara H, Brownlee M. Glucose and aging. *Sci American.* 256:90–96, 1987.

23. Bucala R, Makita Z, Koschinsky T, Cerami A, Vlassara H. Lipid advanced glycosylation: pathway for lipid oxidation in vivo. *Proc Natl Acad Sci USA.* 90:6434–6438, 1993.

24. Vitek MP, Bhattacharya K, Glendening M, Stopa E, Vlassara H, Bucala R, Manogue K, Cerami A. Advanced glycosylation endproducts contribute to amyloidosis in Alzheimer's disease. *Proc Natl Acad Sci USA.* 91:4766–4770, 1994.

25. Bray GA, Popkin BM. Dietary sugar and body weight: have we reached a crisis in the epidemic of obesity and diabetes? Health be damned! Pour on the sugar. *Diabetes Care.* 37(4):950–6, 2014. doi: 10.2337/dc13-2085.

26. Schalkwijk CG, Stehouwer CD, van Hinsbergh VW. Fructose-mediated non-enzymatic glycation: sweet coupling or bad modification. *Diabetes Metab Res Rev.* 20(5): 369–382, 2004.

27. Gensberger S, Glomb MA, Pischetsrieder M. Analysis of sugar degradation products with α-dicarbonyl structure in carbonated soft drinks by UHPLC-DAD-MS/MS. *J Agric Food Chem.* 2013 Oct 30;61(43): 10238–45. doi: 10.1021/jf3048466. Epub 2013 Mar 11.

28. Goldberg T, Cai W, Peppa M, Dardaine V, Gao QD, Baliga BS, Uribarri J, Vlassara H. Advanced glycoxidation endproducts in commonly consumed foods. *J Am Dietetic Assoc.* 104:1287–1291, 2004.

29. Uribarri J, Woodruff S, Goodman S, Cai W, Chen X, Pyzik R, Yong A, Striker GE,

Vlassara H. Advanced glycation end products in foods and a practical guide to their reduction in the diet. *J Am Dietetic Assoc.* 110(6):911–16.e12, 2010.

30. Uribarri J, Cai W, Peppa M, Goodman SM, Ferrucci L, Striker G, Vlassara H. Circulating glycotoxins and dietary AGEs; two links to inflammatory response, oxidative stress and aging. *A J Gerontology Med Sci.* 62A:427–433, 2007.

31. Vlassara H, Cai W, Goodman S, Pyzik R, Yong A, Chen X, Zhu L, Neade T, Beeri M, Ferrucci L, Striker GE, Uribarri J. Protection against loss of innate defenses in adulthood by low AGE intake; role of a new anti-Inflammatory AGE-receptor-1. *J Clin Endocrin Metab.* 94(11): 4483–91, 2009.

32. Makita Z, Vlassara H, Cerami A, Bucala R. Immunochemical detection of advanced glycosylation endproducts in vivo. *J Biol Chem.* 267: 5133–5138, 1992.

33. Mitsuhashi T, Vlassara H, Founds HW, Li YM. Standardizing the immunological measurement of advanced glycation endproducts using normal human serum. *J Immunol Methods.* 207(1): 79–88, 1997.

34. Cai W, Gao GD, Zhu L, Peppa M, Vlassara H. Oxidative stress-inducing carbonyl compounds from common foods: novel mediators of cellular dysfunction. *Mol Med.* 8:337–346, 2002.

35. Scheijen JL, Clevers E, Engelen L, et al. Analysis of advanced glycation endproducts in selected food items by ultra-performance liquid chromatography tandem mass spectrometry: presentation of a dietary AGE database. *Food Chem.* 190:1145–50, 2016.

36. Stirban A, Heinemann L. Skin autofluorescence—a non-invasive measurement for assessing cardiovascular risk and risk of diabetes. *European Endocrinology.* 10(2):106–10, 2014.

37. de Vos LC, Boersema J, Mulder DJ, Smit AJ, Zeebregts CJ, Lefrandt JD. Skin autofluorescence as a measure of advanced glycation end products deposition predicts 5-year amputation in patients with peripheral artery disease. *Arterioscler Thromb Vasc Biol.* 2015 Jun;35(6): 1532–7. doi: 10.1161/ATVBAHA.115.305407.

Chapter 3: AGEs, Aging, and Chronic Disease

1. Illien-Jünger S, Lu Y, Qureshi SA, Hecht AC, Cai W, Vlassara H, Striker GE, Iatridis JC. Chronic ingestion of advanced glycation end products induces degenerative spinal changes and hypertrophy in aging pre-diabetic mice. *PLoS One.* 2015 Feb 10;10(2): e0116625. doi: 10.1371/journal.pone.0116625.

2. Drinda S, Franke S, Canet CC, Petrow P, Bräuer R, Hüttich C, Stein G, Hein G. Identification of the advanced glycation end products N(epsilon)-carboxymethyllysine in the synovial tissue of patients with rheumatoid arthritis. *Ann Rheum Dis.* 2002 Jun;61(6):488–92.

3. Libby P, Ridker PM, Maseri A. Inflammation and atherosclerosis. *Circulation.* 2002 Mar 5;105(9):1135–43.

4. Vlassara H, Bucala R, and Stitt A. *Vascular complications of diabetes. An introduction to vascular biology.* Hunt B, Poston L, Halliday A, Schachter M, Editors. Cambridge University Press (1998), p. 173–194.

5. Lopes-Virella MF, Hunt KJ, Baker NL, Lachin J, Nathan DM, Virella G; Diabetes Control and Complications Trial/Epidemiology of Diabetes Interventions and Complications Research Group. Levels of oxidized LDL and advanced glycation end products-modified LDL in circulating immune complexes are strongly associated with increased levels of carotid intima-media thickness and its progression in type 1 diabetes. *Diabetes.* 2011 Feb;60(2): 582–9. doi: 10.2337/db10-0915. Epub 2010 Oct 27.

6. Uribarri J, Stirban A, Sander D, Cai W, Negrean M, Buenting CE, Koschinsky T, Vlassara H. Single oral challenge by advanced glycation end products acutely impairs endothelial function in diabetic and nondiabetic subjects. *Diabetes Care.* 2007 Oct;30(10): 2579–82. Epub 2007 May 11. PMID:17496238

7. Negrean M, Stirban A, Stratmann B, Gawlowski T, Horstmann T, Götting C, Kleesiek K, Mueller-Roesel M, Koschinsky T, Uribarri J, Vlassara H, Tschoepe D. Effects of low- and high-advanced glycation endproduct meals on macro- and microvascular endothelial function and oxidative stress in patients with type 2 diabetes mellitus. *Am J Clin Nutr.* 2007 May;85(5):1236–43. Erratum in: *Am J Clin Nutr.* 2007 Oct;86(4): 1256. PMID: 17490958.

8. Zimmerman GA, Meistrell M 3rd, Bloom O, Cockroft KM, Bianchi M, Risucci D, Broome J, Farmer P, Cerami A, Vlassara H. Neurotoxicity of advanced glycation end-products during focal stroke and neuroprotective effects of aminoguanidine. *Proc Natl Acad Sci USA.* 1995 Apr 25;92(9): 3744–8.

9. Dickson DW, Sinicropi S, Yen SH, Ko LW, Mattiace LA, Bucala R, Vlassara H. Glycation and microglial reaction in lesions of Alzheimer's disease. *Neurobiol Aging.* 17(No.5):733–743, 1996.

10. Vitek MP, Bhattacharya K, Glendening JM, Stopa E, Vlassara H, Bucala R, Manogue K, Cerami A. Advanced glycation end products contribute to amyloidosis in Alzheimer disease. *Proc Natl Acad Sci USA.* 1994 May 24;91(11): 4766–70.

11. Cai W, Uribarri J, Zhu L, Chen X, Swamy S, Zhao Z, Grosjean F, Simonaro C, Kuchel GA, Schnaider-Beeri M, Woodward M, Striker GE, Vlassara H. Oral glycotoxins are a modifiable cause of dementia and the metabolic syndrome in mice and humans. *Proc Natl Acad Sci USA.* 2014 Apr 1;111(13): 4940–5. doi: 10.1073/pnas.1316013111. Epub 2014 Feb 24.

12. Beeri MS, Moshier E, Schmeidler J, Godbold J, Uribarri J, Reddy S, Sano M, Grossman HT, Cai W, Vlassara H, Silverman JM. Serum concentration of an inflammatory glycotoxin, methylglyoxal, is associated with increased cognitive decline in elderly individuals. *Mech Ageing Dev.* 2011 Nov-Dec;132(11-12): 583–7. doi: 10.1016/ j.mad. 2011.10.007. Epub 2011 Nov 3.

13. Vlassara H, Striker GE. (2010) Intake of advanced glycation endproducts; role in the development of diabetic complications. In *Principles of diabetes mellitus,* Second Edition. L Poretsky, Editor. Springer Publications.

14. Sun JK, Keenan HA, Cavallerano JD, Asztalos BF, Schaefer EJ, Sell DR, Strauch CM, Monnier VM, Doria A, Aiello LP, King GL. Protection from retinopathy and other complications in patients with type 1 diabetes of extreme duration: the joslin 50-year medalist study. *Diabetes Care.* 2011 Apr;34(4): 968–74. doi: 10.2337/dc10-1675.

15. Vlassara H, Striker GE. AGE restriction in diabetes mellitus: a paradigm shift. *Nat Rev Endocrinol.* 2011 May 24;7(9): 526–39. doi: 10.1038/nrendo.2011.74. Review. PMID: 21610689.

16. Leslie RD, Beyan H, Sawtell P, Boehm BO, Spector TD, Snieder H. Level of an advanced glycated end product is genetically determined: a study of normal twins. *Diabetes.* Sep;52(9): 2441–4. 2003. PMID: 12941787.

17. Beyan H, Riese H, Hawa MI, Beretta G, Davidson HW, Hutton JC, Burger H, Schlosser M, Snieder H, Boehm BO, Leslie RD. Glycotoxin and autoantibodies are additive environmentally determined predictors of type 1 diabetes: a twin and population study. *Diabetes.* 61(5):1192–8,2012. doi: 10.2337/db11-0971. Epub 2012 Mar 6.

18. Vlassara H, Cai W, et al. Protection against loss of innate defenses in adulthood by low advanced glycation end products (AGE) intake: role of the anti-inflammatory AGE receptor-1. *J Clin Endocrinol Metab.* 94(11): 4483–4491, 2009.

19. Uribarri J, Cai W, Ramdas M, Goodman S, Pyzik R, Chen X, Zhu L, Striker GE, Vlassara H. Restriction of advanced glycation end products improves insulin resistance in human type 2 diabetes: potential role of AGER1 and SIRT1. *Diabetes Care.* 34:1610–6. 2011 doi: 10.2337/dc11-0091.

20. Vlassara H, et al. Oral AGE restriction ameliorates insulin resistance in obese individuals with the metabolic syndrome: A randomized controlled trial. (Publication pending.)

21. Vlassara H, Uribarri J, Cai W, Goodman S, Pyzik R, Post J, Grosjean F, Woodward M, Striker GE. Effects of sevelamer on HbA1c, inflammation, and advanced glycation end products in diabetic kidney disease. *Clin J Am Soc Nephrol.* 7(6): 934–942, 2012.

22. Koschinsky T, He C, Mitsuhashi T, Bucala R, Liu C, Buenting C, Heitmann K, Vlassara H. Orally absorbed reactive glycation products (glycotoxins): an environmental risk factor in diabetic nephropathy. *Proc Natl Acad Sci USA.* 94: 6474–6479, 1997.

23. He C, Sabol J, Mitsuhashi T, Vlassara H. Dietary glycotoxins: inhibition of reactive products by aminoguanidine facilitates renal clearance and reduces tissue sequestration. *Diabetes.* 48:1308–1315, 1999.

24. Makita Z, Radoff S, Rayfield EJ, Yang Z, Skolnik E, Delaney V, Friedman EA, Cerami A, Vlassara H. Advanced glycosylation endproducts in patients with diabetic nephropathy. *N Engl J Med.* 325: 836–842, 1991.

25. Yubero-Serrano EM, Woodward M, Poretsky L, Vlassara H, Striker GE, AGE-less Study Group. Effects of sevelamer carbonate on advanced glycation end products and antioxidant/pro-oxidant status in patients with diabetic kidney disease. *Clin J Am Soc Nephrol.* 10(5): 759–766, 2015.

26. Striker GE, Vlassara H, Ferrucci L. Aging and the kidney: introduction. *Semin Nephrol.* 29(6): 549–550, 2009.

27. Cai W, He JC, Zhu L, Chen X, Wallenstein S, Striker G, Vlassara H. Reduced oxidant stress and extended lifespan in mice exposed to a low glycoxidant diet: association with increased AGER1 expression. *AJ Pathology.* 170: 1893–1902, 2007.

28. Uribarri J, Peppa M, Cai W, Goldberg T, Lu M, He C, Vlassara H. Restriction of dietary glyctoxins reduces excessive advanced glycation end products in renal failure patients. *JASN.* 14: 728–731, 2003.

29. Mericq V, Piccardo C, Cai W, Chen X, Zhu L, Striker GE, Vlassara H, Uribarri J. Maternally transmitted and food-derived glycotoxins: a factor preconditioning the young to diabetes? *Diabetes Care.* 33(10): 2232–7, 2010.

30. Haus JM, Carrithers JA, Trappe SW, Trappe TA. Collagen, cross-linking, and advanced glycation end products in aging human skeletal muscle. *J Appl Physiol.* 103(6): 2068–2076, 1985.

31. Dalal M, Ferrucci L, Sun K, Beck J, Fried LP, Semba RD. Elevated serum advanced glycation end products and poor grip strength in older community-dwelling women. *J Gerontol A Biol Sci Med Sci.* 64(1): 132–137, 2009.

32. Sandu O, Song K, Cai W, Zheng F, Uribarri J, Vlassara H. Insulin resistance and type 2 diabetes in high-fat-fed mice are linked to high glycotoxin intake. *Diabetes.* 54(8): 2314–2319, 2005.

33. Uribarri J, Cai W, Woodward M, Tripp E, Goldberg L, Pyzik R, Yee K, Tansman L, Chen X, Mani V, Fayad ZA, Vlassara H. Elevated serum advanced glycation endproducts in obese indicate risk for the metabolic syndrome: a link between healthy and unhealthy obesity? *J Clin Endocrinol Metab.* 100(5): 1957–1966, 2015.

34. Guarente L. Franklin H. Epstein Lecture: Sirtuins, aging, and medicine. *N Engl J Med.* 364(23): 2235–2244, 2011.

35. Rosenquist JN, Lehrer SF, O'Malley AJ, Zaslavsky AM, Smoller JW, Christakis NA. Cohort of birth modifies the association between FTO genotype and BMI. *Proc Natl Acad Sci USA.* 112(2): 354–359, 2015.

36. Cai W, Ramdas M, Zhu L, Chen X, Striker G, Vlassara H. Oral advanced glycation endproducts (AGEs) promote insulin resistance and diabetes by depleting the antioxidant defenses AGE receptor-1 and sirtuin 1. *Proc Natl Acad Sci USA.* 109(39): 15888–93, 2012.

37. Karim L, Vashishth D. Heterogeneous glycation of cancellous bone and its association with bone quality and fragility. *PLoS One.* 7(4): e35047, 2012.

38. Illien-Junger S, Grosjean F, Laudier DM, Vlassara H, Striker GE, Iatridis JC. Combined anti-inflammatory and anti-AGE drug treatments have a protective effect on intervertebral discs in mice with diabetes. *PLoS One.* 8(5): e64302, 2013.

39. Peppa M, Brem H, Ehrlich P, Zhang JG, Cai W, Li Z, Croitoru A, Thung S, Vlassara H. Adverse effects of dietary glycotoxins on wound healing in genetically diabetic mice. *Diabetes.* 52(11): 2805–2813,2003.

40. Cerami C, Founds H, Nicholl I, Mitsuhashi T, Giordano D, Vanpatten S, Lee A, Al-Abed Y, Vlassara H, Bucala R, Cerami A. Tobacco smoke is a source of toxic reactive glycation products. *Proc Natl Acad Sci USA.* 94(25): 13915–13920, 1997.

41. Li YM, Steffes M, Donnelly T, Liu C, Fuh H, Basgen J, Bucala R, Vlassara H. Pre-

vention of cardiovascular and renal pathology of aging by the advanced glycation inhibitor aminoguanidine. *Proc Natl Acad Sci USA.* 93: 3902–3907, 1996.

42. Hammes HP, Hoerauf H, Alt A, Schleicher E, Clausen JT, Bretzel RG, Laqua H. N(epsilon)(carboxymethyl)lysin and the AGE receptor RAGE colocalize in age-related macular degeneration. *Invest Ophthalmol Vis Sci.* 40(8): 1855–9, July 1999.

Chapter 4: The AGE-Less Diet

1. Goldberg T, Cai W, Peppa M, Dardaine V, Gao Q-D, Baliga BS, Uribarri J, Vlassara H. Advanced glycoxidation endproducts in commonly consumed foods. *J Am Dietetic Assoc.* 104:1287–1291, 2004.

2. Finot, PA. Historical perspective of the Maillard reaction in food science. *Ann N Y Acad Sci.* 1043: 1–8, 2005.

3. Makita Z, Vlassara H, Cerami A, Bucala R. Immunochemical detection of advanced glycosylation endproducts in vivo. *J Biol Chem.* 267: 5133–5138, 1992.

4. Mitsuhashi T, Vlassara H, Founds HW, Li YM. Standardizing the immunological measurement of advanced glycation endproducts using normal human serum. *Journal of Immunological Methods.* 207:79–88, 1997.

5. Bucala R, Makita Z, Koschinsky T, Cerami A, Vlassara H. Lipid advanced glycosylation: pathway for lipid oxidation in vivo. *Proc Natl Acad Sci USA.* 90:6434–6438, 1993.

6. Scheijen JL, Clevers E, Engelen L, et al. Analysis of advanced glycation endproducts in selected food items by ultra-performance liquid chromatography tandem mass spectrometry: presentation of a dietary AGE database. *Food Chem.* 190:1145–50, 2016.

7. Uribarri J, Cai W, Woodward M, Tripp E, Goldberg L, Pyzik R, Yee K, Tansman L, Chen X, Mani V, Fayad ZA, Vlassara H. Elevated serum advanced glycation endproducts in obese indicate risk for the metabolic syndrome: a link between healthy and unhealthy obesity? *J Clin Endocrinol Metab.* 100(5): 1957–1966, 2015.

8. Brownlee M, Vlassara H, Kooney A, Ulrich P, Cerami A. Aminoguanidine prevents diabetes induced arterial wall protein crosslinking. *Science.* 232:1629–1632, 1986.

9. Wolffenbuttel BH, et al. Breakers of advanced glycation end products restore large artery properties in experimental diabetes. *Proc Natl Acad Sci USA.* 95(8): p. 4630-4, 1998.

10. Nakamura S, Makita Z, Ishikawa S, Yasumura K, Fujii W, Yanagisawa K, Kawata T, Koike T. Progression of nephropathy in spontaneous diabetic rats is prevented by OPB-9195, a novel inhibitor of advanced glycation. *Diabetes.* 46: 895–899, 1997.

11. Thornalley P J. The potential role of thiamine (vitamin B1) in diabetic complications. *Curr Diabetes Rev.* 1: 287–298, 2005.

12. Onorato JM, et al. Pyridoxamine, an inhibitor of advanced glycation reactions, also inhibits advanced lipoxidation reactions. Mechanism of action of pyridoxamine. *J Biol Chem.* 275(28): p. 21177–84, 2000.

13. Williams ME, Bolton WK, Khalifah RG, Degenhardt TP, Schotzinger RJ, McGill JB. Effects of pyridoxamine in combined phase 2 studies of patients with type 1 and type 2 diabetes and overt nephropathy. *Am J Nephrol.* 27: 605–614, 2007.

14. Keavney BD, Dudley CR, Stratton IM, Holman RR, Matthews DR, Ratcliffe PJ, Turner RC. UK prospective diabetes study (UKPDS) 14: association of angiotensin-converting enzyme insertion/deletion polymorphism with myocardial infarction in NIDDM. *Diabetologia.* 38: 948–952, 1995.

15. Yubero-Serrano EM, Woodward M, Poretsky L, Vlassara H, Striker GE; AGE-less Study Group. Effects of sevelamer carbonate on advanced glycation end products and antioxidant/pro-oxidant status in patients with diabetic kidney disease. *Clin J Am Soc Nephrol.* 2015 May 7;10(5):759–66. doi: 10.2215/CJN.07750814. Epub 2015 Feb 20.

16. Wu CH, Huang SM, Lin JA, Yen GC. Inhibition of advanced glycation endproduct formation by foodstuffs. *Food Funct.* 2011 May;2(5):224-34. doi: 10.1039/c1fo10026b. Epub 2011 Apr 8.

17. Peng X, Ma J, Chen F, Wang M. Naturally occurring inhibitors against the formation of advanced glycation end-products. *Food Funct.* 2011 Jun;2(6):289–301. doi: 10.1039/c1fo10034c. Epub 2011 Jun 15.

Chapter 5: Applying the AGE-Less Way to Different Diets

1. Swain JF, McCarron PB, Hamilton EF, Sacks FM, Appel LJ. Characteristics of the diet patterns tested in the optimal macronutrient intake trial to prevent heart disease (Omni-Heart): options for a heart-healthy diet. *J Am Diet Assoc.* 2008 Feb; 108(2): 257–265.

2. National Heart, Lung, and Blood Institute. (September 16, 2015) Description of the DASH eating plan. https://www.nhlbi.nih.gov/health/health-topics/topics/dash

3. U.S. Department of Health and Human Services. Scientific report of the 2015 Dietary Guidelines Advisory Committee. http://health.gov/dietaryguidelines/2015-scientific-report/

4. Lopez-Moreno J, Quintana-Navarro GM, Delgado-Lista J, Garcia-Rios A, Delgado-Casado N, Camargo A, Perez-Martinez P, Striker GE, Tinahones FJ, Perez-Jimenez F, Lopez-Miranda J, Yubero-Serrano EM. Mediterranean diet reduces serum advanced glycation end products and increases antioxidant defenses in elderly adults: a randomized controlled trial. *J Am Geriatr Soc.* 2016 Apr;64(4):901-4. doi: 10.1111/jgs.14062.

5. Sofi F, Macchi C, Abbate R, Gensini GF, Casini A. Mediterranean diet and health status: an updated meta-analysis and a proposal for a literature-based adherence score. *Public Health Nutr.* 2014 Dec;17(12):2769–82.

6. Dinu M, Abbate R, Gensini GF, Casini A, Sofi F. Vegetarian, vegan diets and multiple health outcomes: a systematic review with meta-analysis of observational studies. *Crit Rev Food Sci Nutr.* 2016 Feb 6:0. http://www.ncbi.nlm.nih.gov/pubmed/26853923.

About the Authors

Helen Vlassara, MD, received her medical degree from the Medical School of Athens University in Greece. She has been an Associate Professor at the Rockefeller University in New York, and is Professor Emeritus and former Director of Diabetes and Aging Research at the Mount Sinai School of Medicine. A pioneer in disease-causing advanced glycation end products, her laboratory and clinical research, largely conducted at The Rockefeller University and Mount Sinai School of Medicine, was sponsored by the National Institutes of Health, American Diabetes Association, American Heart Association, and National Institute of Aging, and earned her numerous awards and international renown. She has authored hundreds of publications, including scientific articles and books.

Sandra Woodruff, MS, RD, LD/N, has a master's of science in food and nutrition from Florida State University. She has worked in a variety of settings, including a hospital-based wellness center, dialysis clinic, physician offices, and private practice. She has also taught college health and nutrition courses and served as president of the Florida Dietetic Association. Sandra is now a consultant specializing in culinary nutrition and diet-related health problems. She is the best-selling author of numerous health-related cookbooks, including *Soft Foods for Easier Eating Cookbook.*

Gary E. Striker, MD, received his medical degree from the University of Washington in Seattle. Currently, he is Professor of Medicine and Geriatrics at the Mount Sinai School of Medicine in New York. His focus includes research, medical education, and public service. At the National Institutes of Health, as Director of Kidney Research, he developed national studies on diabetic complications. He has authored over 300 publications, including scientific articles and books, and has collaborated with Dr. Vlassara since 1996.

$\mathcal{I}$ndex

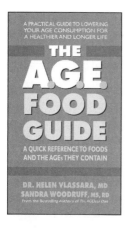

THE AGE FOOD GUIDE
A Quick Reference to Foods and the AGEs They Contain
Helen Vlassara, MD and Sandra Woodruff, RD

All foods contain naturally occurring toxic substances called AGEs—advanced glycation end products. Studies have shown that a buildup of AGEs increases oxidation and free radicals, hardens tissue, and creates chronic inflammation, leading to a host of illnesses. While many foods contain high AGE levels, many others contain very little. By knowing the best foods to choose and their optimal preparation methods, you can lower your consumption of these harmful substances. *The AGE Food Guide* is designed to help. This comprehensive guide lists hundreds of common foods and their AGE levels. In an easy-to-follow format, the foods are listed both alphabetically and within categories for quick and easy access.

With *The AGE Food Guide* in hand, you can confidently make wise food choices that will allow you to enjoy greater health and longevity.

$8.95 • 224 pages • 4 x 7-inch paperback • ISBN 978-0-7570-0429-2

GLYCEMIC INDEX FOOD GUIDE
For Weight Loss, Cardiovascular Health, Diabetic Management, and Maximum Energy
Dr. Shari Lieberman

By indicating how quickly a given food triggers a rise in blood sugar, the glycemic index (GI) enables you to choose foods that can help you manage a variety of conditions and improve your overall health. This easy-to-use guide teaches you about the GI and how to use it. It provides both the glycemic index and the glycemic load for hundreds of foods and beverages. Whether you want to manage your diabetes, lose weight, increase your heart health, or simply enhance your well-being, the *Glycemic Index Food Guide* is the best place to start.

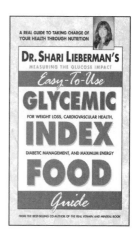

$7.95 • 160 pages • 4 x 7-inch paperback • ISBN 978-0-7570-0245-8

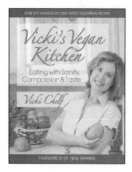

VICKI'S VEGAN KITCHEN
Vicki Chelf

Vegan dishes are healthy and delicious, yet many people are daunted by the idea of preparing meals that contain no animal products. Vicki Chelf presents a comprehensive cookbook designed to take the mystery out of meatless meals.

$17.95 US • 320 pages • 7.5 x 9-inch paperback • ISBN 978-0-7570-0251-9

THE WORLD GOES RAW COOKBOOK
Lisa Mann

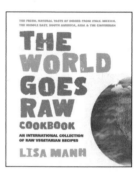

Although raw food can be delicious and improve your well-being, raw cuisine cookbooks have always offered little variety—until now. In *The World Goes Raw Cookbook*, raw food chef Lisa Mann provides a fresh approach to (un)cooking. Lisa first guides you in stocking your kitchen with tools and ingredients, and then presents six chapters of international dishes, including Italian, Mexican, Middle Eastern, Asian, Caribbean, and South American cuisine. Let *The World Goes Raw* add variety to your life while helping you feel healthier and more energized than ever before.

$16.95 US • 176 pages • 7.5 x 9-inch paperback • ISBN 978-0-7570-0320-2

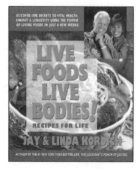

LIVE FOODS LIVE BODIES!
Jay and Linda Kordich

Through years of healthful living, Jay and Linda Kordich have learned that abundant energy, enhanced mental clarity, and a sense of well-being are easily within reach. In *Live Foods Live Bodies!,* they reveal all their secrets, including juice therapy and a living foods diet. This powerful book—lavishly illustrated with beautiful full-color photos—was designed to help you transform the person you are into the person you want to become, and features over 100 kitchen-tested recipes for delectable juices, salad dressings, soups, and much more.

$18.95 US • 240 pages • 7.5 x 9-inch paperback • ISBN 978-0-7570-0385-1